ANNUAL REVIEW OF GERONTOLOGY AND GERIATRICS

VOLUME 36, 2016

Annual Review of Gerontology and Geriatrics

Optimizing Physical Activity and Function Across Settings

VOLUME 36, 2016

Volume Editors

BARBARA RESNICK, PhD, CRNP, FGSA, FAANP, FAAN
MARIE BOLTZ, PhD, RN, GNP-BC, FGSA, FAAN

Series Editor

TONI C. ANTONUCCI, PhD

SPRINGER PUBLISHING COMPANY
NEW YORK

Springer Publishing Company, LLC
11 West 42nd Street
New York, NY 10036
www.springerpub.com

Acquisitions Editor: Sheri W. Sussman
Composition: Exeter Premedia Services

ISBN: 978-0-8261-9815-0
E-book ISBN: 978-0-8261-9816-7
ISSN: 0198-8794
Online ISSN: 1944-4036

16 17 18/ 5 4 3 2 1

Printed in the United States of America by Gasch Printing.

Contents

PART 2: Aerobic Exercises and Stretching

PART 3: Resistance Exercise

PART 4: Balance Exercise

PART 5: Physical Activity as a Determinant of Health

PART 6: Cross-Setting Approaches to Increase Function and Physical Activity

About the Volume Editors

Barbara Resnick, PhD, CRNP, FGSA, FAANP, FAAN, is a professor in the Department of Organizational Systems and Adult Health at the University of Maryland School of Nursing; she codirects the Adult/Gerontological Nurse Practitioner Program and the Biology and Behavior Across the Lifespan Research Center of Excellence, holds the Sonya Ziporkin Gershowitz Chair in Gerontology, and does clinical work at Roland Park Place. Her research program is focused on optimizing function and physical activity among older adults, exploring the impact of resilience and genetics on function and physical activity, and testing dissemination and implementation of interventions in real-world settings. Dr. Resnick has to her credit over 250 published articles, numerous chapters in nursing and medical textbooks, and books on restorative care and resilience in older adults. She has held leadership positions in multiple organizations including the American Academy of Nurse Practitioners, Gerontological Advanced Practice Nurses Association, the Society of Behavioral Medicine, the Gerontological Society of America, and the American Geriatrics Society.

Marie Boltz, PhD, RN, GNP-BC, FGSA, FAAN, is an associate professor at the Connell School of Nursing. She has served as principal investigator (PI) on several studies that examined the trajectory of change in physical function. Some of her recent research has focused on testing system-level interventions to maximize physical and cognitive recovery in older persons in the acute and postacute settings. She has also served as PI, co-PI, and consultant on studies that have examined the geriatric care environment, models of care, and measures of quality around the care of older persons. In her prior role as practice director of the Hartford Institute for Geriatric Nursing, she developed educational resources and project management tools for clinicians, families, and administrators, designed to improve the health and function of older adults. Dr. Boltz contributes to editorial boards, is the lead editor of *Evidence-Based Geriatric Nursing Protocols for Best Practice*, and serves on several national advisory boards informing aging program development and evaluation.

Contributors

Dale Avers, PT, DPT, PhD, FAPTA, Upstate Medical University, Syracuse, NY

Bryan J. Blissmer, PhD, Department of Kinesiology, University of Rhode Island, Kingston, RI

Marie Boltz, PhD, RN, GNP-BC, FGSA, FAAN, Boston College, William F. Connell School of Nursing Chestnut Hill, MA

Shannon S. D. Bredin, PhD, Associate Professor, Director, Cognitive and Functional Learning Laboratory, Physical Activity Promotion and Chronic Disease Prevention Unit, University of British Columbia, Vancouver, BC, Canada

Wojtek Chodzko-Zajko, PhD, Department of Kinesiology and Community Health, University of Illinois at Urbana-Champaign, IL

Leatha A. Clark, DPT, MS, Ohio Musculoskeletal and Neurological Institute, Department of Family Medicine at Ohio University, Athens, Ohio

Brian C. Clark, PhD, Ohio Musculoskeletal and Neurological Institute, Department of Geriatric Medicine, and Department of Biomedical Sciences at Ohio University, Athens, Ohio

Phillip G. Clark, ScD, Program in Gerontology, and the Rhode Island Geriatric Education Center

Zoe Durand, MPH, Department of Public Health Sciences, University of Hawaii at Manoa

Katarina Friberg Felsted, MS, Doctoral Student (Nursing), College of Nursing, University of Utah, Salt Lake City, UT

Elizabeth Galik, PhD, CRNP, University of Maryland School of Nursing, Baltimore, MD

Norman Gledhill, PhD, FACSM, Full Professor/Emeritus, School of Kinesiology and Health Science, York University, Toronto, ON, Canada

Mary L. Greaney, PhD, Department of Kinesiology, University of Rhode Island, Kingston, RI

Tracey E. Howe, PhD, MSc, PGD, CertEd GradDipPhys, MCSP, School of Health and Life Sciences, Glasgow Caledonian University, Glasgow, Scotland

Veronica Jamnik, PhD, Associate Professor, School of Kinesiology and Health Science, York University, Toronto, ON, Canada

James F. Konopack, PhD, Department of Health and Physical Education, Marjorie K. Unterberg School of Nursing and Health Studies, Monmouth University

Timothy D. Law, DO, MBA, Ohio Musculoskeletal and Neurological Institute, Department of Family Medicine, Ohio University, Athens, OH

Faith D. Lees, MS, Program in Gerontology: and the Rhode Island Geriatric Education Center

Carlos Marquez, MA, Doctoral Candidate (Clinical Psychology), Neuropsychology Minor, Ferkauf Graduate School of Psychology, Yeshiva University, New York, NY

Colin Milner, Chief Executive Officer, International Council on Active Aging

Jenifer Milner, Editor-in-Chief, *Journal on Active Aging*, International Council on Active Aging

Claudio R. Nigg, PhD, FSBM, Department of Public Health Sciences, University of Hawaii at Manoa

Barbara Resnick, PhD, CRNP, Professor, University of Maryland School of Nursing, Baltimore, Maryland

Deborah Riebe, PhD, Department of Kinesiology, University of Rhode Island, Kingston, RI

Carol E. Rogers, PhD, RN, College of Nursing/Donald W Reynolds Center Gerontological Nursing, University of Oklahoma, Oklahoma City, OK

Andiara Schwingel, PhD, Department of Kinesiology and Community Health, University of Illinois at Urbana-Champaign, IL

Emerson Sebastião, PhD, Department of Kinesiology and Community Health, University of Illinois at Urbana-Champaign, IL

Roy J. Shephard, MD, PhD, CM, MBBS, DPE, LLD, DSc, Full Professor/Emeritus, Faculty of Kinesiology and Physical Education, University of Toronto, Toronto, ON, Canada

Liza Stathokostas, School of Kinesiology, Faculty of Health Sciences, University of Western Ontario, London, ON, Canada

Anthony A. Vandervoort, School of Physical Therapy, Faculty of Health Sciences, University of Western Ontario, London, ON, Canada

Darren E. R. Warburton, PhD, Full Professor, Director, Cardiovascular Physiology and Rehabilitation Laboratory, Physical Activity Promotion and Chronic Disease Prevention Unit, University of British Columbia, Vancouver, BC, Canada

Danielle M. Wischenka, MA, Doctoral Candidate (Clinical Psychology), Ferkauf Graduate School of Psychology, Yeshiva University, New York, NY

Previous Volumes in the Series

Vol. 35, 2015: Subjective Aging: New Developments and Future Directions

Editors: Manfred Diehl, PhD, and Hans-Werner Wahl, PhD

Vol. 34, 2014: Genetics

Editor: Richard L. Sprott, PhD

Vol. 33, 2013: Healthy Longevity: A Global Approach

Editors: Jean-Marie Robine, DEA, DED, Carol Jagger, PhD, and Eileen M. Crimmins, PhD

Vol. 32, 2012: Emerging Perspectives on Resilience in Adulthood and Later Life

Editors: Bert Hayslip, Jr., PhD, and Gregory C. Smith, PhD

Vol. 31, 2011: Pathways Through the Transitions of Care for Older Adults

Editors: Peggye Dilworth-Anderson, PhD, and Mary H. Palmer, PhD

Vol. 30, 2010: Biobehavioral Perspectives on Health in Later Life

Editor: Keith E. Whitfield, PhD

Vol. 29: Life-Course Perspectives on Late Life Health Inequalities

Editors: Toni C. Antonucci, PhD, and James S. Jackson, PhD

Vol. 28: Gerontological and Geriatric Education

Editors: Harvey L. Sterns, PhD, and Marie A. Bernard, MD

Vol. 27: Biopsychosocial Approaches to Longevity

Editors: Leonard W. Poon, PhD, DPhil, and Thomas T. Perls, MD, MPH

Vol. 26: The Crown of Life Dynamics of the Early Postretirement Period

Editors: Jacquelyn Boone James, PhD, and Paul Wink, PhD

Vol. 25: Aging Health Care Workforce Issues

Editors: Toni Miles, MD, PhD, and Antonio Furino, PhD, JD

Vol. 24: Focus on Intergenerational Relations Across Time and Place

Editors: Merril Silverstein, PhD, and K. Warner Schaie, PhD

Vol. 23: Focus on Aging in Context: Socio-Physical Environments

Editors: Hans Werner Wahl, PhD, Rick J. Scheidt, PhD, and Paul G. Windley, PhD

Foreword

What Will It Take to Motivate Older Adults and Caregivers to Engage in Regular Physical Activity at a Level Sufficient to Result in Benefits?

There is abundant evidence supporting the benefits of a physically active lifestyle, yet the majority of older adults are not engaged in regular physical activity. This is not a simple problem to solve, as outlined by the authors in this book. The key principle of "overload"—doing more than one is accustomed to—can be varied in many ways to observe these benefits. The exercise literature is replete with studies of intensity (how hard), duration (how long), and frequency (how often), and the associated benefits to health and function. These studies have been synthesized to derive the *Physical Activity Guidelines for Older Adults*. While the science is apparent, the accompanying behavior change has not occurred in many older adults. Few older adults seem to be motivated to decrease their risk of cardiovascular disease or hyperlipidemia, and so forth. The functional benefits of exercise and physical activity programs are also abundant, but if the older adult does not have a functional deficit, the motivation for a daily physical activity regime is lessened. Clearly, there is no single approach that can address this question.

An approach to behavior change is one that addresses the heterogeneity of aging. The message behind "Be Active Your Way" (Department of Health and Human Services) embraces the multitude of ways that older adults can be active. This individualized approach is essential because engaging in regular physical activity is as important for the independent 75-year-old who was an avid tennis player in his youth as it is to the 92-year-old woman who uses a walker, has mild dementia, and lives in assisted living. The exercise prescription or activity recommendations will look very different for these people, yet both can engage in evidence-based programs shown to improve health and function.

Another approach to engaging older adults is to talk to them like consumers, as is being promoted by the American Board of Internal Medicine Foundation. Their "Choosing Wisely" initiative aims to help consumers make informed health-care choices by providing procedures that tend to be done frequently, yet whose usefulness is called into question by evidence. Last year, the following was added to their list: "Don't prescribe under-dosed strength training programs for older adults. Instead, match the frequency, intensity and duration of exercise to the individual's abilities and goals."

Recognizing ageism (no, you are not too old to get stronger), combatting ignorance about the benefits of exercise including the positive changes in lifestyle, cognition, and attitude, and sharing resources for community-level involvement are part of the multitude of methods to engage older adults in exercise. It will take many voices over time to convince older adults and caregivers that regular physical activity can be an enjoyable and beneficial part of their life.

Thus, it is with great pleasure that I encourage you all to read and share the amazing wealth of information provided in this edition of *Annual Review of Gerontology and Geriatrics*, Volume 36, 2016: *Optimizing Physical Activity and Function Across Settings*. This volume brings together an incredible amount of work in the area of physical activity, specifically exercise, and the challenges we face in engaging older adults in optimal amounts and intensities of activity. The authors of this book have done a remarkable job at highlighting practical ways to share information that are known to be effective from research trials and clinical practice.

The book has multiple sections and covers different types of exercise activities including those focused on aerobic activity, stretching, resistance, and balance. What is particularly exciting is that across these areas, the chapters move beyond simple recommendations to carefully address challenges in getting individuals to achieve the stated recommendations and provide thoughtful solutions on how to overcome challenges. The authors share positive approaches to motivating and educating older adults and recognize that older adults were not always encouraged to be active.

The book starts with a fascinating history of international policy related to physical activity and how policy impacts practice and activity among older adults. Additional chapters review real-world practical issues in engaging older adults in exercise, such as whether or not one needs to worry about preexercise screening. In addition to exercise programs such as Tai Chi, specific guidelines for resistive and aerobic activity, and activity recommendations for those with specific diseases (e.g., cognitive impairment, arthritis), there are also chapters on theoretical approaches to motivate older adults to exercise and ways in which to integrate physical activity into all routine care interactions. As an educator and provider of innovative approaches to engage the oldest old in exercise and physical activity, I believe this edition can serve as a critical source for students across multiple disciplines including physical therapy, occupational therapy, nursing, medicine, and social work.

Kathleen Mangione, PhD, PT, GCS

Introduction

The decrements in strength, endurance, flexibility, and balance that occur with aging contribute to reduced independence, diminished vitality, and increased risk of disabling injury. A considerable body of research substantiates the benefits of regular exercise and increased physical activity with regard to the health, function, and quality of life of older adults. The purpose of this book is to present the state of the science on various exercise approaches (aerobic, stretching, resistance, and balance) in older adults, as well as salient clinical, programmatic, and policy considerations related to implementation and dissemination of exercise programs across a variety of settings. This book is divided into six sections, each having a focus on a particular type of exercise or aspect of initiatives aimed at promoting physical activity and exercise. Each chapter offers the current evidence, provides suggestions and recommendations to support uptake, and offers recommendations for future research and program development.

Despite the known advantages of regular exercise, physical inactivity continues to be a major public health concern, with many people failing to exercise as recommended. Therefore, Section 1, Policy and Practice Related to Exercise and Function, describes policies and guidelines aimed at increasing physical activity across diverse older adult populations. The goal of Chapter 1 is to describe governmental and organizational policies designed to increase physical activity levels in older adults, their impact to date, and recommendations for future international, national, regional, and local policy development. Chapter 2 provides a synopsis of the evidence linking physical activity with positive outcomes in older persons, and the current U.S. Federal guidelines regarding the frequency, intensity, duration, and type of physical activity recommended. Also discussed is the role that geriatricians and gerontologists can play in helping older adults to learn how to "be active in their own way." Chapter 3 provides a summary of the current consensus on evidence-based best practice guidelines for safe and effective preparticipation screening and risk stratification, including for those living with chronic medical conditions. Next, Chapter 4 examines the evidence base of the effects of physical activity on the prevention, delay, and slowing of cognitive decline.

Section 2 addresses aerobic exercises and stretching. Within this section, Chapter 5 reviews the effects of aging on aerobic capacity, the benefits of aerobic exercise across many common chronic diseases, and an evidence-based exercise prescription based on appropriate screening for a variety of conditions common to older adults. Recognizing the current and predicted future global burden of osteoarthritis (OA), Chapter 6 summarizes the evidence on the effectiveness of land- and water-based exercise programs for people with OA of the hip and knee. Chapter 7 summarizes the role of physical activity levels and exercise interventions in the maintenance and training of range of motion (ROM). The pressing need for high-quality purposive study of flexibility and its impact on function is discussed.

Studies have shown that even those of advanced age can benefit from a regular program of strength-building exercises. Section 3, Resistance Exercise, addresses the clinical utility and practical issues to consider when providing evidence-based interventions to increase muscle strength and endurance. Chapter 8 provides recommendations for the design of safe and effective resistance-training protocols, emphasizing psychosocial considerations to maximize participant adherence to and satisfaction with the exercise regimen. Chapter 9 presents the evidence for the use of resistance exercise in the management and prevention of sarcopenia and dynapenia. Guidelines for a well-rounded resistance exercise training program, including example training programs for the beginner through programs for the advanced senior resistance exerciser, are described.

The *2008 Physical Activity Guidelines for Americans* recommends Tai Chi (TC) as a muscle-strengthening exercise and states that TC may prevent falls. In the fourth section, Chapter 10 describes the effect of TC on static and dynamic balance and other outcomes in healthy adults as well as persons with chronic disease, functional impairment, and those living in long-term care facilities. Section 5, Physical Activity as a Determinant of Health, approaches the theoretical basis for and the psychosocial factors influencing exercise habits. To that end, Chapter 11 explores some of the leading theoretical frameworks that have been applied to older adults' physical activity and place them into a classification system to facilitate understanding. The psychosocial constructs that individuals and groups may want to consider when developing interventions to increase or maintain physical activity participation among older adults, regardless of intervention setting, are presented in Chapter 12.

Finally, Chapter 13 presents a theoretically based intervention, Function Focused Care, wherein caregivers engage older adults in function and physical activity during all care interactions. A four-step practical cost-neutral approach is described. This chapter delineates the ways in which to implement Function Focused Care across all settings, describes outcomes associated with this approach, and provides ways in which to overcome the setting-specific challenges.

Barbara Resnick and Marie Boltz

Acknowledgments

We acknowledge the support and enthusiasm of series editor, Dr. Toni Antonucci; Springer executive editor, Sheri W. Sussman; and the authors who contributed to this volume. We are especially appreciative of the commitment and expertise of the authors who have so graciously and thoroughly shared their knowledge in this critically important work. Finally, we acknowledge the older adults who serve as role models for all of us as they continue to remain physically active despite challenges they encounter.

Barbara Resnick and Marie Boltz

CHAPTER 1

Impact of Policy on Physical Activity Participation and Where We Need to Go

Colin Milner and Jenifer Milner

ABSTRACT

Physical inactivity among adults 60 and older is a global health challenge with a significant economic and human cost. Nearly 50% of older people are physically inactive worldwide. To address this challenge, governmental and organizational policy makers have drafted, adopted, and implemented policies to increase physical activity levels, some targeted specifically at the older adult. This investigation of the impact of policy on physical activity and exercise found gradually rising participation levels. Between 1998 and 2012 in the United States, for example, there was a 116% increase in age 65-plus adults deemed active enough to meet the 2008 Physical Activity Guidelines for Americans—from 5.5% to 11.9%, respectively (Centers for Disease Control and Prevention [CDC], 2014). Policies at a variety of levels have created environments and messages to increase physical activity among the older population while delivering services and advice designed to do the same. Yet, the overall impact has been minimal. Addressing the inactivity challenge will require more international, national, regional, and local responses. Some promising areas of focus for policy makers and influencers include the built environment, translation and implementation of research findings on aging as well as efforts to understand their implications, increased health span, and life course approaches to physical activity.

http://dx.doi.org/10.1891/0198-8794.36.1

INTRODUCTION

The best way to meet the challenges of old age is to prepare for them now, before they arrive.

—Reverend Billy Graham

There is a rising awareness in society of both a new life stage created by increased life expectancy and the opportunities and challenges presented by the longevity of older adults, especially when coupled with population aging. Globally, the impact of this demographic shift has yet to be fully realized. Influencing outcomes is a growing body of research and reports recognizing the challenges of an older population—810 million people aged 60 and beyond in 2012 (United Nations Population Fund [UNFPA] & HelpAge International, 2012, p. 19)—while embracing the opportunities, contributions, and benefits they provide (Beard et al., 2011; UNFPA & HelpAge International, 2012). How society responds to these challenges and opportunities may well dictate the societal impact of this demographic as its numbers continue to grow exponentially in the years to come.

We know that to maximize the opportunities and minimize the challenges of longer life, older adults need to stay healthy and well for as long as possible. A physically active lifestyle has been shown to slow declines in function, both physical and cognitive, and therefore is key to the ability to stay independent with age and preserve or enhance the quality of life (King & King, 2010). Physical activity is generally defined as any bodily movements produced by skeletal muscles that result in energy expenditure above resting level, according to Caspersen, Powell, and Christenson (1985). Exercise, a subset, is a planned, structured, and repetitive activity, with the final or intermediate objective of improving or maintaining physical fitness (Caspersen et al., 1985).

Many health benefits of physical activity accrue when people achieve the levels of activity set out in guidelines created by various groups around the globe (United States Department of Health & Human Services [HHS], 2008; World Health Organization [WHO], 2011b, "Recommendations for 65 years and above"). Despite physical activity's vital influence on how people age, nearly 50% of adults 60 years of age and above are inactive worldwide (Franco et al., 2015). There is a health, social, and economic cost that comes with failing to meet the guidelines (Kraus et al., 2015, p. 1).

Physical inactivity has contributed to the rise in ill-health and noncommunicable diseases (NCDs) such as diabetes that challenges health-care systems worldwide (Lee et al., 2012a, 2012b). Its economic impact is significant on these systems (e.g., US$75 billion a year in the United States [WHO, 2003, p. 4] and

CDN$2.4 billion in Canada in 2009 [Janssen, 2012, p. 805]). The impact of physical inactivity goes well beyond health-care settings, however. In a theoretical example from Europe, if 50% of a population of 10 million failed to achieve the health benefits of regular physical activity, inactivity would result in an estimated economic burden of €910 million a year (WHO Regional Office for Europe, 2007, p. 9). (Indirect costs associated with inactivity included lost economic output due to illness, disease-related work disabilities, and premature death.) A real-world estimate suggested that physical inactivity in the United Kingdom had a UK£8.2 billion impact, once indirect costs were added to those that directly affected the health-care system (Department for Culture, Media & Sport, 2002, p. 48).

In fact, the five leading NCDs alone—cardiovascular disease, chronic respiratory disease, cancer, diabetes, and mental ill-health—could exact a US$47 trillion cost globally by 2030 if left unchecked, according to a report from the World Economic Forum (WEF) and Harvard School of Public Health (Bloom et al., 2011, p. 6). Approximately 40% of these costs would affect areas of society unrelated to health (WEF, 2011). Further, as the population ages, NCDs such as diabetes, heart disease, and arthritis will increase in prevalence (Bloom et al., 2011, p. 7; WHO, 2011a, p. 1), which suggests that growing proportions of expenditures will go toward adults aged 60 years and older.

There is also the human cost. Globally, physical inactivity is the fourth leading risk factor for death (Kraus et al., 2015, p. 1), claiming 5.3 million lives each year (Lee et al., 2012a, 2012b). As it has positive effects on 25 diseases and health conditions, physical activity participation could help change this statistic (Kraus et al., 2015, p. 1). We could prevent 533,000 deaths a year if we lowered physical inactivity rates by just 10% (Lee et al., 2012a, 2012b).

Inactivity with advancing age is not just about death, disease, and economics, however; it is also about people's loss of potential due to declines in health status, function (physical, cognitive and social), independence, and quality of life. Individuals may lose not only the ability to contribute actively to and participate fully in society and the daily life of their families and communities but also to thrive in their later years. As physical activity helps maintain, improve, or restore health and function, participation can transform lives, which has value at all levels (King & King, 2010).

Physical inactivity is now a global health challenge (Kraus et al., 2015, p. 1), particularly in the 60-plus population, the least active of all age groups (HHS, 2008, p. 29). Because of the human and economic costs of inactivity, robust policies, strategies, and solutions that promote physical activity are a public and private health imperative if we are to minimize the impact on this population (Kraus et al., 2015, p. 1; Lee et al., 2012b).

Researchers, governments, businesses, families, and individuals have been responding to the physical inactivity challenge in their own ways. The WHO provided the 2002 framework for national policies around active aging—which includes physical activity—to support continued participation in society and the workforce by older adults (2002). Agencies and organizations have since made many policy recommendations and undertaken important efforts to promote healthy, active aging.

In Europe, one ongoing response has come from the European Commission (EC), which manages and implements European Union (EU) policies. Driven by the implications of demographic change, the EC "identified active and healthy ageing" as a societal challenge and an area of potential for all EU states, and in 2011, created the European Innovation Partnership on Active and Healthy Ageing (2013, p. 4). This partnership unites public and private sector stakeholders in health policy to support active, healthy aging through innovation and research.

Earlier projects set the stage for increased EU engagement in older adult health promotion. For example, under the EU Public Health Programme, the Swedish National Institute of Public Health (2007) embarked upon the Healthy Ageing project [2004–2007], with support from the EC and 12 partners, including the WHO. The project's report, released in 2007, concluded there were "insufficient ageing policies at EU-level and inconsistent focuses on health promotion in national age policies," according to a later report by EuroHealthNet for the Federal Centre for Health Education in Germany (2012, p. 12).

Another EU-funded initiative, the PASEO (Building Policy Capacities for Health Promotion through Physical Activity among Sedentary Older People) Project, sought to build policy capacity for active aging in 15 EU countries (Institute of Sport Science and Sport, 2010). Launched in 2009, PASEO helped address barriers to policy interest, adoption, and implementation. The project, which ended in 2011, focused on strengthening intersectoral and intraorganizational policy capacities, with the goal of improving efforts by agencies and organizations to promote physical activity for older adults (Institute of Sport Science and Sport, 2010). National and/or regional alliances were created in the 15 participating nations. Overall, 114 "specific measures were developed to improve capacities, including dissemination and networking activities, staff training, infrastructures, and pilot projects," according to Rütten, Abu-Omar, Frahsa, and Gelius (2013, p. 151).

In 2013, WHO Member States adopted the goal of reducing the levels of physical inactivity 10% by 2025 (WHO, 2015, "How to increase physical activity?"). About 80% of the Member States now have a physical activity plan or policies in place (WHO, 2015). Even with these and other physical activity developments worldwide, policies are still lacking in implementation (Kohl et al., 2012). In fact, policies were operational in just over half (56%) of the WHO's Member States in 2013 (WHO, 2015).

In the United States, a similar movement to address inactivity is underway. Under its Healthy Aging Program, the CDC funds the Prevention Research Centers Healthy Aging Research Network (PRC-HAN), which was established in 2001. The PRC-HAN's mission is "to better understand the determinants of healthy aging in older adult populations, to identify interventions that promote healthy aging, and to help translate this knowledge into sustainable community-based programs" (the Healthy Aging Research Network Writing Group, 2006, p. 3). The network chose physical activity as its initial focus area for research.

Another major U.S. initiative is the National Physical Activity Plan (NPAP). Released in May 2010, NPAP provides comprehensive policy recommendations, programs, and initiatives intended "to increase physical activity in all segments of the American population" (NPAP, n.d., para. 2). The strategic plan strives "to create a national culture that supports physically active lifestyles. Its ultimate purpose is to improve health, prevent disease and disability, and enhance quality of life" (NPAP, n.d., para. 3). Created through a private–public collaboration, NPAP focuses on physical activity for health, yet it is limited when it comes to the 60-plus population as it does not address older adults' specific needs in its recommended policies, programs, and initiatives.

NPAP aims to increase activity rather than to reduce sedentary behavior, though it recognizes such behavior change as "an important public health goal" (NPAP, n.d., para. 6). Even small amounts of physical activity are beneficial for adults aged 60 and older, according to a growing body of research (CDC, n.d., p. 1). The challenge is that while individuals may engage in some activity, too few achieve participation levels that provide the multiple health benefits associated with recommended amounts of physical activity. In 2012, only 14.8% of adults 65–74 years old, and 7.9% of people 75 years and older met the 2008 Physical Activity Guidelines for Americans (CDC/National Center for Health Statistics [NCHS], 2014, p. 222).

The U.S. guidelines call for 150 minutes of moderate-intensity aerobic activity per week as well as strengthening exercises on at least 2 days a week (HHS, 2008, p. 30). Vigorous aerobic activity requires accumulating just 75 minutes weekly to meet the guidelines, or individuals may perform an equivalent combination of moderate- and vigorous-intensity activity (HHS, 2008, p. 30). Resistance and balance training are also recommended. These exercise modes benefit older adults as they address the declines in muscle strength, cardiovascular capacity, and balance associated with the aging process (HHS, 2008).

It is important to recognize that the guidelines assume the minimal amount of moderate-intensity physical activity for health. Both the U.S. guidelines and the WHO encourage older adults to "be as physically active as their abilities and conditions allow" if health conditions prevent them from doing the recommended amount of activity (HHS, 2008, p. 30; WHO, 2011b, "Recommendations for 65 years and above," point 6).

The good news is that the percentage of older adults who meet the physical activity guidelines has actually risen in the United States, increasing 116% between 1998 and 2012 (from 5.5% to 11.9 %, respectively; CDC/NCHS, 2014, p. 222). The overall rates are still well below desired results but are moving in the right direction. A full 51.7% of adults 65–74 years old and 67.2% of people 75 years and older had not met the overall guidelines in 2012, down from 65.6% and 77.8%, respectively, in 1998 (CDC/NCHS, 2014, p. 222).

The question now is, how do we optimize adoption and participation as well as the levels of physical activity across settings? In this chapter, we look at policy, the role it plays, and the impact it could have on physical activity and exercise now and in the future.

POLICY AND ITS IMPACT

To explore policy and its role and impact on physical activity, we must first define policy. We discover that what constitutes policy varies among agencies and organizations, and at international, national, regional, and local levels, which presents a challenge and a barrier for those who seek to influence it (McKinnon, Bowles, & Trowbridge, 2011; Rütten et al., 2012). One general definition of "policy" includes laws, rules, regulations, organizational guidelines, internal agency decisions/memoranda, and social norms that guide behavior (Brownson, Chriqui, & Stamatakis, 2009).

The WHO defines health policy as referring "to decisions, plans and actions that are undertaken to achieve specific health care goals within a society. An explicit health policy can achieve several things: It defines a vision for the future, which in turn helps to establish targets and points of reference for the short and medium term" (WHO, n.d., para. 1).

However, policies that encourage physical activity are not the purview of health departments only; they cross departments within agencies and organizations. These policy makers and partners play key roles in promoting physical activity through indirect and direct policy methods, including such things as community design (built environment and transportation policies) and business and industry policies and practices (McKinnon et al., 2011). Policy makers and influencers must effectively navigate the overall landscape as an important step toward success with policy development, adoption, and implementation (Rütten et al., 2012, pp. 8, 9).

In South Australia, the state government has recognized the need to bridge the various stakeholders by creating the Department of Health in All Policies. This department ensures that all governmental agencies take health into consideration. It provides opportunities for agencies to work together to help improve the health of South Australia's population through addressing factors that influence health but lie outside the realm of the health sector. In addition, the Department of Health in All Policies works directly with other government departments to examine the implications of these departments' policies on health and well-being—and health and well-being on those departments. Policy options are then posed to improve health outcomes (WHO & Government of South Australia, 2010).

From Finland (Vuori, Lankenau, & Pratt, 2004) to Thailand (Leppo, Ollila, Peña, Wismar, & Cook, 2013, p. 37) to South Australia (WHO & Government of South Australia, 2010), numerous places around the world use a Health in All Policies (HiAP) strategy. The term first appeared in 2006 during the second Finnish EU presidency, with the goal of promoting intersectoral collaboration to accomplish common goals (Leppo et al., 2013, p. 6). HiAP particularly encourages sectors that influence health—transportation, housing, public safety, education, and environment, among others—to consider health factors in their policy-making (Leppo et al., 2013, p. 3). Today, the EC requires all EU policies to incorporate an HiAP approach, states the European Commission Directorate-General for Health and Food Safety (DG SANTE, n.d.). "But to be fully effective, this approach needs to be extended to national, regional and local policies" (DG SANTE, n.d., para. 2).

One regional example is ActNow BC in British Columbia, Canada. Led by the Government of British Columbia's Ministry of Health and involving all provincial government ministries as well as external partners, this health promotion initiative focused on addressing risk factors for and reducing chronic diseases (2006). ActNow BC supported local governments, communities, employers, and schools in developing and promoting programs to "make healthy choices the easy choices for all British Columbians" (Government of British Columbia, 2006, para. 3).

The HiAP strategy "has quickly gained momentum in the US and internationally," noted Wernham and Teutsch (2015, para. 3) For example, health officials in large U.S. cities pointed to HiAP as "a top priority" in a recent survey, the researchers revealed (Wernham & Teutsch, 2015, para. 2). Some cities that use this strategy include San Francisco, Seattle, Los Angeles, Boston, and

Washington, D.C. Wernham and Teutsch added that California provided "an early and influential application" of HiAP with its 2010 executive order (2015, "Tools of HiAP").

Such a rapid embrace of HiAP, including funding allocated for its implementation, suggests that governments at all levels and foundations fully realize the value of intersectoral approaches when it comes to health promotion. Wernham and Teutsch concur. They write, "Creating healthy communities requires building a culture of health, where health is integrated into decisions made in all sectors of society" (2015, para. 6).

Although Switzerland does not have a specific department charged with promoting physical activity, the Swiss Government does use a multisectoral approach to encourage physical activity participation. Approved in January 2013, the Swiss Health 2020 strategy "emphasizes that a person's health is determined by up to 60% through factors outside the health sector. The Swiss Federal Office of Public Health has focused on specific cooperative projects with other federal agencies in order to create opportunities to promote physical activity in urban and regional planning" (WHO Regional Office for Europe, 2015, "Intersectoral collaboration").

This level of coordination between governments, funders, and private stakeholders across sectors is still missing in many places around the world. Calls for increased collaboration are widespread, however. In a European example, the Swedish Association of Local Authorities and Regions (SALAR), EuroHealthNet, and Euregha (n.d., point 2) issued a 2014 recommendation for an HiAP approach "at all levels of government, from local and regional to EU level."

With efforts to encourage new and more widespread collaborations, we are likely to see varying degrees of HiAP implementation as well as success. As HiAP strategies focus on health, we do not know whether they will give enough attention to physical activity in the 60-plus population to change participation levels.

While physical activity has increased in older adults, can we pinpoint the role that policy has played in addressing this challenge? We know that policy makers confront unique challenges in their efforts to increase population activity levels, according to McKinnon et al. (2011). The authors write that physical activity promotion differs in a number of key ways from other public health challenges: Physical activity is an encouraged behavior, rather than a discouraged one; it requires continued commitment to behavior change, rather than momentary action; and it offers myriad ways to participate while appropriate time and intensity vary, "making generic, 'sound-bite' recommendations challenging" (McKinnon et al., 2011, p. S145). The diversity of the older adult population simply adds to these challenges, requiring policy initiatives that provide diverse messages and solutions (Health Canada, 1999, p. 7).

AN AMERICAN PERSPECTIVE

A review of the literature reveals that the United States lacks a dedicated federal policy to increase physical activity adoption and participation levels specifically for adults 60 years of age and older. Still, there are efforts undertaken at various levels of government and business that have had an impact—from policies and programs to priorities and interventions.

In fact, several policies include physical activity for older adults as one or more of their component(s). Additionally, many general policies focused on such areas as the built environment, transportation, health care, and worksites aim to encourage physical activity directly or as a by-product for all populations, not just the old. In the following text are examples of some of the big "P" policies targeted to older adults. These policies "are implementable by public policy makers, rather than small 'p' policies that may be implemented unilaterally by organizations" (McKinnon et al., 2011, S145).

Older Americans Act

In 1965, the U.S. Congress passed the Older Americans Act (OAA) to provide community-based services and programs for older adults. This law also created the Administration on Aging (AoA, n.d.a). Charged with administering the government's new grant programs, this agency was also expected to serve as "the federal focal point on matters concerning older persons" (AoA, n.d.a, para. 1). OAA amendments enacted in 2006 highlighted both the need for, and support of, evidence-based prevention programs (AoA, n.d.b, "Funding and Innovation").

Under "Disease Prevention and Health Promotion Services" (Title IIID), funding is provided to evidence-based health promotion programs, including physical activity (AoA, n.d.b, "Funding and Innovation"). This support has driven government agencies and organizations such as senior centers, hospitals, universities, and many others to seek out evidence-based programs. The National Registry of Evidence-based Programs and Practices (NREPP) facilitates this need (Substance Abuse and Mental Health Services Administration, n.d.). In fiscal year 2013, nearly US$20 million was invested in these programs (AoA, n.d.b, "Funding and Innovation").

As of October 1, 2016, AoA will adopt a new definition for evidence-based programs that requires programs to meet one set of stringent criteria in order to be eligible for Title IIID funds. The first of these criteria will involve showing a program's effectiveness through evaluation (AoA, n.d.b, "Future Definition of Evidence-Based").

The scientific evidence for physical activity benefits in older adults has already played a key role in motivating initiatives and funding to improve participation levels. Part of the credit belongs to the National Institute on Aging (NIA), a component of the National Institutes of Health that focuses on aging research. NIA, established under the OAA, has built an evidence base and also spurred others to examine the effects of physical activity in the older adult.

National Institute on Aging

In 1974, Public Law 93-296 authorized establishing NIA (NIA, n.d., "May 31, 1974"). This law required the institute to "develop a national comprehensive plan to coordinate the HEW (Health, Education, Welfare) agencies involved in aging research" (NIA, n.d., "May 31, 1974"). Since then, NIA's research findings have spurred others to conduct additional research. All told, this research has created a body of evidence that informs everything from physical activity guidelines; to professional services in health care, fitness, and community services; to community design and the built environment. The evidence has supported calls for change and demonstrated that prior perceptions of old age were ill-founded. It has also been the catalyst for change (Beard et al., 2011; United Nations Department of Economic and Social Affairs, 2012).

In the past, people aged 60 and beyond were frequently discouraged from doing exercise and vigorous physical activity (Franco et al., 2015; Ory, Kinney Hoffman, Hawkins, Sanner, & Mockenhaupt, 2003). NIA has provided credible support and evidence that shows that, far from harming older people, a physically active lifestyle is essential to enjoying a healthier, more active life as people age. The research has also shown how to design exercise properly to meet the diversity of older adults' needs and abilities, adding to the success and safety of their activity (NIA, 2009).

Today's new research findings set the stage for tomorrow's policies, services, and environments. They also continue to drive changes in the way society perceives aging. Beyond its research impacts, NIA also promotes health by disseminating information such as *Exercise & Physical Activity: Your everyday guide from the National Institute on Aging!* (NIA, 2009) for older Americans. The institute's influence on physical activity is indisputable—yet we do not know at what level.

Affordable Care Act

The evidence for physical activity in aging adults also influenced the 2010 Patient Protection and Affordable Care Act (more commonly known as the Affordable Care Act, or ACA; HHS, 2009a). Within the ACA, a variety of action plans address physical activity, although indirectly. These include:

- Medicare-covered Annual Wellness Visits (AWVs) offer a personalized prevention plan, with assessment and counseling (HHS, 2009b, pp. 1153–1155). Components include health advice and referral to health education or preventive counseling services or community-based lifestyle interventions to address identified health risk factors (Centers for Medicare & Medicaid Services, 2015; HHS, 2009b, p. 1156). A significant gap exists, however, between the total number of Medicare enrollees (45 million) and the number who have completed a wellness visit (1.35 million; Mancuso, 2013). Poor communication may contribute. One year after launch, 68% of enrollees "had not heard of the benefit or were not sure if they had heard of it" (John A. Hartford Foundation, 2012, "Medicare's Annual Wellness Visit: The benefit nobody knows").

- Creating Healthier Communities includes provisions for developing and promoting programs that boost access to physical activity and other community-based health activities. Programs target various age levels (HHS, 2009c, p. 1184).
- Healthy Aging, Living Well supports intervention activities "to improve nutrition, increase physical activity . . . and promote healthy lifestyles" among adults aged 55–64 years (HHS, 2009d, pp. 1188–1190; Legal Information Institute, n.d., Section 3B[ii]). Included were a demonstration project on individualized wellness plans as well as small business grants to promote workplace wellness programs.

While it is hard to know with any certainty how effective all these policies have been in increasing physical activity adoption and participation levels, they are setting the stage for progress. It is still virtually impossible to pinpoint any one specific thing so far that has had the greatest success with older adults due to the difficulty of evaluating the overall impact of policies.

EVALUATING THE IMPACT

Evaluating policy impact is difficult because of the variability of resources available in different countries, cultures, and settings. Among the things that influence policy efforts are guidance and information, guidelines and recommendations, policy papers, action plans, frameworks, blueprints, and white papers. Evaluation tools are often a work in progress (Rütten et al., 2012, pp. 2, 7). Further, there is a lack of clarity, consistency, and understanding when it comes to terminology (e.g., the difference between physical activity and exercise) and methods (e.g., which physical activity guidelines are used, how older adults are defined; Garcia, Sá, Rezende, & Silva, 2015; Sun, Norman, & White, 2013).

In addition, policy makers with different agendas drive physical activity initiatives. What constitutes success, therefore, may look different to individual policy makers and stakeholders depending on their frames of reference (Rütten et al., 2012, p. 7).

For example, an environmental department may aim to decrease greenhouse gas emissions by increasing cycling and walking, and greater participation in these physical activities may be only one target toward the larger goal. In another example, a transportation department may provide free transportation to older adults to encourage social activity, as the Department of Transport has done in South Australia (Truong & Somenahalli, 2015). Increased physical activity becomes a by-product that is not evaluated as an outcome—even though the science shows that free transportation can increase activity levels as older adults travel more in their communities (Coronini-Cronberg, Millett, Laverty, & Webb, 2012).

While these challenges exist in evaluating the impact of policies that promote physical activity, policy makers and partners can look at the impact on short- and medium-term targets as indicators of whether or not policies are having the desired effect.

The clearest message to date is that individual education and programming are not sufficient for real change in physical activity at the population level (McKinnon et al., 2011). Environmental systems and policy strategies are required (McKinnon et al., 2011; Ory, Jordan, & Bazzarre, 2002).

THE SOCIAL–ECOLOGICAL MODEL

Given that "human behavior is difficult to change, especially in an environment that does not support change" (ParticiPACTION Advisory Groups, 2011, p. 24), embracing a social–ecological model for physical activity promotion allows policy makers and partners to identify more opportunities for diverse, flexible, and inclusive responses. This framework takes into account the impact of social, physical, and policy environments on physical activity participation (King & King, 2010; ParticiPACTION Advisory Groups, 2011, p. 8). To support change and promote activity, approaches must focus not only on individual behavior choices but also on those factors that influence them. The framework begins with the individual level and extends through the interpersonal, organizational, community, and public policy spheres (ParticiPACTION, 2011, p. 24).

We can see a microcosm of how this model works in the many senior living communities in the United States that now provide environments to encourage physical activity and exercise. From cycling and walking paths to outdoor exercise stations and meditation gardens, to swimming pools and golf courses, these residential properties offer a wide range of community features to support lifestyle choices for residents who desire to age well. Also included on many properties are fitness or wellness centers with qualified staff to inspire and support behavior change at individual and organizational levels. Residents who live physically active lifestyles often act as role models and physical activity ambassadors for their peers, while activities and programs foster social networks of individuals who lead fuller, more active lives. A 2014 International Council on Active Aging (ICAA) survey revealed that, in responding organizations, a median 33% of residents in continuing care retirement communities (CCRCs) and 30% in independent living (IL) and active adult communities participated in fitness/physical activity (ICAA, 2014a).

More recently, these senior living communities are increasingly adopting formal programs and cultures where the emphasis is on wellness and living. Formal, structured wellness programs were established in 82% of CCRCs and 76% of IL plus independent/assisted living communities that responded to another ICAA survey (ICAA, 2015). These programs had been in place for an average of 6–7 years (ICAA, 2015). Organizational policies can bolster communities' efforts to support resident wellness in all areas of life, including physical activity. Hiring practices, for example, can include screening to discover the attitudes of job candidates toward older adults, their abilities, and their potential to participate in physical activity. Programs in individual communities may also connect with public policy initiatives intended to encourage active lifestyles.

This environmental shift in senior living has been taking place over the past few decades. It is in the past few years, though, that we have seen this growing focus on prevention, health, lifestyle, and quality of life (ICAA, 2014b). What is behind the increased momentum? Ninety percent of the community owners and managers that ICAA surveyed have accepted the need for, and embraced the benefits of, physical activity in older adults (ICAA, 2014a, pp. 18, 23).

Still, even with such positive environments and multilevel supports for physical activity, efforts will likely enjoy limited success if they fail to address older adults' barriers to participation.

BARRIERS AND FACILITATORS

Older adults know the benefits of regular physical activity (AARP, 2002, p. 8)—yet a significant percentage of this population has yet to change behaviors and embrace an active lifestyle (CDC/NCHS, 2014, p. 222). As previously noted, behavior change requires more than a focus on the individual. It also takes a focus on the factors that influence choices (see "The Social–Ecological Model" section) to set the stage for success (King & King, 2010; McKinnon et al., 2011).

Whether real or perceived, barriers to physical activity adoption and participation are as diverse as the 60-plus population itself, challenging policy makers at all levels to move beyond "one size fits all" solutions to more person-centered approaches. In addition to national, regional, and cultural differences, older people vary in functional levels (physical, cognitive, social), stages of life, life experiences, beliefs, values, expectations, aspirations, incomes, races, capabilities (hearing, vision, touch and speech), and health status (Health Canada, 1999, p. 7; King & King, 2010, p. 412; UNFPA & HelpAge International, 2012, pp. 13, 21). This diversity should not prevent a focused effort on reducing or eliminating barriers to physical activity adoption and participation. Understanding population differences and barriers allows policy makers at all levels of government and business to make better decisions about the direction, design, development, and delivery of their policy initiatives.

The following are some of the barriers and facilitators that commonly influence physical activity adoption and participation in older adults and can be found throughout the social–ecological model (Breen, 2015; Franco et al., 2015; King & King, 2010; Moschny, Platen, Klaaßen-Mielke, Trampisch, & Hinrichs, 2011):

- Public policy (few or ineffective policies and funding to support physical activity participation by older adults; progressive urban-planning policies; confusing messages about physical activity guidelines)
- Community (accessible or inaccessible facilities; access or barriers to moving about in the built environment [e.g., safety, crime, transportation]; walkable neighborhoods [e.g., street connectivity, pedestrian access, sidewalks]; presence of parks and green spaces; lack of local facilities and spaces for physical activity)
- Organizational (lack of workplace or organizational policies to support physical activity, affordability of programs; competing priorities [e.g., work responsibilities, lack of time]; design of physical spaces [e.g., workplace environment]; messages about aging, both implicit and explicit)
- Interpersonal (valuing interaction with peers, encouragement from others, social awkwardness, no exercise companions, competing priorities [e.g., family, friends, other activities]; ageist stereotypes resulting in lack of support)
- Individual (physical, cognitive, and mental health [e.g., physical health status, frailty, chronic pain or discomfort, chronic diseases, depression, fatigue and low energy]; physical and cognitive functional abilities; self-perception [e.g., values, culture, self-confidence, negative stereotypes, fear of falling and injury, unattainable expectations]; lifestyle [e.g., apathy, isolation, independence, socioeconomic status, enjoyment of physical activity])

Ageism and its effects present a pervasive barrier to physical activity participation by age 60-plus adults. Negative stereotypes and myths of aging infuse society's views of what is possible in this life stage, distorting how people understand and respond to aging and older adults. Ageism is manifested in a general disregard that renders older people "invisible" and a lack of societal support for their continued participation as full members of their communities (Ory et al., 2003). When it comes to physical activity, ageist attitudes may influence whether or not older adults are active and to what degree, what kinds of activities they do, where they exercise, and whether they find supportive products, services, and environments, and so forth. On a personal level, individuals may doubt their ability to be active and whether or not they may undertake specific activities (especially more vigorous exercise)—including whether or not it is safe or socially acceptable for them to do so (Langer, 2009; Nelson, 2002). Support, guidance, and information are key to their overcoming this barrier (Bethancourt, Rosenberg, Beatty, & Arterburn, 2014).

Physical activity guidelines may themselves present a barrier. Scientists disagree about current physical activity targets for older people and whether these should increase, decrease, or remain as they are (Merom, Buchner, & Fiatarone Singh, 2015; Sparling, Howard, Dunstan, & Owen, 2015). For a segment of the older population, concerns abound about being able to meet the guidelines. A target of 30 minutes of aerobic activity seems daunting, for example, if 5 minutes is only just within reach. Inconsistent messaging about physical activity may further confuse and discourage individuals who already face numerous obstacles to participation, presenting a real barrier to physical activity (The Robert Wood Johnson Foundation, 2001).

An example of a policy designed to remove barriers is the Americans with Disabilities Act (ADA), enacted in 1990 (U.S. Department of Justice, n.d., "The 2010 Regulations"). Americans now have greater physical and social access to physical activity and health promotion activities through measures such as curb cuts, ramps, and accessible entrances to buildings. Has the reduction of these barriers increased physical activity in older adults? We may intuitively believe the answer to be yes, but we were unable to find evidence to support this view. Policy makers would benefit from access to such information, given the growing interest in improving the built environment to make communities more walkable.

A more comprehensive overview is needed to illuminate environmental barriers to physical activity and the policies and strategies believed to be effective in eliminating them. It is also important to know and understand whether increased physical activity levels did, in fact, follow efforts to address barriers to participation (Gellert et al., 2015).

A comparison of highly designed senior living communities can offer anecdotal evidence. Two communities have ideal settings and have worked to eliminate barriers to participation. One achieves high participation levels in physical activity programs and settings, while the other struggles. Why? Answers may give policy makers at all levels information needed for success. For example, an answer may be found in the culture of the organization and the people who are hired to inspire physical activity adoption and participation. It may also be found in peer-to-peer support and interests. Regardless of the answers, such a comparison shows there is no "magic bullet" when it comes to increasing the levels of physical activity participation, even in ideal circumstances.

Will policy makers and policy efforts drive these initiatives and promising practices, moving forward? Or will these initiatives and promising practices influence policy? The verdict is still out.

POLICY BARRIERS

Similar to the situation faced by older adults, policy makers and influencers encounter many barriers to the adoption and implementation of physical activity policies. In the United States, a key barrier is the small percentage of the country's health-care budget allocated to population-wide approaches (Brownson et al., 2009), even with the overwhelming evidence that demonstrates the benefits of physical activity (McKinnon et al., 2011)—especially for the older population.

We might logically expect scientific evidence to be an important support for any policy decisions. In reality, an evidence base has limited impact when it comes to policy-making. In a systematic review of 107 "model" public health laws over 16 topics, Hartsfield, Moulton, and McKie (2007) found that "sponsors provide[d] details showing that the law was based on scientific information" in only 6.5% of these laws (Brownson et al., 2009).

Researchers do have a key role to play in assuring policy makers of the credibility of the arguments. In many cases, however, the messages and the research supporting them are delivered in a more complex manner than desired by policy makers, who are not researchers. This places a high importance on how scientific information is delivered (Hartsfield et al., 2007). Furthermore, many interest groups are ready to "interpret" the evidence as "good" or "bad" for policy makers, which reinforces the need for policy makers to be connected with the research community. Most researchers, however, do not see such efforts as part of their work (Hartsfield et al., 2007).

One way to minimize the barriers to policy adoption is to enable policy makers to gain a clear understanding of the issues, solutions, and supporting evidence by simplifying the information and the way in which it is presented to them (Brownson et al., 2009; Hartsfield et al., 2007; McKinnon et al., 2011). Partners in a variety of settings can support efforts. These partners may influence this work and ensure it is not done in isolation, as this can limit the range of perspectives (Hartsfield et al., 2007).

To address a lack of resources and funding for aging initiatives, policy makers may need to shift their interests, beliefs, and political agendas (Brownson et al., 2009) in order to accept a life course view of physical activity. Presenting more balanced portrayals of today's older adults may help to address ageist attitudes, which are often unconscious (Ory et al., 2003).

In the end, success in overcoming the multiple barriers to policy adoption may require political support, strong partners, and the ability to demonstrate a desired policy's sustainability and designated timeline (Brownson et al., 2009; McKinnon et al., 2011).

PROMISING PRACTICES

Policy makers are more likely to show interest when initiatives show promise. One promising practice that has gained traction around the globe is physician-prescribed exercise. Managed by the American College of Sports Medicine, Exercise is Medicine (EIM) aims to "[encourage] primary care physicians and other health care providers to include physical activity when designing treatment plans for patients" (EIM, n.d.a, para. 1). This global health initiative educates and supports the medical community in prescribing exercise. It also influences policy at a physician level, with medical professionals adopting exercise prescription as a business or practice policy. As of May 2015, EIM has spread to 43 countries (EIM, n.d.b, para. 2).

Research conducted in New Zealand shows that older adults trust their primary care physicians as sources of information about physical activity (Schofield, Croteau, & McLean, 2005). In fact, older adults, inactive individuals, and those with chronic diseases proved most likely to express trust (Schofield et al., 2005). This dynamic ensures the medical community has a central role to play in promoting physical activity among older adults.

In the United States, only 50% of physicians receive any education on physical activity during their degree training (Cardinal, Park, Kim, & Cardinal, in press). This lack of knowledge can inhibit physicians from prescribing exercise and physical activity. Still, physicians and allied health professionals have increased the percentage of patients of all population groups to whom they recommend exercise participation, according to a study by Barnes and Schoenborn from the CDC (2012). Among adults aged 85 years and older who visited a physician or health professional in 2010, 28.9% of patients received advice to exercise, a significant rise from the 15.3% so counseled in 2000 (Barnes & Schoenborn, 2012).

Physician-prescribed exercise is a practice that has shown promise (Kraus et al., 2015, p. 4) and successfully influenced public policy in other countries.

In New Zealand, more than 80% of New Zealand's general practitioners (primary care physicians) have used the Green Prescription or GRx (New Zealand Ministry of Health, n.d., "Programme administration"). Initiated in 1998, the GRx initiative has increased physical activity in the nation's general population. Research has found that 1 in 10 of these written exercise prescriptions resulted in an individual reaching, and sustaining, recommended amounts of physical activity at 12 months (Elley, Kerse, Arroll, & Robinson, 2003). The funding of this policy initiative started at the national level and, over time, has devolved to local-level governments. Direct supervision has been a key factor in its success.

Finland has based its Movement Prescription Project on New Zealand's model. In 2004, a small proportion of physicians and patients had experience with written exercise prescriptions, resulting in positive "initial experiences," reported Vuori et al. (2004, p. 336). In Canada, the Primary Care Networks (PCN) successfully piloted the Prescription to Get Active program in Leduc, Alberta, in 2011 (Prescription to Get Active, n.d.). Also based on GRx, the program has since expanded to the province's two largest cities, Calgary and Edmonton. More than 2,300 family physicians may prescribe activity through this program, and 50 recreational and wellness facilities recognize these prescriptions, according to PCN (C. Leyte, personal communication, April 28, 2015).

Does the AWV have the potential to become a Green Prescription program for Americans aged 60 and older? Efforts to promote physical activity can point policy makers toward physician-prescribed exercise as a promising practice that has shown results for governments and organizations elsewhere.

WHERE DO WE GO FROM HERE?

Over the past 50 years, a gathering momentum has brought us to where we are today: Regular physical activity and exercise are accepted as important to the health and well-being of people over 60 years of age. The question is: Where do we go from here in our efforts to increase physical activity levels in the older adult? There are so many areas to address, some of which are discussed in the following text.

Research

Research creates the foundation for change and progress. We need more research to better understand aging, and we need a better understanding of the research and its implications in order to translate and implement findings. In a review of the evidence for older adult physical activity for Australia's Department of Health and Ageing, Sims et al. (2006, p. 96) from the National Ageing Research Institute concluded, "A key area for future research is to evaluate innovative strategies to achieve effective translation of the research evidence into widespread practice."

Sims et al. (2006, p. 96) also pointed to "methodological weaknesses" that must be addressed when it comes to finding and evaluating research. Among these were "small sample sizes"; "limited sociodemographic characteristics" of those who participate in studies; "lack of follow-up," especially for longer periods; "inappropriate outcome measurement tools" for the older adult; and "mismatch between intervention focus and outcome measures used" (Sims et al., 2006, p. 96). A further weakness involved older adult research findings aggregated into age groupings, instead of with consideration to "baseline functional status" (Sims et al., 2006, p. 96).

Integrated Approaches

As practices, programs, priorities, and policies accumulate, they amplify the physical activity message and promote physical activity adoption and participation. Success at population-level change requires more, however. A dedicated policy for increasing physical activity must be created and integrated throughout all departments (Chodzko-Zajko & Schwingel, 2009, p. 30) and organizations.

Adopting an integrated and inclusive approach to policy will build physical activity into all government levels, systems, and policies (Chodzko-Zajko & Schwingel, 2009, p. 30) and embrace all ages. Greater implementation of HiAP strategies is desirable, though it does not guarantee a focus on older adults and physical activity. Ideally, an integrated approach will heighten the importance of physical activity throughout society for policy makers. It will also enhance awareness in urban planning, health care, commerce, or myriad other settings of the need to build in physical activity policies and initiatives for older adults.

An integrated approach is also needed to create seamless support for physical activity across the full spectrum of services and care for older adults. In the United States, ACA policies focused on reducing readmissions for specific illnesses have already led hospitals and health-care organizations to work with community agencies and residential communities to improve posthospital transitions (Kilroy, Morgan-Solomon, & Landrum, 2013, pp. 6, 9). In a similar vein, "community health business partnership models" (Kindig & Isham, 2014) would ensure a continuum of supportive services—from primary care provider to physical therapist to personal trainer, for example—that bridges transitions to help individuals start and sustain physical activity for improved health.

Activity Over the Life Course

We have begun to understand the importance of life stages "to health capital and specific disease processes," thanks to epidemiological research (International Longevity Centre-UK [ILC-UK] & WHO, 2000, p. 3). Findings will continue to add to our body of knowledge. The result will allow us to create new or refined "life course models with specific implications for health and social policy interventions" (ILC-UK & WHO, 2000, p. 3).

Globally, physical inactivity is a "pandemic" (Kohl et al., 2012) for populations across the life span. In the United States, for example, 46.6% of the 18-and-older population was insufficiently active to meet the *2008 Physical Activity Guidelines for Americans* in 2012 (CDC/NCHS, 2014, p. 222). Given the health risks this reality represents, a life course approach to physical activity would lay the foundation for healthy aging. By emphasizing the impact of health behaviors throughout life, this approach could enhance efforts by governments and businesses to promote physical activity participation as well as increase adoption by families and individuals. To support physical activity over the life course, health literacy will also require a lifelong approach (ILC-UK & WHO, 2000, p. 3; Kickbusch, Wait, Maag, McGuire, & Banks, 2006, p. 11).

A significant health and economic benefit would result from developing a healthy nation versus one challenged by chronic disease and decline (Janssen, 2012; Lee et al., 2012b; WHO, 2003, p. 4). In addition, addressing physical activity in schools and in the community would help restore active play to lifestyles. A great deal of success would depend on the built environment, however—from safe and accessible parks to neighborhood walking and riding paths and trails (Cooper, Andersen, Wedderkopp, Page, & Froberg, 2005). One important first step toward a society where all citizens may age well is to develop policies and programs that encourage structured and unstructured physical activity for all generations.

Reallocated Funding

With population aging, increasing proportions of the population will fall into the 60-and-older demographic, challenging the current public health model to change (Rütten et al., 2012, p. 7). Reallocation of public health funds can have a significant benefit for nations, businesses, families, and individuals, considering the years of added life, the increase in NCDs, the exponential growth in people moving into old age (Bloom et al., 2011, p. 7), and the increased longevity of older adults (the fastest growing segment of the population is 85 years and older) (Kirkwood, 2013, p. 17).

One example is investing in increased health span. FUTURAGE, a 2-year EU-funded project, created a road map for Europe's aging research for the next decade (The FUTURAGE Project, 2011, p. 5). One EU goal involves expanding people's health span—the period of life spent in good health—by 2 years (The FUTURAGE Project, 2011, p. 9). Efforts focus on how to support individuals in living well and condense the period of ill-health at the end of life. This strategy is among those that would maximize the opportunities and minimize the challenges associated with population aging, as longer health spans allow people to stay in the workplace and reduce expenditures on health. Increased physical activity is a way to help people achieve healthier, active lives for longer.

For those who want to influence policy, efforts to overcome a lack of resources and funding for older adult initiatives must start with policy makers. Shifts to interests, beliefs, and political agendas may need to happen for policy makers to take a life course view of physical activity.

Impact of Function

A greater focus on function—physical, cognitive, and social—would forestall many of the issues we see in the age 60-plus population today. A physically active lifestyle contributes to improved function, which directly correlates with falls management, independence, ability to work, and physical activity. Improved function minimizes disability as well as the rising cost of disease and care. It also enhances self-confidence and quality of life (EC European Innovation Partnership on Active and Healthy Ageing, 2013).

For physicians, physical and occupational therapists, health management organizations, and employers, taking a life course approach to functional assessments allows efforts to address functional declines before their ripple effects are fully felt. Professional education, programs, environments, and policies may best serve the older population through improved understanding of how function impacts society (EC European Innovation Partnership on Active and Healthy Ageing, 2013).

Different Thinking About Aging

Adults aged 60 and older are an extremely diverse population. A better understanding of this diversity would help in addressing older adults' needs and expectations at the national, regional, and local policy levels. Whether initiated by business or government, one size fits all solutions reduce the impact of physical activity interventions, health promotion programs, and environmental efforts. Improved communications and program success would likely follow from better knowledge of older adults' diversity among professionals who work with this population as well as policy makers and influencers (UNFPA & HelpAge International, 2012, pp. 13, 21). This enhanced understanding would also help address ageism—which distorts beliefs about aging, often unconsciously—in how people respond to the older adult population segment (Ory et al., 2003).

Accelerated Responses

No longer a "future event," population aging is a current global occurrence. Yet, even with decades of notice, this demographic shift has elicited sluggish responses to date. Prevention and aging are long-term issues in political and health systems geared to dealing with acute issues. The issue today is whether society will manage or mismanage the opportunities and challenges presented by the burgeoning 60-and-older population (Beard et al., 2011; WEF, 2013, p. 10). A societal impact will be felt either way. Increased response rates are the essential first part of the equation; the second is what the response addresses. Already, a growing call exists for new models to manage the challenges of aging, which will highlight and enhance the possibilities (Beard et al., 2011; World Bank, 2015a, 2015b).

Improved Curriculums for Specialists

To support physical activity participation in older adults, many specialists would benefit from improved education and training in this area. Primary care physicians and allied health professionals, for example, often did not discuss physical activity with patients—much less prescribe exercise to them—because they felt their knowledge was inadequate, according to Walsh, Swangard, Davis, and McPhee (1999). They recommended training physicians in techniques to counsel patients effectively on this topic (Walsh et al., 1999).

An American Heart Association's science advisory on the NPAP also called for training: "For physical activity promotion to be successful in healthcare settings, public health professions should ensure that healthcare providers have the skills and resources necessary to effectively counsel patients on the benefits of regular physical activity" (Kraus et al., 2015, pp. 3–4).

Supportive Environments

The built environment is an area swelling with interest, policies, and initiatives. Globally, nationally, regionally, and locally, this area is seen as holding great promise for improving physical activity levels in older adults. A few examples of policies and initiatives include the WHO's Global Network of Age-friendly Cities and Communities (WHO, 2014b); Complete Communities (Urban Land Institute San Diego-Tijuana, n.d.); AARP Livable Communities (AARP, n.d.); and Blue Zones (Blue Zones, 2014). These policies and initiatives have various policy implications, all with the potential to increase physical activity.

Communities that encourage walking could improve physical activity levels, given that older adults commonly cite walking as a top choice for physical activity (CDC/National Center for Chronic Disease Prevention and Health Promotion & The President's Council on Physical Fitness and Sports, 1999). Recent studies point to associations between walkability and walking for transport (Saelens & Handy, 2008a, 2008b, "Discussion"). The evidence is inconsistent, however, on associations between walkability and leisure-time physical activity and total physical activity (Saelens & Handy, 2008a, 2008b, "Discussion").

Policies that foster safe, accessible environments would be desirable, given the importance of walking and mobility to independence, health, and aging in place. Governments at all levels already see the benefit in individuals "aging in place" in their homes and communities, rather than moving through the more costly continuum of residential long-term care. A supportive built environment would also encourage the policy goal of wide adoption of aging in place (UNFPA & HelpAge International, 2012, pp. 14, 76).

CONCLUSION

Physical activity among the 60-plus population is slowly rising. The increase in adoption and participation levels is low, however, as is the overall percent of the older population deemed active enough to meet physical activity guidelines (CDC/NCHS, 2014, p. 222; WHO, 2014a, p. 34). Policies at a variety of levels have created environments and messages to increase physical activity among the older population while delivering services and advice designed to do the same. The overall impact has been minimal at best (CDC/NCHS, 2014, p. 222). What is lacking?

There are no dedicated national policies and funds aimed at improving physical activity adoption and participation rates among older adults in many countries, including the United States. Models in South Australia and Finland teach us that greater implementation of HiAP strategies may draw attention to the need to develop and implement policies that support physical activity directly and indirectly. To ensure benefits are derived from these approaches, more tools and more effective tools are needed to evaluate, translate, and disseminate research and its findings.

Robust responses at all levels will address the global physical inactivity challenge in older adults. From the WHO to the WEF to the World Bank, numerous international organizations and agencies recognize the potential health, economic, and social risks associated with a population that is physically inactive and lives longer. Interest in strategies and solutions is high. To date, efforts have centered largely on implementing policies and initiatives to address these risks, with action slow to follow. The rapidly growing older population calls for quicker responses.

A dedicated international and national focus on physical activity over the life course will change the number of adults aged 60 and older who are inactive in countries worldwide. Considering the limited success to date, we need new models for and changes to areas such as health care and retirement as well as the way policy makers in government or business approach physical activity and aging. By doing so, we may not only achieve the desired economic and human impacts—including healthier, more active people thriving in their later years—but also determine how society benefits from population aging.

REFERENCES

AARP. (n.d.). *AARP Livable Communities*. Retrieved May 10, 2015, from http://www.aarp.org/livable-communities/

AARP. (2002). *Exercise attitudes and behaviors: A survey of adults age 50–79* (Conducted by RoperASW). Washington, DC: Author. Retrieved April 30, 2015, from http://assets.aarp.org/rgcenter/health/exercise.pdf

Administration on Aging. (n.d.a). *Older Americans act* (para. 1). Retrieved April 25, 2015, from http://www.aoa.gov/AoA_programs/OAA/

Administration on Aging. (n.d.b). *Disease prevention and health promotion services* (OAA Title IIID) ("Funding and Innovation" & "Future Definition of Evidence-Based"). Retrieved April 25, 2015, from http://www.aoa.acl.gov/AoA_Programs/HPW/Title_IIID/index.aspx

Barnes, P. M., & Schoenborn, C. A. (2012). Trends in adults receiving a recommendation for exercise or other physical activity from a physician or other health professional. *NCHS Data Brief* (no. 86, pp. 1–3). Retrieved May 1, 2015, from http://www.cdc.gov/nchs/data/databriefs/db86.pdf

Beard, J. R., Biggs, S., Bloom, D. E., Fried, L. P., Hogan, P., Kalache, A., et al. (Eds.). (2011). *Global population ageing: Peril or promise*. Geneva: World Economic Forum. Retrieved May 3, 2015, from http://www3.weforum.org/docs/WEF_GAC_GlobalPopulationAgeing_Report_2012.pdf

Bethancourt, H. J., Rosenberg, D. E., Beatty, T., & Arterburn, D. E. (2014). Barriers to and facilitators of physical activity program use among older adults [abstract]. *Clinical Medicine & Research*, *12*(1–2), 10–20. http://dx.doi.org/10.3121/cmr.2013.1171

Bloom, D. E., Cafiero, E. T., Jané-Llopis, E., Abrahams-Gessel, S., Bloom, L. R., Fathima, S., et al. (2011). *The global economic burden of non-communicable diseases*. Geneva: World Economic Forum. Retrieved April 30, 2015, from http://www.weforum.org/reports/global-economic-burden-non-communicable-diseases

Blue Zones. (2014). *Blue Zones project*. Retrieved May 10, 2015, from https://www.bluezones.com/services/cities/

Breen, C. (2015). *Keeping active for better ageing: Encouraging physical activity in older adults* (pp. 17, 19). Dublin: Centre for Ageing Research and Development in Ireland. Retrieved May 10, 2015, from http://www.cardi.ie/sites/default/files/publications/CARDI%20Keeping%20Active%20Report%20%5Bweb%5D.pdf

Brownson, R. C., Chriqui, J. F., & Stamatakis, K. A. (2009). Understanding evidence-based public health policy. *American Journal of Public Health*, *99*(9), 1576–1583. http://dx.doi.org/10.2105/ajph.2008.156224

Cardinal, B. J., Park, E. A., Kim, M, & Cardinal, M. K. (in press). If Exercise is Medicine®, where is exercise in medicine? Review of U.S. medical education curricula for physical activity-related content. *Journal of Physical Activity & Health*. http://dx.doi.org/10.1123/jpah.2014-0316

Caspersen, C. J., Powell, K. E., & Christenson, G. M. (1985). Physical activity, exercise, and physical fitness: Definitions and distinctions for health-related research. *Public Health Reports*, *100*(2), 126–131.

Centers for Disease Control and Prevention. (n.d.). *Promoting active lifestyles among older adults*. Retrieved April 30, 2015, from http://www.cdc.gov/nccdphp/dnpa/physical/pdf/lifestyles.pdf

Centers for Disease Control and Prevention, National Center for Chronic Disease Prevention and Health Promotion, & The President's Council on Physical Fitness and Sports. (1999). *A report of the Surgeon General. Physical activity and health. Older adults* ("Facts"). Retrieved May 7, 2015, from http://www.cdc.gov/nccdphp/sgr/olderad.htm

Centers for Disease Control and Prevention, National Center for Health Statistics. (2014). *Health, United States, 2013: With special feature on prescription drugs*. Trend Tables. Table 68. Participation in leisure-time aerobic and muscle-strengthening activities that meet the federal *Physical Activity Guidelines for Americans* among adults aged 18 and over, by selected characteristics: United States, selected years 1998–2012. Hyattsville, MD: US Department of Health and Human Services. Retrieved April 30, 2015, from http://www.cdc.gov/nchs/data/hus/hus13.pdf

Centers for Medicare & Medicaid Services. (2015). *The ABCs of the Annual Wellness Visit (AWV)*. ICN 905706. Retrieved April 30, 2015, from http://www.cms.gov/Outreach-and-Education/Medicare-Learning-Network-MLN/MLNProducts/downloads/AWV_chart_ICN905706.pdf

Chodzko-Zajko, W., & Schwingel, A. (2009). Transnational strategies for the promotion of physical activity and active aging: The World Health Organization model of consensus building in international public health. *Quest*, *61*, 25–38.

Cooper, A. R., Andersen, L. B., Wedderkopp, N., Page, A. S., & Froberg, K. (2005). Physical activity levels of children who walk, cycle, or are driven to school. *American Journal of Preventive Medicine*, *29*(3), 179–184.

Coronini-Cronberg, S., Millett, C., Laverty, A. A., & Webb, E. (2012). The impact of a free older persons' bus pass on active travel and regular walking in England. *American Journal of Public Health*, *102*(11), 2141–2148. http://dx.doi.org/10.2105/AJPH.2012.300946

Department for Culture, Media & Sport Strategy Unit. (2002). *Game plan: A strategy for delivering government's sport and physical activity objectives*. London: Cabinet Office, Government of the United Kingdom. Retrieved May 3, 2015, from http://www.gamesmonitor.org.uk/files/game_plan_report.pdf

Elley, C. R., Kerse, N., Arroll, B., & Robinson, E. (2003). Effectiveness of counselling patients on physical activity in general practice: Cluster randomised controlled trial. *BMJ*, *326*(7393), 793. http://dx.doi.org/10.1136/bmj.326.7393.793

European Commission Directorate-General Health and Food Safety, Public Health. (n.d.) Health in all policies. *Policy* (para. 2). Retrieved April 27, 2015, from http://ec.europa.eu/health/health_policies/policy/index_en.htm

European Commission, European Innovation Partnership on Active and Healthy Ageing, Action Group A3 (Prevention and early decline of frailty and functional decline, both physical and cognitive, in older people). (2013). *A compilation of good practices* (1st ed.). Retrieved May 5, 2015, from http://ec.europa.eu/research/innovation-union/index_en.cfm?section=active-healthy-ageing&pg=documents

Exercise is Medicine. (n.d.a). *Exercise is Medicine: A global health initiative* (para. 1). Retrieved May 9, 2015, from http://www.exerciseismedicine.org

Exercise is Medicine. (n.d.b). *Network* (para. 2). Retrieved May 9, 2015, from http://www.exerciseismedicine.org/support_page.php?p=23

Federal Centre for Health Education [Bundeszentrale für gesundheitliche Aufklärung] & EuroHealthNet. (2012). *Healthy and active ageing*. Retrieved May 5, 2015, from http://www.healthyageing.eu/sites/www.healthyageing.eu/files/featured/Healthy%20and%20Active%20Ageing.pdf

Franco, M. R., Tong, A., Howard, K., Sherrington, C., Ferreira, P. H., Pinto, R. Z., et al. (2015). Older people's perspectives on participation in physical activity: A systematic review and thematic synthesis of qualitative literature [abstract]. *British Journal of Sports Medicine, 49*, 1268–1276. http://dx.doi.org/10.1136/bjsports-2014-094015

The FUTURAGE Project. (2011.). *FUTURAGE: A road map for European ageing research*. Retrieved May 5, 2015, from http://futurage.group.shef.ac.uk/road-map.html

Garcia, L. M. T., Sá, T. H., Rezende, L. F. M., & Silva, K. S. (2015). Recommendations for physical activity: Moving beyond minutes and dose-response. Response to Barreto, P. S. (2015). Global health agenda on non-communicable diseases: Has WHO set a smart goal for physical activity? *BMJ*, *350*, h23. http://dx.doi.org/10.1136/bmj.h23

Gellert, P., Witham, M. D., Crombie, I. K., Donnan, P. T., McMurdo, M. E. T., & Sniehotta, F. F. (2015). The role of perceived barriers and objectively measured physical activity in adults aged 65–100. *Age and Ageing*, *44*(3), 384–390. http://dx.doi.org/10.1093/ageing/afv001

Government of British Columbia Ministry of Health. (2006, March 23). *Backgrounder. About ActNow BC* (para. 1, 3). Retrieved April 28, 2015, from http://www2.news.gov.bc.ca/news_releases_2005-2009/2006HEALTH0017-000253-Attachment1.htm

Hartsfield, D., Moulton, A. D., & McKie, K. L. (2007). A review of model public health laws. *American Journal of Public Health*, *97*(Suppl. 1), S56–S61.

Health Canada, Division of Aging and Seniors. (1999). *Communicating with seniors. Advice, techniques and tips*. Retrieved May 7, 2015, from http://publications.gc.ca/collections/Collection/H88-3-26-1999E.pdf

The Healthy Aging Research Network Writing Group. (2006, January). The Prevention Research Centers Healthy Aging Research Network. *Preventing Chronic Disease* [serial online], 3(1). Retrieved May 9, 2015, from http://www.cdc.gov/pcd/issues/2006/jan/pdf/05_0054.pdf

Institute of Sport Science and Sport, University of Erlangen-Nürnberg. (2010). *The national PASEO alliances for physical activity promotion among older people*. Retrieved May 1, 2015, from http://ec.europa.eu/chafea/documents/news/PASEO_National_Alliances.pdf

International Council on Active Aging. (2014a). *ICAA wellness readiness survey 2014 topline and final report, appendix*. Vancouver, BC: Author.

International Council on Active Aging. (2014b). Growth of the active-aging industry in the United States and Canada. *Active aging in America, 2014* (3rd ed.). Vancouver, BC: Author.

International Council on Active Aging. (2015). *ICAA active-aging industry development survey 2015 topline report*. Vancouver, BC: Author.

International Longevity Centre-UK, & World Health Organization. (2000). *The implications for training of embracing: A life course approach to health*. Retrieved May 5, 2015, from http://www.who.int/ageing/publications/lifecourse/alc_lifecourse_training_en.pdf

Janssen, I. (2012). Health care costs of physical inactivity in Canadian adults. *Applied Physiology, Nutrition and Metabolism*, *37*(4), 803–806. http://dx.doi.org/10.1139/h2012-061

John. A. Hartford Foundation. (2012). *National poll: Low cost, lifesaving services missing from most older patients' health care* ("Medicare's Annual Wellness Visit"). Retrieved May 1, 2015, from http://www.jhartfound.org/images/uploads/resources/120420_JAHF_poll_release_FINAL.pdf

Kickbusch, L., Wait, S., Maag, D., McGuire, P., & Banks, L. (2006). *Navigating health: The role of health literacy*. London: Alliance for Health & The Future, International Longevity Centre-UK. Retrieved May 5, 2015, from http://www.ilcuk.org.uk/index.php/publications/publication_details/navigating_health_the_role_of_health_literacy

Kilroy, C., Morgan-Solomon, D., & Landrum, P. (2013). *White paper: Preventing patient rebounds. Value-based care organizations should focus on more than just readmissions*. Eden Prairie, MN: Optum, Inc. Retrieved May 10, 2015, from https://www.optum.com/content/dam/optum/resources/whitePapers/preventing.patient.rebounds.pdf

Kindig, D. A., & Isham, G. (2014). Population health improvement: A community health business model that engages partners in all sectors [abstract]. *Frontiers of Health Services Management*, *30*(4), 3–20.

King, A. C., & King, D. K. (2010). Physical activity for an aging population. *Public Health Reviews*, *32*(2), 401–426.

Kirkwood, T. (2013). Health after 85—The case of the missing data. In "The global impact of aging: The oldest old." *Public Policy & Aging Report*, *23*(2), 17.

Kohl, H. W., Craig, C. L., Lambert, E. V., Inoue, S., Alkandari, J. R., Leetongin, G., et al. (2012). The pandemic of physical inactivity: Global action for public health. *The Lancet*, *380*(9838), 294–305. http://dx.doi.org/10.1016/S0140-6736(12)60898-8

Kraus, W. E., Bittner, V., Appel, L., Blair, S. N., Church, T., Després, J-P., et al. (2015). The National Physical Activity Plan: A call to action from the American Heart Association. A science advisory from the American Heart Association. *Circulation*, *131*(21), 1932–1940. [Advance online publication]. http://dx.doi.org/10.1161/cir.0000000000000203

Langer, E. J. (2009). *Counter clockwise: Mindful health and the power of possibility*. New York, NY: Ballantine Books.

Lee, I-M., Shiroma, E. J., Lobelo, F., Puska, P., Blair, S. N., Katzmarzyk, P. T., et al. (2012a). Effect of physical inactivity on major non-communicable diseases worldwide: An analysis of burden of disease and life expectancy [abstract]. *The Lancet*, *380*(9838), 219–229. http://dx.doi.org/10.1016/s0140-6736(12)61031-9

Lee, I-M., Shiroma, E. J., Lobelo, F., Puska, P., Blair, S. N., Katzmarzyk, P. T., et al. (2012b). Effect of physical inactivity on major non-communicable diseases worldwide: An analysis of burden of disease and life expectancy. *The Lancet*, *380*(9838), 219–229. http://dx.doi.org/10.1016/s0140-6736(12)61031-9 PMCID: PMC3645500

Legal Information Institute, Cornell University Law School. (n.d.). 42 U.S. Code § 300u–14 – Healthy aging, living well; evaluation of community-based prevention and wellness programs for Medicare beneficiaries. Section 3B(ii). Retrieved April 25, 2015, from https://www.law.cornell.edu/uscode/text/42/300u-14

Leppo, K., Ollilia, E., Peña, S., Wismar, M., & Cook, S. (Eds.). (2013). *Health in All Policies. Seizing opportunities, implementing policies*. Finland: Government of Finland Ministry of Social Affairs and Health. Retrieved May 1, 2015, from http://www.euro.who.int/__data/assets/pdf_file/0007/188809/Health-in-All-Policies-final.pdf

Mancuso, A. M. (2013). Making the most of the Medicare Annual Wellness Visit. *Osteopathic Family Physician*, *5*(3), 102–115.

McKinnon, R. A., Bowles, H. R., & Trowbridge, M. J. (2011). Engaging physical activity policymakers. *Journal of Physical Activity and Health*, *8*(Suppl. 1), S145–S147.

Merom, D., Buchner, B. A., & Fiatarone Singh, M. (2015). A daring proposition to change older adults' aerobic recommendations. Response to Sparling, P. B., Howard, B. J., Dunstan, D. W., & Owen, N., (2015), Recommendations for physical activity in older adults. *BMJ*, *350*, h100. http://dx.doi.org/10.1136/bmj.h100

Moschny, A., Platen, P., Klaaßen-Mielke, R., Trampisch, U., & Hinrichs, T. (2011). Barriers to physical activity in older adults in Germany: A cross-sectional study. *International Journal of Behavioral Nutrition and Physical Activity*, *8*, 121. http://dx.doi.org/10.1186/1479-5868-8-121

National Institute on Aging. (n.d.). *NIA timeline* ("May 31, 1974"). Retrieved April 23, 2015, http://www.nia.nih.gov/about/nia-timeline

National Institute on Aging. (2009). *Exercise & physical activity: Your everyday guide from the National Institute on Aging!*. Publication No. 09-4258. Retrieved May 7, 2015, from http://www.nia.nih.gov/sites/default/files/exercise-guide.pdf

National Physical Activity Plan Alliance. (n.d.). *The plan* (para. 2, 3, 6). Retrieved April 28, 2015, from http://www.physicalactivityplan.org/theplan.php

Nelson, T. D. (Ed.). (2002). *Ageism: Stereotyping and prejudice against older persons*. Cambridge, MA: MIT Press.

New Zealand Ministry of Health. (n.d.). *How the green prescription works* ("Programme administration"). Retrieved April 28, 2015, from http://www.health.govt.nz/our-work/preventative-health-wellness/physical-activity/green-prescriptions/how-green-prescription-works

Ory, M. G., Jordan, P. M., & Bazzarre, T. (2002). The behavior change consortium: Setting the stage for a new century of health behavior-change research. *Health Education Research*, *17*(5), 500–511. http://dx.doi.org/10.1093/her/17.5.500

Ory, M., Kinney Hoffman, M., Hawkins, M., Sanner, B., & Mockenhaupt, R. (2003). Challenging aging stereotypes. Strategies for creating a more active society [abstract]. *American Journal of Preventive Medicine*, *25*(3 Suppl. 2), 164–171. http://dx.doi.org/10.1016/S0749-3797(03)00181-8

ParticiPACTION Advisory Groups. (2011). *Active Canada 20/20. A physical activity strategy and change agenda for Canada. Creating a culture of an active nation. Consultation draft 2011*. Retrieved May 6, 2015, from http://sportbc.com/files/Active-Canada-2020-E.pdf

Prescription to Get Active. (n.d.). *Frequently asked questions*. Retrieved May 10, 2015, from http://prescriptiontogetactive.com/faqs/

The Robert Wood Johnson Foundation. (2001). *National blueprint: Increasing physical activity among adults age 50 and older*. Princeton, NJ: Author. Retrieved May 3, 2015, from http://www.activeforlife.info/about_the_program/files/blueprint.pdf

Rütten, A., Abu-Omar, K., Frahsa, A., & Gelius, P. (2013). Physical inactivity and health promotion: Evidence and challenges. In D. V. McQueen (Ed.), *Global handbook on noncommunicable diseases and health promotion*. New York, NY: Springer.

Rütten, A., Abu-Omar, K., Gelius, P., Dinan-Young, S., Frändin, K., Hopman-Rock, M., et al. (2012). Policy assessment and policy development for physical activity promotion: Results of an exploratory intervention study in 15 European Nations. *Health Research Policy and Systems*, *10*, 14. Retrieved May 8, 2015, from http://www.health-policy-systems.com/content/pdf/1478-4505-10-14.pdf

Saelens, B. E., & Handy. S. L. (2008a). Built environment correlates of walking: A review [abstract]. *Medicine & Science in Sports & Exercise*, *40*(7 Suppl), S550–S566. http://dx.doi.org/10.1249/mss.0b013e31817c67a4

Saelens, B. E., & Handy. S. L. (2008b). Built environment correlates of walking: A review ("Discussion"). *Medicine & Science in Sports & Exercise*, *40*(7 Suppl), S550–S566. PMCID: PMC2921187

Schofield, G., Croteau, K., & McLean, G. (2005). Trust levels of physical activity information sources: A population study [abstract]. *Health Promotion Journal of Australia*, *16*(3), 221–224. Retrieved May 1, 2015, from http://www.ncbi.nlm.nih.gov/pubmed/16375038

Sims, J., Hill, K., Hunt, S., Haralambous, B., Brown A., Engel, L., et al. (2006). *National physical activity recommendations for older Australians: Discussion document*. Canberra: Australian Government Department of Health and Ageing. Retrieved May 2, 2015, from http://www.health.gov.au/internet/publications/publishing.nsf/Content/phd-physical-rec-older-disc/$FILE/National%20physical%20activity%20-%20older%20Australians.pdf

Sparling, P. B., Howard, B. J., Dunstan, D. W., & Owen, N. (2015). Recommendations for physical activity in older adults. *BMJ*, *350*, h100. http://dx.doi.org/10.1136/bmj.h100

Substance Abuse and Mental Health Services Administration. (n.d). *NREPP. SAMHSA's National Registry of Evidence-based Programs and Practices*. Retrieved May 1, 2015, from http://www.nrepp.samhsa.gov/

Sun, F., Norman, I. J., & White. A. E. (2013). Physical activity in older people: A systematic review. *BMC Public Health*, *13*, 449. http://dx.doi.org/10.1186/1471-2458-13-449

Swedish Association of Local Authorities and Regions (SALAR), EuroHealthNet and Euregha. (n.d.). *Recommendations on EU support for local and regional action on health equity*. Retrieved May 2, 2015, from http://eurohealthnet.eu/sites/eurohealthnet.eu/files/publications/Reg-loc-Aut_Recommendations.pdf

Swedish National Institute of Public Health. (2007). *Healthy ageing – A challenge for Europe*. Stockholm: Author. Retrieved April 30, 2015, from http://www.healthyageing.eu/sites/www.healthyageing.eu/files/resources/Healthy%20Ageing%20-%20A%20Challenge%20for%20Europe.pdf

Truong, L. T., & Somenahalli, S. V. C. (2015). Exploring frequency of public transport use among older adults: A study in Adelaide, Australia. *Travel Behaviour and Society*, 2(3), 148–155. http://dx.doi.org/10.1016/j.tbs.2014.12.004

United Nations Department of Economic and Social Affairs. (2012). *UN urges countries to address needs of ageing population*. Retrieved May 1, 2015, from http://www.un.org/en/development/desa/news/nocat-uncategorized/un-urges-countries-to-address-needs-of-ageing-population.html

United Nations Population Fund & HelpAge International. (2012). *Ageing in the twenty-first century: A celebration and a challenge*. Retrieved May 4, 2015, from http://www.unfpa.org/sites/default/files/pub-pdf/Ageing%20report.pdf

United States Department of Health and Human Services (HHS). (2008). *2008 physical activity guidelines for Americans*. (ODPHP Publication No. U0036.) Retrieved April 28, 2015, from http://www.health.gov/paguidelines/pdf/paguide.pdf

United States Department of Health and Human Services. (2009a). *Patient Protection and Affordable Care Act*. Retrieved May 4, 2015, from http://www.hhs.gov/healthcare/rights/law/patient-protection.pdf

United States Department of Health and Human Services. (2009b). Title IV—Prevention of Chronic Disease and Improving Public Health. Sec. 4103. Medicare coverage of annual wellness visit providing a personalized prevention plan. *Patient Protection and Affordable Care Act* (pp. 1153–1156). Retrieved May 4, 2015, from http://www.hhs.gov/healthcare/rights/law/patient-protection.pdf

United States Department of Health and Human Services. (2009c). Title IV—Prevention of Chronic Disease and Improving Public Health. Subtitle C—Creating Healthier Communities. Sec. 4201. Community transformation grants. *Patient Protection and Affordable Care Act* (pp. 1182–1185). Retrieved May 4, 2015, from http://www.hhs.gov/healthcare/rights/law/patient-protection.pdf

United States Department of Health and Human Services. (2009d). Title IV—Prevention of Chronic Disease and Improving Public Health. Subtitle C—Creating Healthier Communities. Sec. 4202. Healthy aging, living well; evaluation of community-based prevention and wellness programs for Medicare beneficiaries. *Patient Protection and Affordable Care Act* (pp. 1188–1190). Retrieved May 4, 2015, from http://www.hhs.gov/healthcare/rights/law/patient-protection.pdf

United States Department of Justice, Civil Rights Division. (n.d.). The Americans with Disabilities Act of 1990 and revised ADA regulations implementing Title II and Title III ("The 2010 regulations"). Retrieved May 5, 2015, from http://www.ada.gov/2010_regs.htm

Urban Land Institute San Diego-Tijuana. (n.d.). *Complete communities*. Retrieved May 2, 2015, from http://sandiego.uli.org/complete-communities/

Vuori, I., Lankenau, B., & Pratt, M. (2004). Physical activity policy and program development: The experience in Finland. *Public Health Reports*, *119*(3), 331–345.

Walsh, J. M., Swangard, D. M., Davis, T., & McPhee, S. J. (1999). Exercise counseling by primary care physicians in the era of managed care [abstract]. *American Journal of Preventive Medicine*, *16*(4), 307–313.

Wernham, A., & Teutsch, S. M. (2015). Health in All Policies for big cities. *Journal of Public Health Management and Practice*, *21*(Suppl. 1), S56–S65. http://dx.doi.org/10.1097/phh.0000000000000130

The World Bank. (2015a). *World Bank: Central Europe and the Baltics need to prioritize active, healthy, and productive aging*. Retrieved May 9, 2015, from http://www.worldbank.org/en/news/press-release/2015/03/10/active-healthy-and-productive-aging-in-central-europe-and-the-baltics

The World Bank. (2015b). *What's next in aging Europe: Aging with growth in central Europe and the Baltics*. Retrieved May 9, 2015, from http://www.worldbank.org/content/dam/Worldbank/Publications/ECA/aging%20europe.pdf

World Economic Forum. (2011). *Non-communicable diseases to cost $47 trillion by 2030, new study released today*. Retrieved April 30, 2015, from http://www.weforum.org/news/non-communicable-diseases-cost-47-trillion-2030-new-study-released-today

World Economic Forum. (2013). *Global risks 2013* (8th ed.). Geneva: Author. Retrieved April 26, 2015, from http://www3.weforum.org/docs/WEF_GlobalRisks_Report_2013.pdf

World Health Organization. (n.d.). *Health policy*. Retrieved April 22, 2015, from http://www.who.int/topics/health_policy/en/

World Health Organization. (2002). *Active ageing: A policy framework*. Geneva: Author. Retrieved April 26, 2015, from http://whqlibdoc.who.int/hq/2002/WHO_NMH_NPH_02.8.pdf?ua=1

World Health Organization. (2003). *Health and development through physical activity and sport*. Geneva: Author. Retrieved April 30, 2015, from http://whqlibdoc.who.int/hq/2003/WHO_NMH_NPH_PAH_03.2.pdf

World Health Organization. (2011a). *Global status report on noncommunicable diseases 2010*. Geneva: Author. Retrieved April 30, 2015, from http://www.who.int/nmh/publications/ncd_report_full_en.pdf

World Health Organization. (2011b). *Global recommendations on physical activity for health*. Retrieved May 2, 2015, from http://www.who.int/dietphysicalactivity/leaflet-physical-activity-recommendations.pdf?ua=1

World Health Organization. (2014a). *Global status report on noncommunicable diseases 2014*. Geneva: World Health Organization. Retrieved May 14, 2015, from http://www.who.int/nmh/publications/ncd-status-report-2014/en/

World Health Organization. (2014b). *WHO global network of age-friendly cities and communities*. Retrieved May 2, 2015, from http://www.who.int/ageing/projects/age_friendly_cities_network/en/

World Health Organization. (2015). *Physical activity*. Fact sheet no. 385. Retrieved April 30, 2015, from http://www.who.int/mediacentre/factsheets/fs385/en/

World Health Organization Regional Office for Europe. (2007). *Steps to health. A European framework to promote physical activity for health*. Copenhagen: World Health Organization Regional Office for Europe. Retrieved May 2, 2015, from http://www.euro.who.int/__data/assets/pdf_file/0020/101684/E90191.pdf

World Health Organization Regional Office for Europe. (2015). *Multisectoral action to promote physical activity in Switzerland*. Retrieved April 30, 2015, from http://www.euro.who.int/en/countries/switzerland/news/news/2015/01/multisectoral-action-to-promote-physical-activity-in-switzerland

World Health Organization, & Government of South Australia. (2010). *Adelaide Statement on Health in All Policies. Report from the international meeting on Health in All Policies, Adelaide 2010*. Adelaide, South Australia, April 13–15, 2010. Retrieved April 29, 2015, from http://www.who.int/social_determinants/hiap_statement_who_sa_final.pdf

CHAPTER 2

Promoting Physical Activity in Later Life

How to Respond to Frequently Asked Questions and Concerns About Physical Activity

Andiara Schwingel, Emerson Sebastião, and Wojtek Chodzko-Zajko

ABSTRACT

Over the past half-century, a substantial body of evidence has accumulated regarding the relationship between physical activity and successful aging. Many chronic diseases and conditions share common preventable causes that are lifestyle related. The World Health Organization has identified regular physical activity as an effective means by which an individual can reduce the risk of developing chronic diseases and conditions and thereby promote independence and aging successfully. Epidemiological research has consistently shown significant decreases in the relative risk of cardiovascular and all-cause mortality among persons who are classified as highly active compared to those in a similar age range who are classified as moderately active or less active. This chapter provides a summary of evidence linking physical activity and the health and quality of life of older persons. A synopsis is provided of current U.S. Federal guidelines regarding the frequency, intensity, duration, and type of physical activity recommended for older adults. Finally, we discuss the role that geriatricians and gerontologists can play in helping older adults to learn how to "be active in their own way." In this chapter, we address a number of questions and concerns frequently raised by older adults about physical activity.

http://dx.doi.org/10.1891/0198-8794.36.33

INTRODUCTION

Over the past half-century, a substantial body of evidence has accumulated regarding the relationship between physical activity and successful aging (Chodzko-Zajko et al., 2009). Avoiding a sedentary lifestyle and eating a healthy diet may be one of the most effective means of postponing the onset of functional decline, promoting independence, and maintaining a high quality of life in old age. Many chronic diseases and conditions share common preventable causes that are both lifestyle related (unhealthy diets, physical inactivity, smoking, and alcohol abuse) and biological (hypertension, obesity, and dyslipidemia; Murray, Lopez, & Jamison, 1994). Despite the complex relationships among the many determinants of chronic disease, the World Health Organization has identified regular physical activity as an effective means by which an individual can reduce the risk of developing chronic diseases and conditions and thereby promote independence and aging successfully (Kalache & Gatti, 2002). Epidemiological research has consistently shown significant decreases in the relative risk of cardiovascular and all-cause mortality among persons who are classified as highly active compared to those in a similar age range who are classified as moderately active or less active (Blair & Wei, 2000).

The goal of this chapter is to provide a succinct summary of evidence linking physical activity and the health and quality of life of older persons. In addition, a synopsis is provided of current U.S. Federal guidelines regarding the frequency, intensity, duration, and type of physical activity recommended for older adults. Finally, we discuss the role that geriatricians and gerontologists can play in helping older adults to learn how to "be active in their own way." In this section, we address a number of questions and concerns frequently raised by older adults about physical activity. Throughout the chapter, the Institute of Medicine definitions of physical activity and exercise and related concepts are adopted, where physical activity refers to body movement that is produced by the contraction of skeletal muscles and that increases energy expenditure. Exercise refers to planned, structured, and repetitive movement to improve or maintain one or more components of physical fitness.

THE BENEFITS OF PHYSICAL ACTIVITY

While a detailed review of the many benefits of regular physical activity for older adults is beyond the scope of this chapter, there are now a very significant number of authoritative reviews that provide summaries of the existing evidence (Chodzko-Zajko et al., 2009; Nelson et al., 2007). The American College of Sports Medicine (ACSM) Position Stand on Exercise and Physical Activity for Older Adults states that although no amount of physical activity can stop the biological aging process, there is evidence that regular physical activity can minimize the physiological effects of an otherwise sedentary lifestyle and increase healthy life expectancy by limiting the development and progression of chronic disease and disabling conditions (Chodzko-Zajko et al., 2009). Importantly, physical activity not only benefits physical health, there is also strong evidence that it can improve psychological health and well-being. Regular physical activity can favorably influence a broad range of physiological systems and may be a lifestyle factor that discriminates between individuals who have and have not experienced successful aging.

The American Medical Association and the ACSM have sponsored a major public and professional education campaign called Exercise is Medicine (EIM). The major goal of the EIM project is to make physical activity and exercise a standard part of a global disease prevention and treatment strategy. The initiative recognizes that regular exercise can be an important element in the management of numerous medical conditions including coronary heart disease (Fletcher et al., 2001; Pollock et al., 2000; Thompson et al., 2003), hypertension (Chobanian et al., 2003; Pescatello et al., 2004; Thompson et al., 2003), peripheral vascular disease (McDermott et al., 2006), type 2 diabetes (Sigal, Kenny, Wasserman, Castaneda-Sceppa, & White, 2006), obesity (U.S. Preventive Services Task Force, 2003), elevated cholesterol (Brewer, 2003; Thompson et al., 2003), osteoporosis (Going et al., 2003), osteoarthritis (Gamble, Wyeth-Ayerst, Johnson, Searle, & Beecham, 2000; Katz et al., 2001), claudication (Stewart, Hiatt, Regensteiner, & Hirsch, 2002), and chronic obstructive pulmonary disease (Wan et al., 2005). A joint statement from ACSM and the American Heart Association (Nelson et al., 2007) concludes that physical activity is valuable in the treatment and management of depression and anxiety disorders (Brosse, Sheets, Lett, & Blumenthal, 2002), dementia (Doody et al., 2001), pain (AGS Panel on Persistent Pain in Older Persons, 2002), congestive heart failure (Remme & Swedberg, 2001), syncope (Brignole et al., 2001), stroke (Gordon et al., 2004), back pain (Hagen, Hilde, Jamtvedt, & Winnem, 2000), and constipation (Locke, Pemberton, & Phillips, 2000). In addition, there is some evidence that physical activity prevents or delays cognitive impairment (Abbott et al., 2004; Larson et al., 2006; Weuve et al., 2004) and disability (Fiatarone Singh, 2002; Keysor, 2003; Penninx et al., 2001) and improves sleep (King, Oman, Brassington, Bliwise, & Haskell, 1997; Singh, Clements, & Fiatarone, 1997).

However, despite the accumulation of evidence about the benefits of physical activity, there has been relatively little success in convincing older adults to adopt physically active lifestyles. For example, the Behavioral Risk Factor Surveillance System data of the Centers for Disease Control and Prevention suggest that less than a third of older individuals engage in regular physical activity, with the proportion meeting recommended guidelines progressively decreasing with advancing age (Chodzko-Zajko et al., 2009). Physical inactivity levels are still higher for some groups; for example, in women over 75 years of age, the percentage of sedentary individuals may be as high as 53% (Chodzko-Zajko et al., 2009). In response to the clear evidence of the benefits of physical activity and the need to better educate and inform the public about how much physical activity is needed to achieve health benefits, the Department of Health and Human Services (DHHS) has developed Physical Activity Guidelines for Americans that provide recommendations for the frequency, intensity, and duration of exercise and physical activity for older adults (DHHS, 2008).

Current Physical Activity Recommendations for Older Adults

The Physical Activity Guidelines recommend 150 minutes per week of moderate-intensity aerobic activity for health benefits. However, the DHHS guidelines note that additional benefits accrue as the amount of physical activity increases through higher intensity, greater frequency, and/or longer duration. The DHHS Physical Activity Guidelines stress that if older adults cannot do 150 minutes of moderate-intensity aerobic activity a week because of chronic conditions, they should be as physically active as their abilities and conditions allow. The following recommendation for older adults (Table 2.1) describes the amounts and types of physical activity including aerobic and resistance exercise.

MOTIVATING OLDER ADULTS TO BUILD MORE PHYSICAL ACTIVITY INTO THEIR LIVES

If older adults have been sedentary for many years, it may be necessary to start out slow when beginning a new exercise program, particularly for older adults who are frail or who have chronic conditions that affect their ability to perform physical tasks. Increases in exercise intensity and duration should be gradual and tailored to tolerance and preference. Taking it easy and being patient are good strategies for deconditioned seniors. For some older adults, muscle-strengthening activities and/or balance training may need to precede aerobic-training activities. If chronic conditions prevent activity at the recommended minimum amount, older adults should perform physical activities as tolerated so as to avoid being sedentary. ACSM has summarized the Best Practices for Physical Activity Programs and Behavior Counseling in Older Adult Populations (Cress et al., 2005). The ACSM Best Practice Statement suggests that incorporating a comprehensive behavioral management strategy in physical activity interventions can help maximize recruitment, increase motivation for exercise progression, and minimize attrition.

TABLE 2.1
Physical Activity Recommendations for Older Adults

	Aerobic Exercise	Resistance Exercise
Frequency	For moderate-intensity activities, accumulate at least 30 or up to 60 (for greater benefit) minutes per day in bouts of at least 10 minutes each to total 150–300 minutes per week, or at least 20–30 minutes per day or more of vigorous-intensity activities to total 75–150 minutes per week or an equivalent combination of moderate and vigorous activity	At least 2 days per week
Intensity	On a scale of 0 to 10 for level of physical exertion, 5 to 6 for moderate intensity and 7 to 8 for vigorous intensity	Between moderate (5–6) and vigorous (7–8) intensity on a scale of 0 to 10
Duration	For moderate intensity activities accumulate at least 30 minutes per day in bouts of at least 10 minutes each or at least 20 minutes per day of continuous activity for vigorous intensity activities	
Type	Any modality that does not impose excessive orthopedic stress; walking is the most common type of activity. Aquatic exercise and stationary cycle exercise may be advantageous for those with limited tolerance for weight-bearing activity	Progressive weight-training program or weight-bearing calisthenics (8–10 exercises involving the major muscle groups of 8–12 repetitions each), stair climbing, and other strengthening activities that use the major muscle groups

It is important that professionals who work closely with older adults help them to understand that there are many different ways for older adults to be physically active. For some individuals, structured exercise programs led by certified exercise professionals will be the preferred option, whereas others may wish to find other ways to build physical activity into their everyday lives. The notion that there is one best way to exercise is no longer tenable and it is increasingly clear that individuals will need to select the form of physical activity that works best for them. The DDHS *Be Active Your Way* guide that accompanies the Physical Activity Guidelines invites members of the public to select physical activities that meet their personal needs and preferences. The steps outlined in the *Be Active Your Way* guide (DHHS, 2008) provide an excellent framework around which to initiate discussions related to exercise and physical activity.

DHHS *Be Active Your Way* Step One—Getting Started

Before beginning an exercise or physical activity program, the *Be Active Your Way* guide recommends that older adults first focus on identifying a personally meaningful motive for increasing their activity levels. Health professionals should discuss with older adults physical activity goals that are personally meaningful to them. The possible reasons identified for increasing physical activity are listed in Table 2.2.

DHHS *Be Active Your Way* Step Two—Making Physical Activity Part of Your Life

It is important to encourage older adults to think about reasons why they have not been physically active in the past and to try to develop strategies for overcoming these barriers. The *Be Active Your Way* guide encourages people who have been sedentary for many years to choose something they already like to do and to try to build a physical activity component into the activity. For example, many people like to go shopping or to attend dances and other social events; by

TABLE 2.2
Common Motives to Increase Physical Activity Participation Among Older Adults

Be healthier
Increase my chances of living longer
Feel better about myself
Have less chance of becoming depressed
Sleep better at night
Help me look good
Be in shape
Get around better
Have stronger muscles and bones
Help me stay at or get to a healthy weight
Be with friends or meet new people
Enjoy myself and have fun

TABLE 2.3
Strategies Recommended When Choosing Physical Activity

Pick an activity you like and one that fits into your life
Find the time that works best for you
Be active with friends and family. Having a support network can help you keep up with your program.

increasing the time they spend walking (or dancing), they can gradually combine their fun activity with a healthy dose of physical activity. Older adults should be encouraged to select an activity program that is personally meaningful. Some of the strategies recommended are listed in Table 2.3.

DHHS *Be Active Your Way* Step Three—Keeping It Up, Stepping It Up

Once older adults have managed to integrate physical activity into their everyday lives, health professionals should encourage them gradually increase the intensity and duration of physical activity until they are meeting the physical activity recommendations for older adults. Table 2.4 lists different ways in which this can be achieved.

DHHS *Be Active Your Way* Step Four—Being Active For Life

Once older adults are successfully meeting the Physical Activity Guidelines, they should be encouraged to consider adding new elements to their physical activity regimen in order to keep physical activity interesting and fun. For example, once older adults are comfortable sustaining moderate-intensity activities on a regular basis, they could begin to add higher intensity activities. The *Be Active Your Way* guide lists a number of moderate and vigorous physical activity options that are available to older adults (Table 2.5).

TABLE 2.4
Ways to Gradually Increase the Intensity and Duration of Physical Activity

By being active longer each time. Older adults already walking for 30 minutes, 3 times a week, could go longer—walking for 50 minutes, 3 times a week.
By being active more often. If an older adult is biking lightly 3 days a week for 25 minutes each time, he/she could build up to riding 6 days a week for 25 minutes each time.

TABLE 2.5
Be Active Your Way Guide Moderate and Vigorous Physical Activity Options

Moderate Physical Activity Options
Biking slowly
Canoeing
Dancing
General gardening (raking, trimming shrubs)
Tennis (doubles)
Using your manual wheelchair
Using hand cyclers—also called arm ergometers
Walking briskly
Water aerobics
Vigorous Physical Activity Options
Aerobic dance
Basketball
Fast dancing
Martial arts (such as karate)
Race walking, jogging, or running
Riding a bike on hills or riding faster
Team sports
Swimming fast or swimming laps
Tennis (singles)

ANSWERING QUESTIONS AND CONCERNS ABOUT PHYSICAL ACTIVITY

For many health professionals, it may come as a surprise to realize how little many older adults know about physical activity. Most older adults were educated at a time and in a culture in which little was known about the health benefits of physical activity. Professionals and members of the public alike were often skeptical about the need to remain physically active after retirement. In the final section of this chapter, we address some frequently articulated questions and concerns that older adults raise about exercise and physical activity with the goal of assisting health professionals to provide succinct but authoritative responses that will serve to motivate and inform their older adult clients.

Question and Concern: Why Should I Be Physically Active?

Response to Older Client

There are many reasons you should build physical activity into your everyday life. Regular physical activity can help to improve quality of life in old age.

Physical activity can help you stay active and engaged with your family and community. It can help you to manage or postpone some of the chronic diseases and conditions many of us have come to expect from old age. Aging does not have to be something that "happens to us"—on the contrary, being physically active can help us to play a more active role in our own aging. Physical activity can help us to live happier, healthier, and more productive lives.

Advice to Health Professionals

Health professionals often focus on the health or medical benefits of exercise and physical activity when trying to motivate sedentary individuals to become more active. For some individuals, motives such as decreasing cholesterol levels, improving cardiac output, and increasing bone mineral density are effective motivators, but for many seniors they are not. As a clinician, you should also stress that regular physical activity can be fun, can increase quality of life, and can help seniors continue to do the things that they like to do. It is doubtful that a single motivational strategy will work for all older adults. You should ensure that your clients are exposed to a variety of different motivational strategies in order to find the technique that works best.

Question and Concern: What Is the Best Exercise for Older Adults?

Response to Older Client

There is no single best exercise that works for all older persons. Depending on how you define it, *old age* can cover as much as a 50-year age span, ranging from 50 to 100 years of age and older. For this reason, it is impossible to recommend a single set of activities that is best for all older persons. Some seniors can run marathons or compete in triathlons, whereas others may be more comfortable walking, gardening, or doing tai chi. Still others will get their exercise in a chair or in bed! The most important thing to do, regardless of your age, is to avoid inactivity.

Advice to Health Professionals

The best exercise or physical activity program is the one that your clients are willing and able to do regularly, that they enjoy, and that adds to their quality of life. For some individuals, this will be a structured group exercise program at the local senior center or YMCA, but for others, it will be something much less structured, possibly involving activities such as healthy commuting, gardening, or walking the dog. Many health professionals grew up enjoying games and sports and are extremely comfortable "working out" in traditional exercise environments. It is important to remember that not all older adults have enjoyed similar positive experiences with traditional exercise programs. Work with your clients to understand their goals, aspirations, and personal preferences.

Question and Concern: How Much Physical Activity Do I Need?

Response to Older Client

Ideally, you should aim to do at least 150 minutes of moderate-intensity aerobic activity per week as well as 2 days per week of resistance exercises. However, start by doing what you can and gradually look for ways to do more. If you have not been active for a while, start out slowly. After several weeks or months, build up your activities—do them longer and more often.

Advice to Health Professionals

The current Physical Activity Guidelines for Americans summarize the best available scientific recommendations. Health professionals should be prepared to summarize this information for their patients. However, it is important to understand that, for many older adults, 150 minutes of moderate-intensity aerobic activity per week can be an intimidating target that may leave them discouraged or unwilling to even try to increase their physical activity. It is important that clinicians help patients understand that it is perfectly acceptable to gradually increase physical activity levels, starting at easily achievable, nonthreatening levels and slowly increasing as they become more comfortable with exercise and physical activity.

Question and Concern: How Often Should I Exercise?

Response to Older Client

Generally, it is better to spread physical activity throughout the week with a goal of being active at least 3–5 days per week. By choosing activities that you enjoy, that are convenient and affordable, you may be able to find a way to be active on almost all days of the week. Try to mix up your physical activity program so you are not doing the same thing every day. On some days, you might go for a walk in your neighborhood with a friend or family member; on other days, you might take advantage of a more structured exercise program at the senior center or church. Many people find that wearing a step counter can help them keep track of their activity levels. On days where you have not accumulated many steps, an after-dinner walk can help you maintain your commitment to maintain an active lifestyle.

Advice to Health Professionals

As a clinician, one of the most important things you can do for your clients is to empower them to be independently physically active and not to depend solely on you or other health professionals for advice about their physical activity. Clinicians should work with patients to help them develop activities that they can do in their own time and their own space. By helping seniors understand that there are many different ways to be active, health professionals can help them develop a well-rounded, personalized activity program that selects from a menu of physical activity choices and helps them to be active on most, if not all, days of the week.

Question and Concern: I Have Not Exercised for Many Years, Where Should I Start?

Response to Older Client

Forget the old saying, "No pain, no gain"—it is simply not true! Too many of us learned in childhood that physical activity has to be painful or exhausting if it is going to do us any good. There are many excellent options for those of us who cannot or do not want to exercise vigorously. Walking is a wonderful way to increase your activity level. Stretching, tai chi, and water exercise are also good options. For example, the Arthritis Foundation offers excellent aqua exercise programs designed especially for those with arthritis and joint disorders. Gardening and working outdoors can also be a good form of physical activity. Remember—the most important thing is not what you do—rather—it is most important to avoid complete inactivity.

Advice to Health Professionals

Prescribing exercise and physical activity is as much an art as it is a science. The most successful clinicians are those who have mastered both of these elements. Simply informing patients about the current scientific guidelines may not be sufficient to motivate them to change their behavior. Understanding some of the principles of behavioral change discussed earlier in this chapter can help you develop greater insight into how to identify the right place for an individual to start on the journey toward an active lifestyle.

Question and Concern: Will Physical Activity Help to Reduce My Risk for Specific Diseases and Conditions?

Response to Older Client

Physical inactivity is a major risk factor for many physical and psychological conditions. Sedentary living is associated with heart disease, obesity, diabetes, and many other conditions. Inactivity is also linked to low self-esteem and psychological depression. Regular physical activity can positively influence all of the above conditions. Many studies have shown that activity can also help slow the loss of muscle and bone mass that often occurs with advancing age. In addition to these physical and psychological benefits, physical activity can often have significant social benefits. Many seniors enjoy group exercise programs where they have a chance to interact with fellow exercisers of all ages. Even for those individuals who prefer to be active alone or with a partner, physical activity can help them retain the strength and stamina necessary for playing an active role in everyday life.

Advice to Health Professionals

One of the areas in which more scientific research is needed pertains to the specific mode, intensity, and duration of exercise and physical activity needed to bring about a particular clinical outcome. When approached by an older person with a specific disease or condition, it is especially important for a clinician to recommend an exercise or activity regimen that has been shown to be effective in the treatment and management of that particular condition. For example, when approached by an older woman with osteoporosis who is looking for an exercise program to increase her bone mineral density, it would not be optimal to recommend a low-intensity walking and calisthenics program conducted at the local senior center. Clinicians should familiarize themselves with the variety of exercise and physical activity options available in their community and be prepared to work together with their patients to help identify the most appropriate choice for each individual. The online Exercise Assessment and Screening for You (EASY, 2008) is an excellent resource for clinicians wishing to tailor physical activity to the needs of a particular client.

Question and Concern: Is Exercise Safe?

Response to Older Client

Yes! Almost everyone can find a safe and effective exercise program tailored toward his or her health status, physical activity goals, and personal preferences. It is far more risky for your health to be sedentary than it is to begin a program of light- to moderate-intensity physical activity. The greatest risk is that your muscles will be sore in the first few weeks of an exercise program. There are some things that you can do to reduce these risks. Learn to read your body's signals. On days that your body feels tired or weary—take it easy. On good days, take advantage of your body and enjoy yourself! Once we learn how to read our body's signals and respect its needs, we get a better sense of how to adjust our activity programs as we grow older. Very few individuals will be able to (or would want to) run or dance as energetically in their seventies as they could in their twenties. Many believe that the secret of successful aging is learning how to adjust to changing needs and circumstances while remaining an active and vibrant member of society.

Advice to Health Professionals

While there are some risks associated with participation in regular physical activity, the risks of being sedentary are much greater! Physical activity risks are related to the level of intensity, with lower intensity physical activity being associated with the lowest risk. Low-intensity physical activity reduces the risks of injury and muscle soreness and may be perceived as less threatening than moderate- to high-intensity routines. While lower risk is associated with lower intensity exercise, the consensus is that moderate physical activity has a better risk–benefit ratio, and moderate-intensity physical activity should be the goal for older adults. Although speaking with a health-care provider is always a good idea, the involvement of a primary care provider prior to beginning a program of physical activity may not always be necessary and would depend on a person's health condition, the level of intensity, and mode of physical activity he or she plans to pursue. The ACSM Best Practice Statement recommends that before starting or increasing their level of physical activity, older adults should have a strategy for risk management and prevention of activity-related injuries.

The online risk assessment tool EASY can help older individuals, their health-care providers, and/or exercise professionals identify different types of exercise/physical activity regimens that can be tailored to meet the existing health conditions, illnesses, or disabilities of older adults (Resnick et al., 2008). The EASY tool includes six screening questions that were developed based on an expert roundtable and follow-up panel activities. The philosophy behind EASY is that screening should be a dynamic process in which participants learn to appreciate the importance of engaging in regular exercise, attending to health changes, recognizing a full range of signs and symptoms that might indicate potentially harmful events, and becoming familiar with simple safety tips for initiating and progressively increasing physical activity patterns. The EASY screening philosophy represents a paradigm shift from traditional screening that excludes individuals from participating in exercise in favor of a more inclusive approach that tailors physical activity to meet the needs of virtually all older adults.

Question and Concern: Am I Too Old to Exercise?

Response to Older Client

No! You are never too old to exercise! Physical activity has been shown to be of benefit for individuals of all ages including persons as old as 90 and 100 years of age. Many people just like you are active on a daily basis. You can find a physical activity program that you will enjoy, that will make you feel better, and that will increase your quality of life. Think about what you most like to do in life and what you hope to gain from being active. An exercise professional can help you to develop a physical activity program that will help you to achieve these goals.

Advice to Health Professionals

It is increasingly clear that beneficial effects of regular physical activity can be observed at all stages of the life course, ranging from the very young to the oldest old. In recent years, many excellent and well-publicized studies have focused our attention on the benefits of regular physical activity in those cohorts of seniors who were previously thought to be "too old" or "too frail" to partake in physical activity. There are a number of reasons why the frail and the oldest old tend to be the most sedentary members of society. First, many of the oldest old do not think of themselves as candidates for physical activity. They are unaware of the many benefits that can accrue to them if they increase their physical activity levels, and they do not realize that many people just like them enjoy activity on a regular basis. Second, for many years, exercise and physical activity professionals were reluctant to expose the oldest old to the rigors of even the most modest physical activity regimens. It is only recently that professional organizations and institutional review boards have begun to recognize that the benefits of physical activity are much greater than the very small risks they pose. Third, many of the exercise and physical activity programs traditionally employed with the middle-aged and young old are poorly suited for use with the frail and the oldest old. However, there are now an ample number of effective evidence-based programs that have been proven to work in frail and older adult populations.

Question and Concern: Is This for Me? Addressing Concerns of Minorities and Underrepresented Seniors

Response to Older Client

Yes! This is for everyone! You may not have seen many people like you being physically active on TV, in your neighborhood, or even in your family! You may also think a person your age exercising in public may look silly or embarrassing. There is nothing silly or embarrassing about being active. Many people just like you have found ways to increase their physical activity. Physical activity can help you to feel more energized and to keep doing things you enjoy most (e.g., play with your grandchildren, walk to the church, participate in social events in your community). You do not need to "work out" or go to the gym. Try to find activities that you identify with so that physical activity can be fun and become a part of your routines. If you have any questions about physical activity or exercise, check for support in your community (e.g., health care, senior centers, churches). If they are unable to help you, they certainly will be able to redirect you to people or places where you can get the information you need to get started.

Advice to Health Professionals

Despite considerable research and programmatic efforts to alleviate racial/ethnic disparities in physical activity, disparities in physical activity among minorities and underrepresented groups persist (Macera et al., 2005). It is likely that many older minorities and underrepresented seniors lack basic knowledge about physical activity and exercise. Lack of physical activity–related health education is a common barrier to being more active in older minority groups (Gordon, 2005; Siddiqi, Tiro, & Shuval, 2011). It is important to emphasize that physical activity is beneficial for people from all ages and racial/ethnic groups. Older people from minority groups often suffer a disproportionate burden of distress related to financial issues, living in neighborhoods that lack infrastructure, neighborhood safety issues, immigration status, and so forth (Belza et al., 2004; Siddiqi et al., 2011). It is important to provide these groups with a wide range of choices on how they can build physical activity into their lives. Furthermore, it is also important to match the cultural characteristics of minority populations with interventions to enhance receptivity to, acceptance of, and salience of health programs. Belief systems, religious and cultural values, life experiences, and group identity are powerful filters that influence lifestyle choices (Thomas, Fine, & Ibrahim, 2004). Traditionally, most physical activity interventions for older adults have not considered the unique culture features of elders from diverse cultural backgrounds. Targeting or tailoring a physical activity intervention to make it more appropriate for minority and underrepresented groups necessitates careful understanding of and attention to the community's cultural characteristics and beliefs as well as barriers and facilitators faced by the community or individual (Gordon, 2004). Health professionals can work with this cultural knowledge, to develop a culturally sensitive approach that integrates the intervention with the cultural characteristics and needs of the target population. In doing so, a physical activity intervention becomes more accessible and empowering and better fits the lived reality of the group.

Question and Concern: Do I Need Special Clothing and Equipment?

Response to Older Client

No! Special clothing and equipment are seldom needed. Safe and effective physical activity can be performed wearing comfortable street shoes and loose-fitting everyday clothes. Effective strength training can be achieved with inexpensive equipment such as elastic bands and water-filled jugs.

Advice to Health Professionals

Many older adults have significant discretionary income and are ready and willing to spend it on club memberships and exercise equipment and clothing;

however, many others are in less fortunate financial circumstances and do not have a lot of money to invest in physical activity. Clinicians should be sensitive to the resources available to their patients and tailor their advice and recommendations accordingly. Probably the most important equipment needed to maintain an active lifestyle is a well-fitting pair of shoes that are both comfortable and provide adequate cushioning to minimize the risk of muscle and joint injuries.

SUMMARY

Although no amount of physical activity can stop the aging process, there is strong evidence that regular physical activity can minimize the physiological effects of aging, increase active life expectancy by limiting the development and progression of noncommunicable diseases, and promote independency and quality of life in older age. A combination of aerobic- and resistance-training activities appears to be more effective than either form of training alone in counteracting the detrimental effects of a sedentary lifestyle on the health and functioning of the cardiovascular system and skeletal muscles. While there are clear fitness, metabolic, and performance benefits associated with higher intensity exercise training programs in healthy older adults, it is now evident that such programs do not need to be of high intensity to reduce the risks of developing chronic cardiovascular and metabolic disease. Social support, self-efficacy, perceived safety, and regular feedback are important behavioral factors that can help increase the likelihood of an individual initiating and maintaining a regular program of physical activity. Physical activity risks are often related to the level of intensity, but the risks associated with a sedentary lifestyle far exceed them.

REFERENCES

Abbott, R. D., White, L. R., Ross, G. W., Masaki, K. H., Curb, J. D., & Petrovitch, H. (2004). Walking and dementia in physically capable elderly men. *Journal of the American Medical Association*, *292*(12), 1447–1453.

AGS Panel on Persistent Pain in Older Persons. (2002). The management of persistent pain in older persons. *Journal of the American Geriatric Society*, *50*(6 Suppl), S205–S224.

Belza, B., Walwick, J., Shiu-Thornton, S., Schwartz, S., Taylor, M., & LoGerfo, J. (2004). Older adult perspectives on physical activity and exercise: Voices from multiple cultures. *Preventive Chronic Disease*, *1*(4), A09.

Blair, S. N., & Wei, M. (2000). Sedentary habits, health, and function in older women and men. *American Journal of Health Promotion*, *15*(1), 1–8.

Brewer, H. B. (2003). New features of the national cholesterol education program adult treatment panel III lipid-lowering guidelines. *Clinical Cardiology*, *26*(4 Suppl. 3), III19–III24.

Brignole, M., Alboni, P., Benditt, D., Bergfeldt, L., Blanc, J. J., Thomsen, P. E., et al. (2001). Guidelines on management (diagnosis and treatment) of syncope. *European Heart Journal*, *22*(15), 1256–1306.

Brosse, A. L., Sheets, E. S., Lett, H. S., & Blumenthal, J. A. (2002). Exercise and the treatment of clinical depression in adults. *Sports Medicine*, *32*(12), 741–760.

Chobanian, A. V., Bakris, G. L., Black, H. R., Cushman, W. C., Green, L. A., Izzo Jr, J. L., et al. (2003). The seventh report of the joint national committee on prevention, detection, evaluation, and treatment of high blood pressure: The JNC 7 report. *Journal of the American Medical Association*, *289*(19), 2560–2572.

Chodzko-Zajko, W. J., Proctor, D. N., Fiatarone Singh, M. A., Minson, C. T., Nigg, C. R., Salem, G. J., et al. (2009). American College of Sports Medicine position stand. Exercise and physical activity for older adults. *Medicine and Science in Sports and Exercise*, *41*(7), 1510–1530. http://dx.doi.org/10.1249/mss.0b013e3181a0c95c

Cress, M. E., Buchner, D. M., Prohaska, T., Rimmer, J., Brown, M., Macera, C., et al. (2005). Best practices for physical activity programs and behavior counseling in older adult populations. *Journal of Aging Physical Activity*, *13*(1), 61–74.

DHHS. (2008). *2008 Physical activity guidelines for Americans*. Retrieved October 2, 2008 from http://www.health.gov/PAGuidelines

Doody, R. S., Stevens, J. C., Beck, C., Dubinsky, R. M., Kaye, J. A., Gwyther, L., et al. (2001). Practice parameter: Management of dementia (an evidence-based review) report of the quality standards subcommittee of the American Academy of Neurology. *Neurology*, *56*(9), 1154–1166.

EASY. (2008). *Exercise and Screening for You*. Retrieved March 30, 2015 from http://www.easyforyou.info/

Fiatarone Singh, M. A. (2002). Exercise to prevent and treat functional disability. *Clinics in Geriatric Medicine*, *18*(3), 431–462.

Fletcher, G. F., Balady, G. J., Amsterdam, E. A., Chaitman, B., Eckel, R., Fleg, J., et al. (2001) Exercise standards for testing and training a statement for healthcare professionals from the American Heart Association. *Circulation*, *104*(14), 1694–1740.

Gamble, R., Wyeth-Ayerst, J., Johnson, E. L., Searle, W.-A., & Beecham, S. (2000). Recommendations for the medical management of osteoarthritis of the hip and knee. *Arthritis & Rheumatism*, *43*(9), 1905–1915.

Going, S., Lohman, T., Houtkooper, L., Metcalfe, L., Flint-Wagner, H., Blew, R., et al. (2003). Effects of exercise on bone mineral density in calcium-replete postmenopausal women with and without hormone replacement therapy. *Osteoporosis International*, *14*(8), 637–643.

Gordon, C. (2004). Cultural approaches to promoting physical activity for older adults. *The Journal on Active Aging*, November/December, 22–28.

Gordon, C. (2005). *National roundtable on increasing physical activity among adults of color age 50 and older: Findings and re commendations*. San Francisco, CA: American Society on Aging.

Gordon, N. F., Gulanick, M., Costa, F., Fletcher, G., Franklin, B. A., Roth, E. J., et al. (2004). Physical activity and exercise recommendations for stroke survivors an American heart association scientific statement from the council on clinical cardiology, subcommittee on exercise, cardiac rehabilitation, and prevention; the council on cardiovascular nursing; the council on nutrition, physical activity, and metabolism; and the stroke council. *Stroke*, *35*(5), 1230–1240.

Hagen, K. B., Hilde, G., Jamtvedt, G., & Winnem, M. F. (2000). The Cochrane review of bed rest for acute low back pain and sciatica. *Spine (Phila Pa 1976)*, *25*(22), 2932–2939.

Kalache, A., & Gatti, A. (2002). Active ageing: A policy framework. *Advances in Gerontology*, *11*, 7–18.

Katz, P., O'Grady, M., Davis, G. A., Rojas-Fernandez, C. H., Ferrell, B., Levy, R., et al. (2001). Exercise prescription for older adults with osteoarthritis pain: Consensus practice recommendations-A supplement to the AGS clinical practice guidelines on the management of chronic pain in older adults. *Journal of the American Geriatrics Society*, *49*(6), 808–823.

Keysor, J. J. (2003). Does late-life physical activity or exercise prevent or minimize disablement?: A critical review of the scientific evidence. *American Journal of Preventive Medicine*, *25*(3), 129–136.

King, A. C., Oman, R. F., Brassington, G. S., Bliwise, D. L., & Haskell, W. L. (1997). Moderate-intensity exercise and self-rated quality of sleep in older adults: A randomized controlled trial. *Journal of the American Medical Association*, *277*(1), 32–37.

Larson, E. B., Wang, L., Bowen, J. D., McCormick, W. C., Teri, L., Crane, P., et al. (2006). Exercise is associated with reduced risk for incident dementia among persons 65 years of age and older. *Annals of Internal Medicine*, *144*(2), 73–81.

Locke, G. R., 3rd, Pemberton, J. H., & Phillips, S. F. (2000). American Gastroenterological Association medical position statement: Guidelines on constipation. *Gastroenterology*, *119*(6), 1761–1766.

Macera, C. A., Ham, S. A., Yore, M. M., Jones, D. A., Ainsworth, B. E., Kimsey, C. D., et al. (2005). Prevalence of physical activity in the United States: Behavioral Risk Factor Surveillance System, 2001. *Preventive Chronic Disease*, 2(2), A17.

McDermott, M. M., Liu, K., Ferrucci, L., Criqui, M., Greenland, P., Guralnik, J. M., et al. (2006). Physical performance in peripheral arterial disease: A slower rate of decline in patients who walk more. *Annals of Internal Medicine*, *144*(1), 10–20.

Murray, C., Lopez, A. D., & Jamison, D. T. (1994). The global burden of disease in 1990: Summary results, sensitivity analysis and future directions. *Bulletin of the World Health Organization*, *72*(3), 495–509.

Nelson, M. E., Rejeski, W. J., Blair, S. N., Duncan, P. W., Judge, J. O., King, A. C., et al. (2007). Physical activity and public health in older adults: Recommendation from the American College of Sports Medicine and the American Heart Association. *Circulation*, *116*(9), 1094–1105. http://dx.doi.org/10.1161/circulationaha.107.185650

Penninx, B. W., Messier, S. P., Rejeski, W. J., Williamson, J. D., DiBari, M., Cavazzini, C., et al. (2001). Physical exercise and the prevention of disability in activities of daily living in older persons with osteoarthritis. *Archives of Internal Medicine*, *161*(19), 2309–2316.

Pescatello, L. S., Franklin, B. A., Fagard, R., Farquhar, W. B., Kelley, G. A., Ray, C. A., et al. (2004). American College of Sports Medicine position stand. Exercise and hypertension. *Medicine and Science in Sports and Exercise*, *36*(3), 533–553.

Pollock, M. L., Franklin, B. A., Balady, G. J., Chaitman, B. L., Fleg, J. L., Fletcher, B., et al. (2000). Resistance exercise in individuals with and without cardiovascular disease benefits, rationale, safety, and prescription an advisory from the committee on exercise, rehabilitation, and prevention, council on clinical cardiology, American Heart Association. *Circulation*, *101*(7), 828–833.

Remme, W. J., & Swedberg, K. (2001). Guidelines for the diagnosis and treatment of chronic heart failure. *European Heart Journal*, *22*(17), 1527–1560. http://dx.doi.org/10.1053/euhj.2001.2783

Resnick, B., Ory, M. G., Hora, K., Rogers, M. E., Page, P., Bolin, J. N., et al. (2008). A proposal for a new screening paradigm and tool called Exercise Assessment and Screening for You (EASY). *Journal of Aging and Physical Activity*, *16*(2), 215–233.

Siddiqi, Z., Tiro, J. A., & Shuval, K. (2011). Understanding impediments and enablers to physical activity among African American adults: A systematic review of qualitative studies. *Health Education Research*, *26*(6), 1010–1024. http://dx.doi.org/10.1093/her/cyr068

Sigal, R. J., Kenny, G. P., Wasserman, D. H., Castaneda-Sceppa, C., & White, R. D. (2006). Physical activity/exercise and Type 2 diabetes A consensus statement from the American Diabetes Association. *Diabetes Care*, *29*(6), 1433–1438.

Singh, N. A., Clements, K. M., & Fiatarone, M. A. (1997). A randomized controlled trial of the effect of exercise on sleep. *Sleep*, *20*(2), 95–101.

Stewart, K. J., Hiatt, W. R., Regensteiner, J. G., & Hirsch, A. T. (2002). Exercise training for claudication. *New England Journal of Medicine*, *347*(24), 1941–1951.

Thomas, S. B., Fine, M. J., & Ibrahim, S. A. (2004). Health disparities: The importance of culture and health communication. *American Journal of Public Health*, *94*(12), 2050.

Thompson, P. D., Buchner, D., Pina, I. L., Balady, G. J., Williams, M. A., Marcus, B. H., et al. (2003). Exercise and physical activity in the prevention and treatment of atherosclerotic cardiovascular disease: A statement from the Council on Clinical Cardiology (Subcommittee on Exercise, Rehabilitation, and Prevention) and the Council on Nutrition, Physical Activity, and Metabolism (Subcommittee on Physical Activity). *Circulation*, *107*(24), 3109–3116.

U.S. Preventive Services Task Force. (2003). Screening for obesity in adults: Recommendations and rationale. *Annals of Internal Medicine*, *139*(11), 930–932.

Wan, C. T., Mahayiddin, A. A., Charoenratanakul, S., Zhong, N. S., Seale, P., Ip, M., et al. (2005). Global initiative for chronic obstructive lung disease strategy for the diagnosis, management and prevention of chronic obstructive pulmonary disease: An Asia-Pacific perspective. *Respirology*, *10*(1), 9–17.

Weuve, J., Kang, J. H., Manson, J. E., Breteler, M. M., Ware, J. H., & Grodstein, F. (2004). Physical activity, including walking, and cognitive function in older women. *Journal of the American Medical Asoociation*, *292*(12), 1454–1461.

CHAPTER 3

Consensus on Evidence-Based Preparticipation Screening and Risk Stratification

Darren E. R. Warburton, Shannon S. D. Bredin, Veronica Jamnik, Roy J. Shephard, and Norman Gledhill

ABSTRACT

This chapter is designed to provide a summary of the current consensus on evidence-based, best practice guidelines for safe and effective preparticipation screening and risk stratification. We summarize briefly the irrefutable body of evidence supporting the health benefits of routine physical activity/exercise (particularly in the elderly and at-risk populations). We also highlight the benefit-to-risk paradox, wherein routine physical activity decreases the long-term risk for premature mortality and at least 25 chronic medical conditions, while acute bouts of activity (particularly vigorous-intensity exercise) increase transiently the risk for adverse potentially life-threatening events (such as sudden cardiac death). We examine the various risk factors associated with the transient risks after exercise testing or training, identifying how low the risks are and how regular physical activity participation reduces these transient risks. We highlight current advances in preparticipation-screening and risk stratification strategies and the implications for the elderly (including those living with chronic medical conditions). These advances have resulted in very few participants being sent

http://dx.doi.org/10.1891/0198-8794.36.53

to see a physician prior to participating in a physical activity program. As such, innovations in preparticipation screening and risk stratification have significantly reduced the barriers for physical activity participation so that the vast majority of society can reap the health benefits of routine physical activity.

INTRODUCTION

The health benefits of habitual physical activity are irrefutable; at least 25 chronic medical conditions are associated with a lack of physical activity (Shephard & Johnson, 2015; Warburton, Nicol, & Bredin, 2006a). Moreover, there is overwhelming evidence that the health benefits of routine physical activity and exercise far outweigh the transient risks associated with participating in physical activity or exercise (Goodman, Thomas, & Burr, 2011; Warburton et al., 2011a). The international promotion of habitual physical activity participation is an important cornerstone of the World Health Organization's integrated approach to the primary and secondary prevention of noncommunicable disease (Shephard et al., 2004).

Despite the clear health benefits of routine physical activity, there is also strong evidence demonstrating transient risks for adverse exercise-related events, particularly in individuals who are unaccustomed to physical activity (Albert et al., 2000; Franklin, 2014; Franklin & Billecke, 2012; Goodman et al., 2011; Mittleman et al., 1993; Siscovick, Weiss, Fletcher, & Lasky et al., 1984; Thompson et al., 2007; Whang et al., 2006). Several non-life-threatening adverse exercise-related events are commonly observed (such as musculoskeletal injury); however, the greatest concern resides with potentially life-threatening events (such as heart attack and sudden cardiac death; Bredin, Gledhill, Jamnik, & Warburton, 2013; Bredin, Jamnik, Gledhill, & Warburton, 2013; Shephard, 1988, 1994). Owing to the risk for life-threatening events, many agencies and leading experts have advocated for effective preparticipation-screening strategies designed to help predict those individuals at risk for adverse exercise-related events. This chapter addresses the risks associated with exercise testing and/or training and the latest advances in safe and effective preparticipation screening and risk stratification.

BENEFITS AND RISKS ASSOCIATED WITH EXERCISE TESTING AND TRAINING FOR PERSONS OF ALL AGES

There is a clear dose–response relationship between routine physical activity and health status (Warburton, Charlesworth, Ivey, Nettlefold, & Bredin, 2010) such that most active/fit individuals generally have the lowest overall risk for premature mortality and chronic disease. Moreover, the largest relative health gains are seen when the least active/fit become more physically active (Figure 3.1). This dose–response relationship is generally developed using data from apparently healthy or "normal" individuals, with limited data from the extremes of the health and fitness continuum (such as those living with chronic medical conditions and elite endurance-trained athletes; Warburton, Charlesworth et al., 2010; Warburton et al., 2006a).

In apparently healthy individuals, risk reductions of 25%–50% have been observed for premature mortality and various chronic medical conditions (such as cardiovascular disease, type 2 diabetes, hypertension, various forms of cancer) in those individuals who engage routinely in moderate-to-vigorous physical activities (Warburton, Charlesworth, et al., 2010; Warburton et al., 2006a). For the elderly client, it is important to highlight that marked health benefits can occur at volumes of physical activity that are well below current international physical activity recommendations (Paterson & Warburton, 2010; Warburton et al., 2006a). Similarly, secondary prevention programs have demonstrated marked changes in health status and functional ability in persons living with chronic medical conditions at remarkably low volumes of physical activity. As such, caution should be employed when applying generic physical activity guidelines to the secondary prevention of chronic medical conditions (Bredin, Jamnik, et al., 2013; Bredin & Warburton, 2013).

As shown in Figure 3.1, there is a growing body of evidence that suggests that individuals who engage in extreme endurance training may experience an attenuation of the health benefits of physical activity (George, Shave, Warburton, Scharhag, & Whyte, 2008; La Gerche & Heidbuchel, 2014; La Gerche & Prior, 2007). This is consistent with the early postulations of Gledhill and Jamnik in Canada's primary health-related assessment (the Canadian Physical Activity and Lifestyle Approach), wherein caution was provided to those individuals at the upper end of the fitness continuum (Gledhill & Jamnik, 2003). The optimal level of physical activity has yet to be determined; however, certain endurance athletes (particularly those who engage in repeat ultraendurance events) may be at an increased risk for arrhythmias, sudden cardiac death, pathological myocardial remodeling, and cardiovascular disease (George et al., 2008; La Gerche & Heidbuchel, 2014; La Gerche & Prior, 2007), negating (at least in part) some of the health benefits commonly associated with habitual physical activity. This is currently an area of considerable research and debate, as data from these individuals is seldom included in epidemiological analyses. Conversely, emerging evidence suggests that prolonged sedentary time may attenuate the health benefits of routine exercise participation (Biswas et al., 2015).

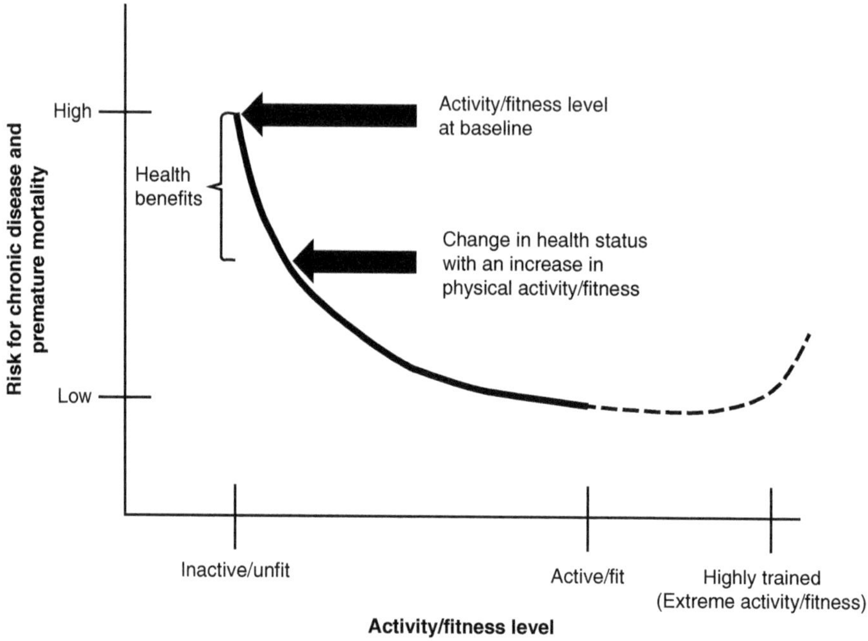

FIGURE 3.1 Dose–response relationship between physical activity/fitness and health status. In individuals who are physically inactive/unfit, a small change in physical activity/fitness will lead to a significant improvement in health status including a reduction in the risk for chronic disease and premature mortality. Dashed line represents the potential attenuation in health status seen in highly (extremely) trained endurance athletes. Adapted with permission from Bredin et al. (2013).

There is strong evidence that engaging in physical activity can increase transiently the risk for potentially life-threatening events. As such, a “risk paradox” exists wherein routine physical activity decreases the long-term risk for premature mortality and chronic disease; however, acute bouts of vigorous-intensity physical activity increase transiently the risk for a cardiovascular event or sudden cardiac death (Goodman et al., 2011; Thompson et al., 2007). Balancing this benefit-to-risk ratio has been an important mandate for various international authorities to ensure the safety and effectiveness of exercise testing/training. As such, current risk stratification and preparticipation screening strategies are designed largely in an attempt to mitigate the risks for adverse exercise-related events particularly cardiovascular events and sudden cardiac death.

In men, approximately 6%–17% of all sudden cardiac deaths are associated with acute physical exertion (Albert et al., 2000; Siscovick et al., 1984) and 4%–10% of myocardial infarction cases occur within 1 hour of vigorous exercise

(Corrado, Basso, Schiavon, & Thiene, 2006). In women, the relative risk of sudden cardiac death during moderate-to-vigorous exercise is 2.38 (1.23–4.60 [95% CI]) versus the risk seen during (light) lesser or no physical exertion (Whang et al., 2006). Similarly, there is a 2.8-fold increased risk for sudden cardiac death in adolescents and young adults during competitive and vigorous sports (Corrado, Basso, Rizzoli, Schiavon, & Thiene, 2003).

Adverse exercise-related events are more frequently observed in physically inactive individuals who engage in vigorous-intensity activities (i.e., ≥6 metabolic equivalents [METs]; ≥21 $mL{\cdot}kg^{-1}{\cdot}min^{-1}$; Albert et al., 2000; Goodman et al., 2011; Siscovick et al., 1984). However, other lower intensity activities have been associated with an increased risk (Bredin, Jamnik, et al., 2013; Reddy et al., 2009). For instance, Reddy and colleagues (2009) reported that only 5% of sudden cardiac arrest cases were associated with vigorous physical activity participation prior to the fatal event. The majority of sudden cardiac deaths occurred during light activities (63%) and other activities such as sleeping (17%), moderate-intensity activities (13%), and sexual activities (2%; Reddy et al., 2009).

The risks associated with engaging in physical activity and exercise training are remarkably low. Goodman and colleagues (2011) revealed that the risk of a cardiovascular event for adults is approximately 0.01 to 0.03 per 10,000 participant hours (lower risks are seen in children and adolescents). Similarly, maximal exercise stress testing is relatively safe (Goodman et al., 2011; Warburton, Bredin, Charlesworth, et al., 2011). The risks for fatal and nonfatal events during a maximal exercise stress test are 0.2–0.8 and 1.4 per 10,000 tests, respectively, in apparently healthy individuals (Goodman et al., 2011). Similar risks are also observed in persons living with established heart disease (Warburton, Bredin, Charlesworth, et al., 2011).

Several studies have revealed that habitual physical activity reduces markedly the acute risk for adverse exercise-related events. Therefore, although an episode of activity/exercise is associated with an increased risk over baseline, habitually physically active individuals have a lower risk. For instance, Mittleman and Mostofsky (2011) demonstrated that habitually active individuals had a lower long-term risk for myocardial infarction at rest and a significantly lower transient risk with episodic exercise. A recent meta-analysis (Dahabreh & Paulus, 2011) revealed that episodic physical activity was associated with an increased risk for myocardial infarction and sudden cardiac death; however, habitual physical activity attenuated the risk greatly. For every additional physical activity episode per week, the relative risk decreased by 45% for myocardial infarction and 30% for sudden cardiac death. Similarly, the transient acute risks seen with vigorous physical activity/exercise are markedly reduced in individuals who are accustomed to this intensity of activity/exercise, as shown in Figure 3.2 (Albert et al., 2000; Siscovick et al., 1984; Whang et al., 2006).

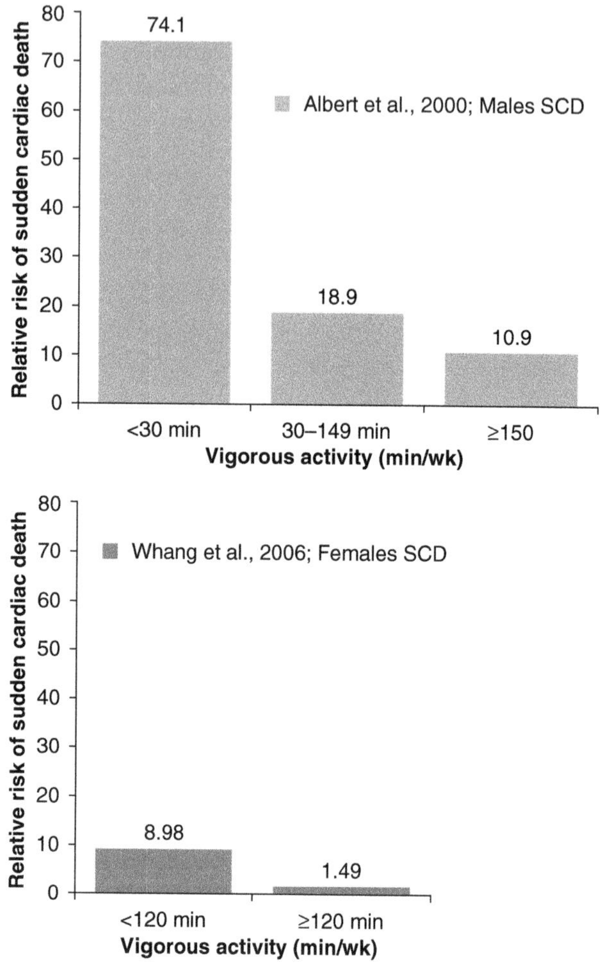

FIGURE 3.2 Relative risk of sudden cardiac death according to previous experience with moderate-to-vigorous activity. Prior participation in moderate-to-vigorous physical activities significantly reduced the transient risks of sudden cardiac death during vigorous exercise in both men and women. In women, the risk was no longer significantly increased in those individuals who exercised for 2 or more hours per week.

Note: Figures generated from information provided by Albert et al. (2000) and Whang et al. (2006). For the Albert et al. (2000) paper, the median duration of 30 minutes was used to calculate the corresponding total time of vigorous physical activity performed per week.

CAUSES OF SUDDEN CARDIAC DEATH

Several seminal reviews have examined the causes of sudden cardiac death and serious cardiovascular events following physical activity or exercise in apparently healthy individuals (e.g., Thompson et al., 2007). The majority of exercise-related sudden cardiac deaths are associated with underlying cardiovascular disease. Unfortunately, in many of these instances, sudden cardiac death is the first observed clinical event. Participation in physical activity/exercise is generally regarded as the trigger and not the cause of the event (Corrado et al., 2006).

The etiology of sudden cardiac death varies according to the age of the participants. In younger individuals (under the age of 35), sudden cardiac death is generally related to hereditary or congenital cardiovascular abnormalities (Goodman et al., 2011; Maron & Pelliccia, 2006; Thompson et al., 2007). In individuals aged 35 or older, sudden cardiac death during or following a bout of activity/exercise is generally secondary to underlying cardiovascular disease (Goodman et al., 2011; Maron & Pelliccia, 2006; Thompson et al., 2007).

RISK FACTORS FOR LIFE-THREATENING ADVERSE EXERCISE-RELATED EVENTS

Several risk factors have been associated with an increased risk for adverse exercise-related events (Goodman et al., 2011). Important risk factors for sudden cardiac death include

- Vigorous-intensity exercise (in particular, activities that are ≥6 METs)
- Male sex
- The absence of or limited previous involvement in physical activity
- Increasing age
- The presence and/or symptoms of chronic medical conditions

These risk factors have often been included (in varying degrees) within preparticipation-screening strategies in an attempt to stratify participants for risk and decrease the potential for adverse exercise-related events.

For persons working with elderly clients, it is important to recognize that the 6 MET criterion is an arbitrary cutoff (Thompson et al., 2007) based on the estimated metabolic requirements of activities such as jogging in younger adults (Bredin et al., 2013; Bredin, Jamnik, et al., 2013). As outlined previously by Shephard (2003), standardized estimates of metabolic costs of various activities are particularly limited for use with middle-aged and older individuals who are unaccustomed to physical activity. For instance, an exercise requiring 4 METs (approximately 14 $mL \cdot kg^{-1} \cdot min^{-1}$) would be potentially near maximal for many elderly people or for someone who is inactive or unfit (Shephard, 2003; Warburton, Nicol, & Bredin, 2006b). For many elderly clients, brisk walking at 3 mph (3–5 METs) would have a relative intensity that would be considered vigorous. The risk for adverse exercise-related events appears to be more related to the relative intensity of effort for each individual participant (Shephard, 2001; Thompson et al., 2007; Warburton et al., 2006b). Moreover, the myocardial oxygen demand of exercise appears to be more closely related to the relative oxygen requirements of exercise (i.e., in relation to the maximal exercise capacity of the individual client; Thompson et al., 2007). Therefore, it is important to consider the relative intensity of effort of each activity/exercise based on the unique characteristics of each client. It is often not feasible to determine the baseline fitness level of elderly clients entering an exercise program; therefore, many risk stratification strategies assess whether the individual is routinely physically active and/or accustomed to higher intensities of activity/exercise.

PREPARTICIPATION-SCREENING AND RISK STRATIFICATION STRATEGIES

The reduction of barriers to physical activity participation is considered to be an important public health approach owing to the associated significant health benefits and small transient risks of physical activity. Shephard (1994) summed up this sentiment when stating

> Ideally, regular physical activity should be conceived as a simple, safe, and natural part of healthy living, a lifestyle to which the human body has adapted over many centuries of evolutionary struggle as a hunter and primitive agriculturalist, rather than as a dangerous medical intervention that requires extensive, high-technology pre-exercise evaluation.

Originally, an exceptionally conservative approach was taken for preparticipation screening and exercise prescription. In the 1970s, physicians in the United States often recommended a stress electrocardiogram (ECG) for men over the age of 35 years who wished to become more physically active (Shephard, 1994, 2014). This was based largely on the belief that further medical testing (such as ECG, echocardiography, and/or medically supervised exercise stress testing) could help predict and thus prevent an exercise-related cardiovascular event (Shephard, 1994, 2014). Moreover, this conservative approach was thought to address concerns regarding the safety of engaging in vigorous exercise testing in large cohorts that had not been cleared with a prior medical examination (Shephard, 2014). However, this approach was deemed to be too costly and prohibitive (Shephard, 1994, 2014).

As discussed by Shephard (2014), the creation of simple and standardized methods for preparticipation screening was founded on the need to promote an increased physical activity on a population basis and conduct large-scale fitness surveys (Shephard, 2014). At this time, misconceptions still existed regarding the risks of exercise, and the logistics and costs associated with physician clearance posed significant barriers to physical activity participation (particularly for the inactive elderly; Shephard, 2014). As such, leading physicians and exercise physiologists sought to create effective risk stratification strategies to ultimately ensure the safety of participants while reducing the barriers to physical activity participation.

Various preparticipation-screening and risk stratification strategies are currently available, ranging from self-administered protocols to those incorporating health-care professionals (Bredin et al., 2013; Bredin, Jamnik, et al., 2013). Landmark recommendations have been provided from agencies such as the American Heart Association (AHA) and the American Association of Cardiovascular and Pulmonary Rehabilitation (AACVPR; Balady et al., 2007; Fletcher et al., 2001; Maron et al., 2001). In the remainder of this chapter, we outline three key preparticipation strategies that have been adopted throughout North America and many international regions.

From a medicolegal standpoint, the completion of an effective and evidence-based preparticipation-screening protocol is now considered to be best practice and a standard of care for effective physical activity programming and exercise testing and intervention (Herbert, 1996; Warburton, Bredin, Jamnik, et al., 2011). Drs. JoAnnn Eickhoff-Shemek and David Herbert and colleagues have conducted a series of innovative liability-related investigations of the practices of exercise professionals, the need for effective preparticipation screening, and the reasons for not including evidence-based preparticipation screening (Eickhoff-Shemek, 2010; Herbert, 1987, 1988a, 1988b, 1993; Herbert & Eickhoff-Shemek, 2010). A growing body of literature and legal case law indicates that exercise professionals who fail to adhere to the best practice standards for preparticipation screening (e.g., do not screen a client prior to starting an exercise program) place themselves and/or their clients at unnecessary medicolegal liability (Herbert, 1987, 1988a, 1996). Despite this clear information, many health and wellness centers and organizations do not endorse and/or employ preparticipation screening (Springer et al., 2009a, 2009b). Varied reasons have been provided for the low adherence to national and international standards related to preparticipation cardiovascular screening including a lack of clarity/understanding regarding the need for screening, inadequate time and staffing to conduct effective screening, the perception of an unnecessary barrier to physical activity participation, legal concerns/issues, company policies that deviate from international standards, and personal responsibility for health behaviors (Springer et al., 2009b). The net effect in the United States is that many fitness centers do not appear to employ preactivity screening procedures or require a physician to clear at-risk clients despite strong messaging indicating the need for this standard of care from leading agencies such as the AHA and the American College of Sports Medicine (ACSM; Springer et al., 2009a).

THE PHYSICAL ACTIVITY READINESS QUESTIONNAIRE AND THE PHYSICAL ACTIVITY READINESS MEDICAL EXAMINATION

The original Physical Activity Readiness Questionnaire (PAR-Q) and the Physical Activity Readiness Medical Examination (PARmed-X) are preparticipation-screening tools designed for individuals (between the ages of 15 & 69 years) who are interested in becoming more physically active or engaging in a fitness appraisal (Shephard, 2014, 2015; Warburton et al., 2011b; Warburton, Jamnik, Bredin, & Gledhill, 2010). The PARmed-X is used as a follow-up to a positive response to one or more questions on the PAR-Q. The PARmed-X was designed to assist physicians in addressing medical concerns regarding physical activity participation (Shephard, 2014, 2015; Warburton et al., 2011a; Warburton et al., 2011b).

The history of the PAR-Q and PARmed-X is quite an interesting story (Shephard, 1988, 1994, 2014, 2015). Readers of this chapter are recommended to consult the recent review chronicling the history of the PAR-Q and its evolution to an evidence-based document (Shephard, 2014). Importantly, Dr. Roy Shephard has played an important role in all versions of the PAR-Q.

The laboratory of Dr. Shephard was provided the opportunity to create and evaluate standardized screening tools in two surveys of population fitness in Canada (Shephard, 2014). The first survey was conducted in August 1966 at the Canadian National Exhibition in Toronto (Shephard & Pelzer, 1966) and the second survey was conducted in the summer of 1973 in Saskatoon (Bailey, Shephard, Mirwald, & McBride, 1974). In developing the screening procedures for these surveys, the research team conducted a review of the various reports on adverse exercise-related events (fatal and nonfatal), providing a summary of various warning signs (see Table 3.1).

Based on these factors, the participants involved in both surveys were asked two simple questions upon initial contact:

1. Have you ever had heart trouble?
2. Have you ever had or do you now have persistent chest pains?

Participants who answered "YES" to either question were excluded from the study. Following the initial screening, participants were then asked a six-item medical questionnaire by a registered nurse. The ultimate goal of these probing questions was to exclude individuals with responses that (suggested) were symptomatic of chronic disease (i.e., hypertension, heart disease, or angina), individuals who were taking prescribed medication on a regular basis, and anyone who had been hospitalized within the previous 6 months (Shephard, 2014). Owing to the exploratory nature of these questions, all participants were also monitored

TABLE 3.1
Factors Increasing the Risk of an Exercise-Related Catastrophe

A history of fainting or chest pain during exercise
A family history of cardiac death at an early age
Undertaking a greater intensity and duration of activity than recently experienced
Competition, publicity or pride encouraging continuation of exercise in the face of warning symptoms
Exercising under pressures of time, or when facing business or social problems
Engaging in activity that required heavy lifting or prolonged isometric effort
Adverse weather conditions (either heat or cold)
A viral infection, a sense of chest discomfort, cardiac irregularity, or a feeling of being "unwell"

Table reproduced with permission from Shephard (2014).

by ECG before and during exercise, with a physician (Dr. John Merriman) being present throughout (Shephard, 2014).

This early work sparked a great deal of interest in screening tests in Canada. The British Columbia Ministry of Health completed another research trial under the direction of Dr. David Chisholm and colleagues at a large agricultural fair at the Pacific National Exhibition in Vancouver, British Columbia (Shephard, 2014). Chisholm, Collis, Kulak, Davenport, and Gruber (1975) used a 19-question self-screening battery similar to the earlier work conducted in Saskatoon. The results from the self-assessment were compared to clinical examinations including measurements of resting blood pressure and resting and exercise ECGs on 1,253 participants (Shephard, 2014). Based on expert opinion, seven questions were identified that had the most relevance for exercise screening prior to increasing physical activity participation (Chisholm et al., 1975; Chisholm et al., 1978), as shown in Table 3.2. The original PAR-Q was created from these seven questions and the PARmed-X (a 4-page form) was created to assist physicians in the clearance of clients who failed the PAR-Q test (Chisholm et al., 1975; Chisholm et al., 1978; Shephard, 2014).

The original PAR-Q has undergone various modifications with Dr. Shephard and Dr. Norman Gledhill playing key roles in their revisions (Table 3.3). The revised 2002 PAR-Q is a self-administered survey that is designed such that when a positive response is made to one of seven questions (Table 3.3), the participant is referred to a physician for clearance to engage in either unrestricted or restricted physical activity. The seven questions of the PAR-Q focus largely on symptoms related to chest pain (angina pectoris) and the presence of heart

TABLE 3.2

Original Questions in the 1975 PAR-Q (Chisholm et al., 1975)

1. Has your doctor ever said that you have heart trouble?
2. Do you frequently have pains in your heart or chest?
3. Do you often feel faint or have spells of severe dizziness?
4. Has a doctor ever said your blood pressure was too high?
5. Has your doctor ever told you that you have a bone or joint problem such as arthritis that has been aggravated by exercise, or might be made worse by exercise?
6. Is there a good physical reason not mentioned here why you should not follow an activity program even if you wanted to?
7. Are you over 65 and not accustomed to vigorous exercise?

Note: PAR-Q = Physical Activity Readiness Questionnaire.

Table reproduced with permission from Shephard (2014).

disease, while examining dizziness and musculoskeletal issues that may require further medical evaluation prior to starting an exercise program (Bredin et al., 2013; Bredin, Jamnik, et al., 2013; Shephard, 2015).

Importantly, age or cigarette smoking does not affect the outcome of the PAR-Q strategy, contrasting the physical activity preparticipation strategy created by the ACSM, as discussed later (Shephard, 2014). It was accepted that both factors increase the risk of sudden cardiac death; however, the experts responsible for the creation and ongoing revision of the PAR-Q argued that neither age nor

TABLE 3.3

Seven Questions That Make up the Revised PAR-Q (Gledhill, 2002; Thomas, Reading, & Shephard, 1992).

1. Has your doctor ever said that you have a heart condition and that you should only do physical activity recommended by a doctor?
2. Do you feel pain in your chest when you do physical activity?
3. In the past month, have you had chest pain when you were not doing physical activity?
4. Do you lose your balance because of dizziness or do you ever lose consciousness?
5. Do you have a bone or joint problem (for example, back, knee or hip) that could be made worse by a change in your physical activity?
6. Is your doctor currently prescribing drugs (for example, water pills) for your blood pressure or heart condition?
7. Do you know of any other reason why you should not do physical activity?

Note: PAR-Q = Physical Activity Readiness Questionnaire.

Table reproduced with permission from Bredin et al. (2013).

smoking (considered in isolation) warranted physician referral prior to physical activity as the benefits of physical activity far outweigh the risks (Shephard, 2014; Warburton, 2013; Warburton et al., 2006a; Warburton et al., 2011b; Warburton, Jamnik, Bredin, & Gledhill, 2011).

Since its creation in the 1970s, the PAR-Q has been used extensively throughout the world and promoted widely by various agencies (Scheinowitz, Dankner, Goldbourt, & Marom-Klibansky, 2008; Shephard, 2014; Warburton et al., 2011a). The use of the PAR-Q by a person prior to becoming more physically active or engaging in a fitness appraisal is considered "best practice" (Eickhoff-Shemek, 2010; Herbert & Eickhoff-Shemek, 2010). In Canada, until the recent (2010) release of the new Physical Activity Readiness Questionnaire for Everyone (PAR-Q+), an estimated 2.5 million Canadians completed the PAR-Q screening process annually. Of these individuals, roughly 400,000 Canadians were required to complete the PAR-Q as part of the Canadian Physical Activity and Fitness Lifestyle Approach (Gledhill & Jamnik, 2003). The PAR-Q was (and often remains to be) used as the primary screening form in various settings such as those that involve fitness-testing batteries, occupational testing, recreation and community-based programs, summer camps, university and college courses involving physical activity, and athletic programs (Gledhill & Jamnik, 1992; Warburton et al., 2011a; Warburton et al., 2011b).

Approximately 40 years of experience have demonstrated the remarkable safety and effectiveness of the PAR-Q for preparticipation screening (Shephard, 1988, 1994, 2014; Warburton et al., 2011a; Warburton, Jamnik, Bredin, & Gledhill, 2011). The PAR-Q reduced greatly the barriers to physical activity participation (Shephard, 1988; Thomas et al., 1992). In Canada, prior to the creation of the PAR-Q, individuals who sought to engage in a fitness appraisal or become more physically active were required to receive medical clearance from a physician (Shephard, 1988, 1994). The PAR-Q has been estimated to reduce the number of required physician clearances in Canada by up to 90% (Warburton et al., 2011a; Warburton, Jamnik, Bredin, & Gledhill, 2011). The PARmed-X has received limited adoption in comparison to the PAR-Q (Warburton et al., 2011a).

Limitations of the Approach

The opinion-based nature of the PAR-Q and PARmed-X has been viewed as a major limitation to the process, despite the established ability for safely and effectively screening large numbers of clients (Bredin, Jamnik, et al., 2013). Most medical and wellness programs are currently required to adhere to evidence-based best practice, placing a significant barrier to the continued usage of the PAR-Q and PARmed-X. Influential medical associations (e.g., the College of

Family Physicians Canada) have also failed to endorse the PARmed-X (Warburton et al., 2011a; Warburton, Jamnik, Bredin, & Gledhill, 2011).

The purposively conservative nature of the PAR-Q and PARmed-X remains a significant barrier to adopting a physically active lifestyle for many individuals (Bredin, Jamnik, et al., 2013). By design, there is an increased likelihood for false-positives, particularly in young children, the elderly, and those living with chronic medical conditions (individuals who stand to receive the greatest benefits from becoming more physically active; Jamnik et al., 2011; Warburton, Jamnik, et al., 2010; Warburton et al., 2011a; Warburton, Jamnik, Bredin, & Gledhill, 2011). It is estimated that the PAR-Q will exclude 10%–30% of the general population (Shephard, 1994; Warburton, Bredin, Jamnik, & Gledhill, 2011; Warburton, Jamnik, Bredin, & Gledhill, 2014), with recent reports of much higher exclusion rates (68%; Whitfield, Pettee Gabriel, Rahbar, & Kohl, 2014). Very high exclusion rates (e.g., 55%) are also often observed in those between the ages of 60 and 69 years (Shephard, 1994).

The early studies that formed the foundation of the PAR-Q (as outlined previously) established the current age restrictions for the PAR-Q screening process (i.e., 15–69 years). Owing to these expert opinion-based age restrictions, many children and elderly are often unnecessarily excluded from fitness appraisals and/or physical activity/exercise programming until medical clearance is provided. In particular, the PAR-Q has led to a significant exclusion of older and clinical populations (Bull, Kreuter, & Scharff, 1999). For instance, Bull et al. revealed that 70% of primary care patients were excluded from participating in a moderate-intensity physical activity program, despite the knowledge that these individuals would benefit greatly from this intervention. This has resulted in programs involving the elderly to either not use any type of preparticipation screening or create their own screening strategy (often involving medical oversight).

The benefit-to-risk ratio for physical activity is clear; routine physical activity should be recommended for the majority of the population and the risks of activity/exercise are remarkably low (including those living with chronic medical conditions; Thomas, Goodman, Burr, 2011; Warburton, Bredin, Jamnik, et al., 2011). Unfortunately, persons living with hypertension or heart disease by default receive the recommendation to visit a physician for medical clearance, increasing greatly the barriers for physical activity participation for these individuals (Warburton, Bredin, Jamnik, et al., 2011).

Marked health benefits can be achieved at low- to moderate-intensity exercise (Balady et al., 1998; Warburton et al., 2006a) where the risks of adverse exercise-related events are relatively low (Goodman et al., 2011). Thus, the PAR-Q often creates a barrier to physical activity programming that is of significant health benefit with minimal risk (Bredin et al., 2013; Bredin, Jamnik, et al., 2013). Acknowledging this contradiction, Jamnik, Gledhill, and Shephard (2007) created a process for qualified exercise professionals (with advanced university training) in Canada to work with persons who answered YES to one or more of the PAR-Q questions, allowing these professionals to clear clients for unrestricted physical activity (without further referral to physicians). Qualified exercise professionals employed this interim strategy (Jamnik et al., 2007) until the development of the new evidence-based PAR-Q+ and the electronic Physical Activity Medical Readiness Questionnaire (ePARmed-X+; www.eparmedx.com).

Despite its conservative nature, there is also the potential for the original PAR-Q to allow higher risk individuals into physical activity programs (Bredin et al., 2013; Bredin, Jamnik, et al., 2013). For instance, persons living with cancer or diabetes may answer NO to all of the PAR-Q questions; however, these individuals may require further probing related to their disease state and/or medical treatment (Bredin et al., 2013; Bredin, Jamnik, et al., 2013). Therefore, it is possible that the original PAR-Q process may inadvertently clear participants who are classified as intermediate to high risk in other risk stratification strategies (as discussed later).

Various other important limitations have been identified including (a) inconsistent and often improper use of the clearance tools, (b) a lack of recognition for the training and expertise of qualified exercise professionals and their critical role in preparticipation screening, (c) inadequate training of practitioners who make use of the tools, (d) increasing demand for preparticipation clearance for individuals from across the life span, and (e) the fact that clearance via the PARmed-X could only be provided by physicians (Warburton et al., 2011a; Warburton, Jamnik, et al., 2010). These limitations create unnecessary barriers to physical activity participation for many individuals, particularly for the elderly and those living with chronic medical conditions. Accordingly, these limitations were addressed with the creation of the new evidence-based PAR-Q+ and ePARmed-X+ preparticipation screening and risk stratification strategy (Warburton et al., 2011a).

AHA/ACSM HEALTH/FITNESS FACILITY PREPARTICIPATION SCREENING QUESTIONNAIRE

In the late 1990s, the AHA and ACSM created a self-guided one-page questionnaire designed to allow individuals to determine whether or not they should consult a physician prior to engaging in physical activity (Balady et al., 1998). This survey (Table 3.4) was designed for health and fitness facilities and is often used in concert with the revised 2002 PAR-Q (Gledhill, 2002). The AHA/ACSM Health/Fitness Facility Preparticipation Screening Questionnaire is more

TABLE 3.4

AHA/ACSM Health/Fitness Facility Preparticipation Screening Questionnaire

Assess your health needs by marking all true statements.

History

You have had

_____a heart attack
_____heart surgery
_____cardiac catheterization
_____coronary angioplasty (PTCA)
_____pacemaker/implantable
_____cardiac defibrillator/rhythm disturbance
_____heart valve disease
_____heart failure
_____heart transplantation
_____congenital heart disease

If you marked any of the statements in this section, consult your health-care provider before engaging in exercise. You may need to use a facility with a medically qualified staff.

Symptoms

_____You experience chest discomfort with exertion.
_____You experience unreasonable breathlessness.
_____You experience dizziness, fainting, blackouts.
_____You take heart medications.

Other Health Issues

_____You have musculoskeletal problems.
_____You have concerns about the safety of exercise.
_____You take prescription medication(s).
_____You are pregnant.

Cardiovascular Risk Factors

_____You are a man older than 45 years.
_____You are a woman older than 55 years or you have had a hysterectomy or you are postmenopausal.

(*Continued*)

TABLE 3.4

AHA/ACSM Health/Fitness Facility Preparticipation Screening Questionnaire (Continued)

_____You smoke.	*If you marked 2 or more of the statements in this section, consult your health-care provider before engaging in exercise. You might benefit by using a facility with a professionally qualified exercise staff to guide your exercise program.*
_____Your blood pressure is greater than 140/90.	
_____You do not know your blood pressure.	
_____You take blood pressure medication.	
_____Your blood cholesterol level is > 240 mg/dL.	
_____You do not know your cholesterol level.	
_____You have a close blood relative who had a heart attack before age 55 (father or brother) or age 65 (mother or sister).	
_____You are diabetic or take medicine to control your blood sugar.	
_____You are physically inactive (i.e., you get less than 30 min of physical activity on at least 3 days per week).	
_____You are more than 20 pounds overweight.	
_____None of the above is true.	*You should be able to exercise safely without consulting your health-care provider in almost any facility that meets your exercise program needs.*

Note: ACSM = American College of Sports Medicine; AHA = American Heart Association.

Adapted from Balady et al. (1998).

complicated than the PAR-Q, considering patient history, symptoms, and various risk factors to determine whether further medical advice is required (Balady et al., 1998).

There are two primary sections to the questionnaire relating to (a) the history of health issues and (b) cardiovascular disease risk factors. If a participant answers yes to any of the statements in the first section, he/she is recommended to contact a health-care provider prior to engaging in exercise. Similarly, if the participant identifies two or more cardiovascular disease risk factors, he/she is recommended to contact a health-care provider (Bredin, Jamnik, et al., 2013). High-risk individuals are recommended to consult a physician (or appropriate health-care provider) and directed to seek a facility that has appropriately trained staff. Highly qualified health-care professionals play an important role in the effective risk stratification of clients, minimizing the number of referrals to physicians for preparticipation screening. This approach is consistent with the interim solution put in place by Jamnik and et al. (2007) for qualified exercise professionals using the 2002 PAR-Q. This strategy has several advantages including quick administration (within 5 min), clear documentation of screening results, and important health background information (reducing potential medicolegal liability), leading to a reduction in unnecessary medical referrals (Balady et al., 1998; Bredin, Jamnik, et al., 2013).

Similar to the PAR-Q, the opinion-based nature of the document is a key limitation. Also, this form can present a significant barrier to physical activity participation for individuals who have two or more risk factors for heart disease. As discussed later, several recent systematic reviews have established clearly that the risk of life-threatening exercise-related events is low in appropriately designed physical activity/exercise programs for persons with established cardiovascular disease. Fortunately, there are various other screening strategies that can assist in the risk stratification and preparticipation-screening process. The PAR-Q and the AHA/ACSM Health/Fitness Facility Preparticipation Screening Questionnaire are first-step approaches to physical activity screening, particularly for apparently healthy individuals (Bredin, Jamnik, et al., 2013).

THE PHYSICAL ACTIVITY QUESTIONNAIRE FOR EVERYONE (PAR-Q+) AND THE ELECTRONIC PHYSICAL ACTIVITY MEDICAL READINESS QUESTIONNAIRE (EPARMED-X+)

In 2007, a collaboration of international authorities and health and fitness organizations sought to reduce barriers for participation in low- to moderate-intensity physical activity and more exactly identify those persons who may require additional screening prior to becoming more physically active. The overall aim was to simplify the follow-up of traditional physical activity participation clearance and minimize or expedite the involvement of physicians, allied health-care professionals, and/or qualified exercise professionals, thereby reducing both the barriers to physical activity participation as an adjunct treatment of chronic conditions and the health-care costs associated with traditional medical clearance (Bredin et al., 2013; Bredin, Jamnik, et al., 2013). The result of this process was the development of a new, evidence-based risk stratification and preparticipation clearance strategy that reduces markedly the barriers to physical activity participation for everyone. There are both paper and online versions of the new PAR-Q+ and the online electronic ePARmed-X+ (www.eparmedx.com; Bredin et al., 2013; Bredin, Jamnik, et al., 2013).

The PAR-Q+ and ePARmed-X+ were formulated, designed, and written by a team of investigators from the PAR-Q+ Collaboration. A working group of the PAR-Q+ Collaboration (i.e., Dr. Darren Warburton, Dr. Norman Gledhill, Dr. Veronica Jamnik, & Dr. Shannon Bredin) was tasked with creating and updating the PAR-Q+ and ePARmed-X+ with ongoing feedback from members of the PAR-Q+ Collaboration and international authorities. The PAR-Q+ and ePARmed-X+ were created using the Appraisal of Guidelines for Research and Evaluation (AGREE) process, relying on evidence-based best practice recommendations emanating from up-to-date systematic reviews of the literature, evidence-based clinical practice guidelines, and current research practice (AGREE Collaboration, 2001, 2003). The PAR-Q+ Collaboration was formalized to ensure the ongoing evaluation and refinement of the PAR-Q+ and related documents. Importantly, Dr. Shephard and Dr. Gledhill played key roles in the new PAR-Q+, building upon their work with the PAR-Q to ensure that the new PAR-Q+ was true to the original and revised PAR-Q strategy.

The new PAR-Q+ preparticipation clearance and risk stratification strategy is based on a very high level of evidence, including several systematic reviews of the literature that established the risks associated with exercise and effective risk stratification for various prominent chronic medical conditions (orthopedic conditions, cancer, heart or cardiovascular conditions, metabolic conditions, psychological conditions, respiratory conditions, spinal cord injury, and stroke). Other systematic reviews also examined the risks associated with exercise training and testing in the general population, the role and requisite training of qualified exercise professionals (to work with persons who have varied chronic medical conditions), and the risks associated with exercise during pregnancy (Bredin et al., 2013; Warburton et al., 2011b; Warburton, Jamnik, Bredin, Burr, et al., 2011). In addition to these systematic reviews, the primary authors of the PAR-Q+ and ePARmed-X+ conducted a critical analysis of best practices in clinical exercise rehabilitation and other allied health professions.

More than 540,000 citations were retrieved during the systematic reviews, with approximately 1,000 specific articles leading to the more than 60 evidence-based recommendations that formed the foundation of the new PAR-Q+ and ePARmed-X+ (Bredin et al., 2013; Warburton et al., 2011a; Warburton et al., 2011b). The process adhered to the international standards established by the AGREE Instrument.

An international research team and a consensus panel are continually evaluating the PAR-Q+ and ePARmed-X+. Any changes to these documents go through a systematic and consensus-based approach. The international research team and consensus panel convene every 6 months to update and revise (if necessary) the PAR-Q+ and ePARmed-X+ based on the current evidence and the various international research initiatives that are utilizing these documents. The current consensus panel–approved plus evidence-based PAR-Q+ and ePARmed-X+ are based on the feedback from users from around the world including the direct research evaluation with tens of thousands of participants in various trials. The most recent versions of the PAR-Q+ and ePARmed-X+ can be found at www.eparmedx.com.

The systematic reviews and international consensus process established clearly that the benefits of routine physical activity far outweigh the transient risks seen after acute exercise and/or exercise training (Bredin et al., 2013) for both apparently healthy (asymptomatic) and symptomatic individuals across the life span (Warburton et al., 2006a). This process also revealed that there was no evidence-based need to incorporate an age restriction into the new PAR-Q+ and ePARmed-X+ (unlike the original opinion-based PAR-Q). A key feature of this new risk stratification and preparticipation clearance strategy was the development of an evidence-based risk continuum (Figure 3.3) such that

- Low-risk persons may exercise at low-to-moderate intensities with minimum supervision.
- Intermediate-risk persons should exercise under the guidance of an appropriately trained qualified exercise professional with advanced specialized university training.
- High-risk persons should exercise in a medically supervised setting that includes a qualified exercise professional with advanced specialized university training.

The international consensus process established the important role of qualified exercise professionals in effective preparticipation clearance and risk stratification for exercise testing/training (Bredin et al., 2013; Jamnik et al., 2007). The need for clinical exercise prescriptions (not guidelines) for persons with prominent medical conditions was also confirmed, establishing that generic physical

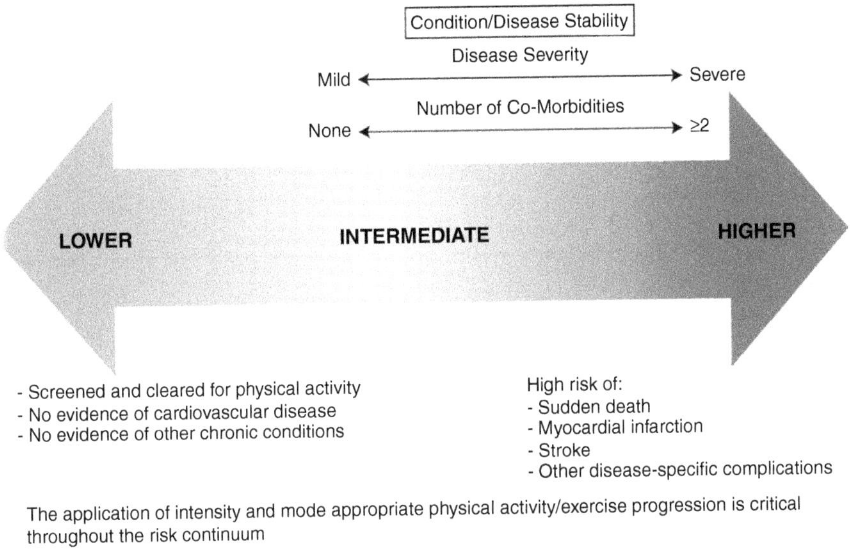

FIGURE 3.3 Risk continuum for the PAR-Q+ and ePARmed-X+ risk stratification process. Reproduced with permission from Bredin et al. (2013).

Note: PAR-Q+ = Physical Activity Readiness Questionnaire for Everyone; ePARmed-X+ = electronic Physical Activity Medical Readiness Questionnaire.

activity guidelines (developed for apparently healthy individuals) are often not appropriate for persons living with certain chronic conditions. The systematic evaluation of the literature revealed that marked health benefits occur at exercise volumes and intensities that are well below those currently recommended for the general population (i.e., 150 minutes of moderate-to-vigorous physical activity on a weekly basis).

Using the PAR-Q+ is as Easy as 1, 2, 3

The new evidence-based PAR-Q+ and ePARmed-X+ preparticipation-screening and risk stratification strategy is meant for EVERYONE regardless of age, sex, or health status (Bredin et al., 2013; Bredin, Jamnik, et al., 2013). The new preparticipation screening and risk stratification strategy has several strengths over other strategies. It is evidence based, self-administered, has no age restrictions, recognizes the importance of qualified exercise professionals (in preparticipation clearance and exercise training), and makes use of a stratification process that takes into account the risks for adverse exercise-related events in a wide range of both healthy and clinical populations (Bredin et al., 2013; Bredin, Jamnik, et al., 2013).

The PAR-Q+ is available in both paper (4 pages) and online formats, while the ePARmed-X+ is completely online. Using the PAR-Q+ is quite straightforward (i.e., "as simple as 1, 2, 3"; see Table 3.5; Bredin, Gledhill, Jamnik, &

TABLE 3.5

Brief Summary of the Steps of the New PAR-Q+ Risk Stratification and Preparticipation Clearance Strategy

Step 1

- Client completes seven new evidence-based questions.
  - Client who answers **NO** to all questions on Page 1 is cleared for **UNRESTRICTED PHYSICAL ACTIVITY**.
    - Client completes the Participant Declaration on Page 4.
- Client who answers **YES** to one or more questions on Page 1 is directed to answer follow-up questions on Pages 2 and 3.

Step 2 (If Required)

- Client completes a series of follow-up questions regarding specific chronic medical conditions.
  - Client who answers NO to all questions on Pages 2 and 3 is cleared for physical activity participation as lower risk (Unrestricted, Minimal Supervision).
    - Client completes the Participant Declaration on Page 4.
- A client who answers YES to one or more questions on Pages 2 or 3 is directed to receive further information before becoming more physically active.
  - Recommend that the client complete the specially designed online screening and exercise recommendations program (i.e., the ePARmed-X+; www.eparmedx.com) and/or visit a qualified exercise professional for further information.
  - Client completes the Participant Declaration on Page 4.

Step 3 (If Required)

- Client contacts a qualified exercise professional and/or completes the ePARmed-X+.
  - Client is stratified into low-, intermediate-, or high-risk categories.
  - Low risk = unrestricted physical activity with minimal supervision.
  - Intermediate risk = low- to moderate-intensity exercise under consultation/supervision of qualified exercise professional.
  - High risk = low-intensity physical activity until the client has received clearance from a physician. Recommendation to exercise under the direct supervision of a qualified exercise professional.

Note: PAR-Q+ = Physical Activity Readiness Questionnaire for Everyone.

Adapted with permission from Bredin et al. (2013).

Warburton, 2015). On Page 1, the client answers seven evidence-based questions. If the client answers "No" to all of the questions, he or she is cleared for physical activity (Bredin et al., 2013) and given general physical activity recommendations for healthy asymptomatic populations (Tremblay et al., 2011; Warburton, Charlesworth, et al., 2010; Warburton, Katzmarzyk, Rhodes, & Shephard, 2007). The client is directed to go to Page 4 of the document and sign the "Participant Declaration." The Participant Declaration is to be stored by the client or with the client's designate such as a community fitness program (with approval from the client). These results are not to be shared with anyone else without the expressed written permission of the client, adhering to international privacy mandates (Bredin et al., 2013; Bredin, Jamnik, et al., 2013).

If the client answers YES to one of more of the questions on the first page of the PAR-Q+, the client is directed to complete Pages 2 and 3 of the PAR-Q+ that contain a series of follow-up questions related to various chronic medical conditions (Bredin et al., 2013). The goal of these questions is to determine whether persons living with a chronic medical condition can be cleared for unrestricted physical activity participation or referred to a qualified exercise professional and/or the online ePARmed-X+ for further probing questions. If a client answers NO to all of the follow-up questions on Pages 2 and 3, the client is then cleared to become more physically active. With this new strategy, a person living with a chronic medical condition can often be cleared (often self-cleared) for physical activity participation without further medical referral (an important distinction from the original PAR-Q; Bredin et al., 2013).

The new PAR-Q+ provides advice regarding developing safe and effective exercise plans including general recommendations (i.e., 20–60 min of low- to moderate-intensity exercise, 3–5 times per week progressing toward 150 min per week). Importantly, these progressive recommendations are based on the knowledge that health benefits often occur in clinical populations at much lower volumes than generic population physical activity guidelines (Adams, 2013; Bronstad et al., 2012; Freyssin et al., 2012; Gjellesvik, Brurok, Hoff, Torhaug, & Helgerud, 2012; Holleran, Straube, Kinnaird, Leddy, & Hornby, 2014; Stefanelli et al., 2013; Warburton et al., 2005; Weston, Wisloff, & Coombes, 2014).

If the client answers YES to one or more follow-up questions on Page 2 or 3, he or she is referred to the ePARmed-X+ and/or a qualified exercise professional. At the end of this process, the client may be cleared with specific restrictions and given a tailored low-intensity exercise prescription until additional medical clearance information is obtained (Bredin et al., 2013; Bredin, Jamnik, et al., 2013). Ultimately, the new PAR-Q+ and ePARmed-X+ clearance process results in a remarkably small referral rate to physicians (approximately 1%) versus the 15%–30% referral rate seen with the original PAR-Q (Warburton, Bredin,

Jamnik, et al., 2011). Accordingly, persons normally restricted from participating in a physical activity program are now screened (often self-screened) back into physical activity (Bredin et al., 2013; Warburton, Jamnik, Bredin, Burr, et al., 2011). Importantly, the new PAR-Q+ strategy has reduced markedly the barriers to physical activity participation for elderly patients.

The new PAR-Q+ and ePARmed-X+ clearances are valid for 12 and 6 months, respectively (Bredin et al., 2013). Importantly, the exercise recommendations contained in the ePARmed-X+ and available at www.eparmedx.com are evidence based from a systematic review and consensus-based AGREE process. These new clinical exercise prescriptions have been shown to lead to marked improvements in a wide range of clientele (including persons living with breast cancer, chronic kidney disease, bariatric obesity, major mental illness; Bailey, 2010; Bredin, Warburton, & Lang, 2013; Flesher et al., 2011; West Coast Bariatric Surgery, 2012).

ACSM RISK STRATIFICATION

The ACSM risk stratification (and more recently a *risk classification*) process is based on the opinions of leading physical activity and exercise medicine specialists. This process is used around the world, particularly in the United States by ACSM-certified health and fitness professionals (ACSM, 2006). In 2013, the ACSM revised its preparticipation health-screening recommendations, reflecting a significant change in our understanding of the risks associated with exercise and the health benefits of physical activity participation (Thompson, Arena, Riebe, & Pescatello, 2013).

It should be highlighted that various international authorities (including Dr. Warburton) participated in a scientific roundtable convened by the ACSM in June 2014 to evaluate the current ACSM exercise preparticipation health-screening recommendations. It is anticipated that the new health-screening process and related recommendations will be released formally in November 2015. The 10th edition of *ACSM's Guidelines for Exercise Testing and Prescription* will contain updated information on ACSM's exercise preparticipation health-screening process (Riebe et al., 2015).

Prior to the 2013 ACSM strategy, the ACSM recommended that all individuals interested in participating in a formal exercise program should be evaluated for various cardiovascular disease risk factors and signs or symptoms of cardiovascular, metabolic, or pulmonary disease (ACSM, 2006; Thompson et al., 2013). Also, clients at risk for cardiovascular disease who are interested in engaging in vigorous exercise were recommended to have a medical examination and symptom-limited exercise test as part of the preparticipation-screening process.

Within the original ACSM recommendations, persons who were considered to be at risk were men ≥ 45 years and women ≥ 55 years, individuals with two or more major risk factors for cardiovascular disease, individuals with signs and symptoms of cardiovascular disease, and individuals with known heart, pulmonary, or metabolic disease. This risk stratification allows for the classification into low-, moderate-, or high-risk categories (ACSM, 2006).

The ninth edition of *ACSM's Guidelines for Exercise Testing and Prescription* was released in 2014 (Pescatello, Riebe, Arena, & American College of Sports Medicine, 2014) containing new preparticipation health-screening recommendations (Thompson et al., 2013). As reviewed by Dr. Paul Thompson and colleagues (2013), the 2013 ACSM recommendations made important changes to previous strategies including

- Reducing the emphasis on the need for medical examination and exercise testing as part of the preparticipation-screening process in apparently healthy (asymptomatic) individuals
- Using the term *risk classification* of persons as low, moderate, or high risk based on
  - Known cardiovascular, metabolic, or pulmonary disease
  - Signs or symptoms of cardiovascular, metabolic, or pulmonary disease
  - Risk factors for cardiovascular disease
- Emphasizing how those with established chronic disease are at the greatest risk for an adverse exercise-related cardiac event
- Adopting the AACVPR risk stratification for persons with cardiovascular disease (as discussed later)
- Promoting the message that *all* individuals should adopt a physically active lifestyle

The 2013 ACSM recommendations for exercise training and testing in asymptomatic individuals are less conservative than previous versions (Bredin et al., 2013; Bredin, Jamnik, et al., 2013). Low-risk individuals are asymptomatic apparently healthy with ≤ 1 risk factor for heart disease having a relatively low risk for an acute cardiovascular event. Moderate-risk individuals have two or more risk factors for cardiovascular disease with a somewhat increased risk for an acute cardiovascular event. A medical examination is recommended for those moderate-risk individuals who wish to engage in vigorous-intensity exercises. High-risk individuals have known cardiovascular, metabolic, or pulmonary disease OR one or more signs and symptoms of these conditions (Table 3.6). Medical examination and clearance is required prior to the initiation of exercise for the high-risk participants owing to the risk of an acute cardiovascular event.

TABLE 3.6

The 2013 ACSM Identification of Individuals at High Risk for an Exercise-Related Cardiac Event

Factors Leading to a High-Risk Classification

Diagnosed cardiovascular disease

Unstable or new or possible symptoms of cardiovascular disease

Diabetes mellitus and at least one of the following criteria:

- Age > 35 years or
- Type 2 diabetes > 10-year duration or
- Type 1 diabetes > 15-year duration or
- Hypercholesterolemia (total cholesterol ≥ 240 mg/L)
- Hypertension (systolic blood pressure ≥ 140 or diastolic blood pressure ≥ 90 mmHg) or
- Smoking or
- Family history of coronary artery disease in first-degree relative <60 years or
- Presence of microvascular disease or
- Peripheral vascular disease or
- Autonomic neuropathy

End-stage renal disease

Patients with diagnosed or symptomatic pulmonary disease (including asthma, chronic obstructive pulmonary disease, interstitial lung disease, or cystic fibrosis)

Note: ACSM = American College of Sports Medicine.

Adapted from Thompson et al. (2013).

The 2013 ACSM guidelines also provide recommendations for medical examination prior to initiating a physical activity program and/or engaging in a submaximal or maximal exercise test (Bredin et al., 2013; Bredin, Jamnik, et al., 2013; Table 3.7). These recommendations will be updated with the release of the 2015 ACSM guidelines (Riebe et al., 2015). Implicit within the 2013 ACSM strategy is the recommendation to use appropriate screening tools (such as the new evidence-based PAR-Q+/ePARmed-X+ and AHA/ACSM Health/Fitness Facility Preparticipation Screening Questionnaire). Moderate-risk individuals (i.e., with ≥2 risk factors for heart disease) are recommended to consult a physician prior to engaging in a vigorous intensity exercise program (Table 3.7). High-risk clients (i.e., with symptoms or diagnosed disease) should consult a physician prior to initiating an exercise program. Exercise stress testing prior to engaging in a vigorous-intensity physical activity program is only recommended

TABLE 3.7

2013 ACSM Recommendations Regarding Medical Examination and Medical Supervision of Exercise Stress Testing Prior to the Initiation of Exercise Training

	ACSM Risk Categorization		
Level of Exercise	**Low Risk (Asymptomatic <2 Risk Factors)**	**Moderate Risk (Asymptomatic ≥ 2 Risk Factors)**	**High Risk (Symptomatic or Known Cardiovascular, Pulmonary, Renal, or Metabolic Disease)**
Moderate (3–5 METs)	Medical exam and exercise testing are **NOT** required before exercise	Medical exam and exercise testing are **NOT** required before exercise	Medical exam and exercise testing **ARE** recommended
Vigorous (≥ 6 METs)	Medical exam and exercise testing are **NOT** required before exercise	Medical exam **IS** recommended before vigorous exercise, but exercise testing is **NOT** necessary	Medical exam and exercise testing **ARE** recommended
Submaximal exercise test (if done)	MD supervision of exercise testing is **NOT** necessary	MD supervision of exercise testing is **NOT** necessary	MD supervision of exercise testing **IS** recommended
Maximal exercise test (if done)	MD supervision of exercise testing is **NOT** necessary	MD supervision of exercise testing is **NOT** necessary	MD supervision of exercise testing **IS** recommended

Note: ACSM = American College of Sports Medicine; MET = metabolic equivalent.

Adapted with permission from Bredin et al. (2013). Created from information provided by the American College of Sports Medicine (2013); Thompson et al. (2013).

for high-risk individuals (Bredin et al., 2013; Bredin, Jamnik, et al., 2013). The 2013 ACSM recommendations are consistent with the recommendations of the PAR-Q+ Collaboration (Bredin et al., 2013; Warburton, Bredin, Jamnik, et al., 2011; Warburton et al., 2011b; Warburton, Jamnik, Bredin, Burr, et al., 2011; Warburton, Jamnik, Bredin, & Gledhill, 2011). A common goal of all modern risk stratification strategies is to reduce unnecessary barriers to physical activity participation (Bredin et al., 2013; Bredin, Jamnik, et al., 2013; Thompson et al., 2013).

RISK STRATIFICATION FOR PATIENTS WITH HEART DISEASE

Two important risk stratification strategies for persons living with heart disease have been created by leading American organizations (i.e., AHA and AACVPR). The ACSM has recently advocated the adoption of the AACVPR risk stratification strategy.

AHA Guidelines

The AHA guidelines provide recommendations for asymptomatic and symptomatic populations, as shown in Table 3.8 (Fletcher et al., 2001) with either no physical activity restrictions or ECG and blood pressure monitoring during

TABLE 3.8

AHA Risk Classification for Apparently Healthy Individuals

Risk Classification for Apparently Healthy Individuals (Class A)
Class A1
• Children, adolescents, men < 45 years, and women < 55 years who have no symptoms or known presence of cardiovascular disease or major risk factors for heart disease.
Class A2
• Men ≥ 45 years and women ≥ 55 years with no symptoms or known presence of cardiovascular disease and with <2 major risk factors for heart disease.
Class A3
• Men ≥ 45 years and women ≥ 55 years with no symptoms or known presence of cardiovascular disease and with ≥2 major risk factors for heart disease.

Note: AHA = American Heart Association.

Adapted from Fletcher et al. (2001).

exercise prior to engaging in training for apparently healthy individuals. Class A2 and Class A3 participants are recommended to undergo a medical examination and potentially a supervised exercise test prior to engaging in vigorous intensity exercise training (Fletcher et al., 2001).

The risk stratification process is slightly more complicated for individuals with heart disease (see Table 3.9). Persons with heart disease are classified according to the perceived risk for adverse exercise-related events: Class B (lower risk), Class C (moderate-to-higher risk), and Class D (highest risk). A risk continuum is established wherein Class B participants are considered to be a low risk for vigorous exercise-related adverse events, Class C participants have a risk of adverse event that is slightly higher than seen in apparently healthy individuals, while Class D patients are considered to have an increased risk for adverse exercise-related events.

An individualized exercise prescription provided by qualified exercise professionals (and approved by a primary health-care provider) is recommended for Class B patients (Fletcher et al., 2001). Medical supervision is recommended during the initial exercise prescription session and subsequent sessions until the participant is able to monitor his or her activity. Blood pressure and ECG monitoring are also recommended during the early phases of training (i.e., the first 6–12 sessions). Nonmedical personnel (e.g., qualified exercise professionals) should be trained and certified in basic life support (including cardiopulmonary resuscitation; Fletcher et al., 2001).

Moderate- to high-risk individuals (Class C) are considered to be at an increased risk for adverse cardiac complications during exercise and/or unable to appropriately manage activity levels (Table 3.9). Class C participants should receive individualized exercise prescriptions (approved by a primary health-care provider) from qualified individuals (Fletcher et al., 2001). Medical supervision (including ECG and blood pressure monitoring) during all exercise-training sessions (usually for 12 or more sessions) is recommended until safety can be assured.

Class D patients are considered at the greatest risk for an adverse exercise-related event. These individuals would be considered to be unstable and, as such, no exercise prescription would be recommended for conditioning purposes. Daily activity guidelines will be provided by the patient's personal physician, with the ultimate goal of returning the patient to Class C or better (Fletcher et al., 2001).

The opinion-based AHA guidelines have been used extensively in exercise prescription and risk stratification (particularly with elderly patients with heart disease). This risk stratification strategy is designed such that the qualified exercise professional works closely with a physician.

TABLE 3.9

Criteria for Risk Classification

Class B Risk Classification

Individuals within this classification include those with any of the following diagnoses:

- Stable coronary artery disease (i.e., coronary artery bypass graft surgery, percutaneous transluminal coronary angioplasty, myocardial infarction, angina pectoris, abnormal exercise test, and abnormal coronary angiograms) with clinical characteristics as outlined below.
- Valvular heart disease, excluding severe valvular stenosis or regurgitation with clinical characteristics as outlined below.
- Congenital heart disease.
- Cardiomyopathy: ejection fraction ≤ 30%; includes stable patients with heart failure with clinical characteristics as outlined below. Does not include hypertrophic cardiomyopathy or recent myocarditis.
- Exercise stress findings/abnormalities that do not meet any of the criteria associated with the high-risk categorization (i.e., Class C).

Clinical characteristics must include *ALL* of the following:

- New York Heart Association Class 1 or 2.
- Exercise capacity/tolerance ≤ 6 METs.
- No evidence of congestive heart failure.
- No evidence of angina or myocardial ischemia at rest or during the exercise test at or below 6 METs.
- Appropriate increase in systolic blood pressure during exercise.
- Absence of sustained or nonsustained ventricular tachycardia at rest or with exercise.
- Satisfactory ability to self-monitor the intensity of exercise.

Class C Risk Classification (Moderate-to-High Risk)

Individuals within this classification include those with any of the following diagnoses:

- Coronary artery disease with the clinical characteristics outlined below.
- Valvular heart disease, excluding severe valvular stenosis or regurgitation with the clinical characteristics as outlined below.
- Congenital heart disease.
- Cardiomyopathy: ejection fraction < 30%, including stable patients with heart failure with clinical characteristics as outlined below (but not hypertrophic cardiomyopathy or recent myocarditis).
- Complex ventricular arrhythmias that are not well controlled.

(*Continued*)

TABLE 3.9
Criteria for Risk Classification (Continued)

Clinical characteristics (must include *ALL* of the following):

- New York Heart Association Class 3 or 4.
- Exercise-specific findings:
  - Exercise capacity/tolerance < 6 METs.
  - Angina or ischemia ST depression at an exercise intensity < 6 METs.
  - A fall in systolic blood pressure below resting levels during exercise.
  - Nonsustained ventricular tachycardia with exercise.
- A medical problem that the physician deems as potentially life-threatening.

Class D Risk Classification (Highest Risk)

Individuals within this classification include those with any of the following diagnoses:

- Unstable ischemia.
- Severe and symptomatic valvular stenosis or regurgitation.
- Congenital heart disease. In these individuals, exercise conditioning would be prohibited according to the risk criteria established by the 27th Bethesda Conference recommendations (Fuster, Gotto, Libby, Loscalzo, & McGill, 1996).
- Uncompensated heart failure.
- Other medical conditions that could be worsened by exercise.

Note: MET = metabolic equivalent.
Adapted from Fletcher et al. (2001).

AACVPR Guidelines

The AACVPR risk stratification strategy is designed for persons living with cardiovascular disease. Similar to the AHA and PAR-Q+ strategies, the AACVPR process allows for the stratification of patients into low-, moderate-, and high-risk categories (Table 3.10). The AACVPR risk stratification process provides clear instructions regarding the amount and type of exercise supervision provided and how patients may move from one risk category to the other. This stratification process is enhanced greatly by clinical competency guidelines for working with cardiac patients (Hamm et al., 2011). These guidelines were created with the understanding that qualified exercise professionals have attained appropriate training and possess the requisite skills to deal with patients living with heart disease (Bredin et al., 2013; Bredin, Jamnik, et al., 2013). This strategy was not designed to be used with individuals who do not possess established clinical competencies for work with cardiac patients.

TABLE 3.10

American Association of Cardiovascular and Pulmonary Rehabilitation Risk Stratification Guidelines and Exercise Supervision Recommendations for Cardiac Patients

Risk Stratification	Exercise Supervision
Low-Risk Classification (All Criteria Must Be Present)	**Low Risk**
Exercise-Specific Findings • No complex ventricular arrhythmias during exercise testing or recovery from exercise testing. • Absence of angina or other significant symptoms (such as abnormal shortness of breath, lightheadedness, or dizziness during exercise and/or recovery. • Normal hemodynamic response to exercise testing and recovery (i.e., appropriate increases [and decreases] in heart rate and blood pressure). • Functional capacity ≥ 7 METs. *Non-Exercise-Specific Findings* • Resting ejection fraction > 50%. • Uncomplicated myocardial infarction or revascularization procedure. • Absence of complicated ventricular arrhythmias at rest. • Absence of congestive heart failure. • Absence of signs or symptoms of postevent/postprocedure ischemia. • Absence of clinical depression.	• Direct supervision of exercise is recommended for a minimum of 6–18 exercise sessions or 30 days after event/procedure. • Supervision should begin with continuous ECG monitoring (for 6–12 sessions) decreasing to intermittent monitoring.

Moderate-Risk Classification (One or More Criteria Must Be Present)	**Moderate Risk**
Exercise-Specific Findings • Presence of angina or other significant symptoms (such as abnormal shortness of breath, lightheadedness, or dizziness during exercise of higher intensity (i.e., 7 METs). • Silent ischemia (mild to moderate) during exercise testing or recovery (i.e., ST segment depression of <2 mm from baseline). • Functional capacity < 5 METs. *Non-Exercise-Specific Findings* • Resting ejection fraction between 40% and 50%.	• Direct supervision of exercise for a minimum of 12–14 exercise sessions or 60 days after event/procedure. • Supervision should begin with continuous ECG monitoring (for 12–18 sessions) decreasing to intermittent monitoring. • Movement to low- or high-risk categories will depend on the patient's response to the training program. Movement to the lowest risk category requires normal exercise ECG and hemodynamic responses, no abnormal signs and symptoms (within or away from the exercise program), and an appropriate progression of the exercise program. It is possible for a patient to remain within the moderate-risk category or move to a higher risk category.
High-Risk Classification (One or More Criteria Must Be Present)	**High Risk**
Exercise-Specific Findings • Complex ventricular arrhythmias (ventricular tachycardia, frequent [>6/min] multiform PVCs) at rest, during exercise, or recovery. • Presence of angina or other significant symptoms (such as abnormal shortness of breath, lightheadedness, or dizziness during low-intensity exercise [i.e., <5 METs] or during recovery.	• Direct supervision of exercise for a minimum of 18–36 exercise sessions or 90 days after event/procedure. • Supervision should begin with continuous ECG monitoring decreasing to intermittent monitoring as appropriate (e.g., at 18, 24, or 30 sessions).

(Continued)

TABLE 3.10

American Association of Cardiovascular and Pulmonary Rehabilitation Risk Stratification Guidelines and Exercise Supervision Recommendations for Cardiac Patients (Continued)

• Significant silent ischemia (high level) during exercise testing or recovery (i.e., ST segment depression of ≥ 2 mm from baseline). • Abnormal hemodynamic response with exercise testing (i.e., failure of heart rate and systolic blood pressure to increase with increasing workload, severe postexercise hypotension). • Functional capacity < 5 METs. *Non-Exercise-Specific Findings* • Resting ejection fraction < 40%. • History of cardiac arrest or sudden death. • Complex arrhythmias at rest. • Complicated myocardial infarction or revascularization procedure. • Presence of chronic heart failure. • Presence of signs or symptoms of postevent/postprocedure ischemia. • Clinical depression or depressive symptoms.	• Movement to moderate-risk category will depend on the patient's response to the training program (including normal hemodynamic and ECG response during exercise and no abnormal signs within or away from the exercise program). • Discontinuation of the training may be warranted when abnormal ECG or hemodynamic findings during exercise, the development of abnormal signs and symptoms within or outside of the training program, or significant limitations in the ability to participate in the exercise prescription.

Note: ECG = electrocardiogram; MET = metabolic equivalent; PVC = premature ventricular complex.

Adapted from Williams (2001) and the 2012 AACVPR Risk Stratification Algorithm for Risk of Event.

EXERCISE TESTING AND PREPARTICIPATION SCREENING

Various international groups recommend the use of exercise testing in the preparticipation-screening process according to the risk stratification of the client and the intensity of exercise to be engaged in (Bredin et al., 2013; Bredin, Jamnik, et al., 2013). For instance, with the 2013 ACSM risk classification system, exercise stress testing is not required prior to the initiation of moderate-to-vigorous exercise training in both low-risk and moderate-risk individuals. Physician-supervised exercise testing is only recommended for high-risk individuals interested in moderate-to-vigorous exercise. It is recommended that physicians monitor both submaximal and maximal exercise tests in high-risk patients. This recommendation is consistent with the recommendations of the new PAR-Q+ and ePARmed-X+ preparticipation clearance and risk stratification strategy (Bredin et al., 2013; Bredin, Jamnik, et al., 2013).

Various agencies have endorsed the medical supervision of maximal exercise testing (particularly in high-risk individuals; Gibbons et al., 2002). However, a wide range of practice and standard of care is acknowledged (Goodman et al., 2011). Many academics and clinicians advocate for the inclusion of exercise stress testing across the health and fitness continuum (Mezzani et al., 2012, 2013; Stone, McCartney, Millar, Tremblay, & Warburton, 2007; Warburton et al., 2006a, 2006b). However, others believe that exercise testing is not warranted in low-risk individuals (Carneiro, 2004; Fowler-Brown et al., 2004). Fowler-Brown and colleagues (2004) recommended that clinical exercise stress testing should not be conducted in low-risk patients owing to lower likelihood of coronary artery disease in these individuals and the inability of participants to attain a maximal effort, resulting in a lower test sensitivity to detect electrophysiological (ST segment) changes (Fowler-Brown et al., 2004). Also, there is concern related to the inappropriate labeling of participants as high risk as the result of increased false-positives leading to unnecessary medical referral (including invasive procedures) and/or worry. Carneiro (2004) stated that exercise stress tolerance testing in low-risk patients "does more harm than good, and should not be performed."

The new evidence-based PAR-Q+ and ePARmed-X+ preparticipation-screening and risk stratification strategy has not explicitly outlined the role of exercise stress testing. However, implicit within this strategy is the need for moderate-risk individuals to exercise under the guidance of a qualified exercise professional and for high-risk individuals to exercise in a medically supervised environment. Also, contained on the first page of the PAR-Q+ is a recommendation for individuals over the age of 45 years who are unaccustomed to vigorous exercise (i.e., ≥6 METs) to consult a qualified exercise professional prior to performing this level of exercise. Low-risk clients are free to engage in physical activities and exercise testing of varying intensities (including moderate-to-vigorous intensity; Bredin et al., 2013; Bredin, Jamnik, et al., 2013).

Symptom-limited graded exercise stress testing in patients entering traditional cardiac rehabilitation programs has been a standard of care since the 1970s (Mezzani et al., 2012, 2013). Recently there has been a trend for cardiac rehabilitation programs in Canada, Europe, and the United States to not incorporate exercise stress testing. However, a recent joint position paper from the major international cardiovascular disease prevention and rehabilitation bodies (i.e., the European Association for Cardiovascular Prevention and Rehabilitation, the AACVPR, and the Canadian Association of Cardiovascular Prevention and Rehabilitation) recommended strongly the inclusion of exercise stress testing prior to engaging in cardiac rehabilitation (Mezzani et al., 2012, 2013). Exercise testing is viewed as important for effective risk stratification, identifying the presence and severity of arrhythmias and/or signs and symptoms of myocardial ischemia, establishing functional capacity or work tolerance and the chronotropic and inotropic responses to exercise, determining the level of supervision required, and the creation of effective individualized exercise prescriptions (Mezzani et al., 2012, 2013). The exercise stress test is also beneficial for determining the long-term risk for various chronic medical conditions and assessing the effectiveness of an exercise (or lifestyle) intervention (Visich, 2009; Warburton et al., 2006a).

RECOMMENDATIONS FOR REDUCING THE RISKS OF ADVERSE EXERCISE-RELATED EVENTS

In an attempt to reduce the risk of adverse exercise-related events, the AHA and ACSM have established expert opinion-based recommendations for both absolute and relative contraindications to exercise (Gibbons et al., 2002). Similarly, specific recommendations have been made for health and fitness facilities to reduce the potential risks associated with exercise training and/or testing (Balady et al., 1998).

Absolute and Relative Contraindications to Exercise

The AHA and ACSM have led the international community in the creation of absolute and relative contraindications to exercise training and testing (Gibbons et al., 2002; Table 3.11). For the vast majority of persons, the benefits of exercise far outweigh the small transient risks associated with exercise (Goodman et al., 2011; Thomas et al., 2011; Warburton, Jamnik, Bredin, Burr, et al., 2011).

Therefore, reducing the barriers to physical activity is widely advocated. However, careful consideration of the relative and absolute contraindications to

TABLE 3.11

AHA and ACSM Contraindications to Exercise Training and Testing

Absolute Contraindications
Recent marked change in resting electrocardiogram suggesting ischemia, acute/recent myocardial infarction (within 2 days), or other acute cardiac event
Unstable angina
Uncontrolled cardiac arrhythmias causing symptoms or hemodynamic compromise
Symptomatic severe aortic stenosis
Uncontrolled symptomatic heart failure
Acute pulmonary embolus or pulmonary infarction
Acute myocarditis or pericarditis
Suspected or known acute aortic dissecting aneurysm
Acute systemic infection (associated with fever, body ache, or swollen lymph glands)
Relative Contraindications
Left main coronary stenosis
Moderate stenotic valvular heart disease
Electrolyte abnormalities (such as hypokalemia, hypomagnesemia)
Severe arterial hypertension (i.e., systolic blood pressure of > 200 mmHg and/or a diastolic blood pressure of > 110 mmHg)
Tachyarrhythmias or bradyarrhythmias
Hypertrophic cardiomyopathy and other forms of outflow tract obstruction
Mental or physical impairment leading to inability to exercise adequately
High-degree atrioventricular block
Neuromuscular, musculoskeletal, or rheumatoid disorders that are worsened by exercise
Ventricular aneurysm
Uncontrolled metabolic disease (e.g., diabetes, thyrotoxicosis, or myxedema)
Chronic infectious disease (e.g., mononucleosis, hepatitis, AIDS)

Modified from Gibbons et al. (2002); American College of Sports Medicine (2006).

exercise is advisable to ensure safety. An effective and thorough preparticipation-screening process and review of the medical history of persons living with chronic medical conditions will assist in determining each client's benefit-to-risk ratio.

Recommendations for Health and Fitness Facilities

The AHA and ACSM released a series of recommendations for appropriate cardiovascular screening, staffing, and emergency procedures at health and fitness facilities (ACSM & AHA, 1998; Balady et al., 1998). In 1998, Balady and colleagues revealed that approximately 40% of health/fitness facilities (in a subsample within the United States) did not routinely use preparticipation-screening process, with 10% conducting no initial cardiovascular health history screening. Based on this evidence, the AHA and ACSM (led by Dr. Balady et al.) created an official position statement regarding cardiovascular health screening of all individuals (including children, adolescents, and adults) within health and fitness facilities. These recommendations have become the international standard for health and fitness facilities (see Balady et al., 1998 for further information).

The expert advice of Balady and colleagues provided very important recommendations for the training of professionals working with a wide range of clientele including the recommendation to use effective screening tools such as the revised PAR-Q (Gledhill, 2002; Shephard, Thomas, & Weller, 1991; Thomas et al., 1992) and the AHA/ACSM Health/Fitness Facility Preparticipation Screening Questionnaire. The innovative work of Dr. Eickhoff-Shemek and Dr. Herbert also supported the need for including effective screening questionnaires in health and fitness facilities through a critical evaluation of negligence lawsuits against personal trainers and other exercise professionals (Eickhoff-Shemek, 2010; Eickhoff-Shemek & Herbert, 2007, 2008a, 2008b; Herbert, 1987, 1988b, 1993, 1996, 1999; Herbert & Eickhoff-Shemek, 2010). Our recent systematic review of the literature also supported the need for qualified exercise professionals to employ effective preparticipation-screening and risk stratification processes (Warburton, Bredin, Charlesworth, et al., 2011). With the introduction of the evidence-based PAR-Q+ and ePARmed-X+, these screening strategies should be integrated into the recommendations for Health and Fitness Clubs.

The Role of the Qualified Exercise Professional in the Preparticipation Screening and Risk Stratification Strategy

With advances in training, qualified exercise professionals have assumed a greater role in the effective risk stratification and exercise testing and training of asymptomatic and symptomatic populations (Jamnik et al., 2007; Warburton, Bredin, Charlesworth, et al., 2011; Warburton et al., 2011b). Qualified exercise professionals play key roles in new preparticipation-screening and risk stratification strategies (such as the PAR-Q+; Warburton, Bredin, Charlesworth, et al., 2011; Warburton et al., 2011b). They are required to adhere to the international standards established by other allied health professions and must possess a series of discipline-specific core competencies before working with moderate- to high-risk conditions (Warburton, Bredin, Charlesworth, et al., 2011; Warburton et al., 2013). For individuals working with moderate- to high-risk clinical populations, we recommended *advanced postgraduate training in the exercise sciences and clinical internships with appropriate practical and written evaluations* (Warburton, Bredin, Charlesworth, et al., 2011; Warburton et al., 2013). For further information, please see Warburton, Bredin, Charlesworth, et al. (2011a). These recommendations are founded on the fact that the vast majority of studies demonstrating the health benefits and safety of exercise testing and training in clinical populations employed qualified exercise professionals with advanced clinical training (Bredin, Jamnik, et al., 2013). These recommendations are supported by several high-profile lawsuits against inappropriately trained "personal trainers" and "fitness professionals" who worked with clinical populations and did not adhere to evidence-based best practice within a clearly defined scope of practice (Warburton, Bredin, Charlesworth, et al., 2011).

The increased role of the qualified exercise professional in the preparticipation screening has decreased markedly the barriers to physical activity participation while also reducing the burden to already overworked physicians who often complained that the risk stratification process was cumbersome and onerous (Bredin et al., 2013; Bredin, Jamnik, et al., 2013). For instance, in the new PAR-Q+ and ePARmed-X+ preparticipation-screening and risk stratification strategy, the qualified exercise professional assumes a great deal of the burden previously placed on physicians and patients alike. Only 1% of persons using these forms are now sent to physicians (in comparison to 15%–30% with previous risk stratification processes; Bredin et al., 2013; Bredin, Jamnik, et al., 2013).

Qualified exercise professional have been warmly welcomed by physicians (and other health-care professionals) in exercise screening, testing, and training (Bredin & Warburton, 2013). For instance, qualified exercise professionals (who have completed advanced university education, training, and clinical internships) play the key role in preparticipation screening, risk stratification, and exercise prescription for the Physical Activity Line (a free telehealth program in the province of British Columbia, Canada; www.physicalactivityline.com). These qualified exercise professionals interact on a daily basis with physicians, the general public, allied health professionals, and persons living with chronic medical conditions (Bredin & Warburton, 2013). Physicians have welcomed the increased responsibility afforded by qualified exercise professionals, recognizing the advancements in training and instruction within the exercise sciences (Bredin & Warburton, 2013). It is anticipated that that the greater role of qualified exercise professionals will enhance patient-centered care and reduce the burden of physical activity clearance and counseling often placed on physicians (Warburton et al., 2013).

POINTS TO CONSIDER WHEN ASSESSING THE RISK FOR ADVERSE EXERCISE-RELATED EVENTS

There are various points to consider and practical steps that can be taken by health-care providers and qualified exercise professionals to mitigate the risks associated with exercise:

- Activities of all intensities have been associated with a transient increase in the risk for cardiac-related events related to rest; however, the risk appears to be greater in vigorous-intensity exercise. The absolute cutoff of ≥6 METs has been associated with an increased risk; however, health-care providers (particularly those working with the elderly and clinical populations) should recognize that the relative intensity of effort appears to be the key factor related to the increased exercise-related risk.
- The acute risks for adverse exercise-related cardiac events are mitigated by previous experience with physical activity/exercise (particularly vigorous-intensity activities/exercises) (Albert et al., 2000; Siscovick et al., 1984; Whang et al., 2006).
- Vigorous-intensity exercise training can lead to significant health benefits in apparently healthy individuals and persons living with chronic medical conditions (Adams, 2013; Bronstad et al., 2012; Freyssin et al., 2012; Gjellesvik et al., 2012; Holleran et al., 2014; Stefanelli et al., 2013; Warburton et al., 2005; Weston et al., 2014). However, the following special precautions should be employed to minimize the risk of vigorous-intensity programs.
  - Ensure appropriate preparticipation screening and risk stratification.
  - Ensure careful monitoring of heart rate (using ECG as appropriate) and rating of perceived exertion.
  - Avoid exercising in extremes of temperature (i.e., hot or cold environments).
  - Include appropriate warm-up and cooldown.
- Preparticipation screening (such as the PAR-Q+) is the standard of practice for exercise testing/screening. EVERY person regardless of age or clinical status should complete a preparticipation-screening process and provide a written informed consent.
- Health-care professionals must be aware of the unique limitations and clinical status of each client.
- Every client should receive an individualized, progressive, and evidence-based exercise prescription that is appropriate for his/her functional status.
- Exercise stress testing (submaximal or maximal) will assist in the design of effective and individualized exercise prescriptions.

- Individuals classified as being at high risk for an adverse exercise-related event should exercise in a medically supervised environment (under the direct supervision of a qualified exercise professional and overseen by a physician).
- Health and fitness facilities should have appropriate safeguards, emergency plans, and resuscitation equipment in place. Appropriate training of staff is essential for a safe and effective practice.

CONCLUSIONS

An acute bout of activity/exercise (particularly of vigorous intensity) increases transiently the risk of an adverse potentially life-threatening event. However, the benefits of routine physical activity outweigh greatly the transient risks of acute bouts of physical activity (Goodman et al., 2011; Warburton et al., 2011a). In fact, the health benefits of physical activity are irrefutable; routine physical activity decreases markedly the risk for premature mortality and morbidity (Warburton et al., 2006a). In the elderly and clinical populations, relatively small volumes of physical activity/exercise have been associated with marked improvements in health status.

Reducing barriers to physical activity/exercise participation is of great importance for individuals from the across the life span (Warburton, Charlesworth, et al., 2010; Warburton et al., 2006a, 2006b; Warburton et al., 2007). Various preparticipation screening and risk stratification strategies have been used throughout the world including expert opinion-based questionnaires (such as the PAR-Q and the AHA/ACSM Health/Fitness Facility Preparticipation Screening Questionnaire). These documents have been shown to be highly effective at preparticipation screening; however, these strategies may also increase the barriers to physical activity participation for those individuals who may serve to benefit the most from becoming more physically active (i.e., the elderly and persons living with chronic medical conditions). It is recommended that health-care and qualified exercise professionals incorporate new preparticipation-screening and risk stratification strategies to ensure the adherence to evidence-based best practice and a reduction in the barriers to physical activity participation.

The new evidence-based PAR-Q+ and ePARmed-X+ preparticipation and risk stratification strategy has led to a marked decrease in the number of persons directed to see a physician, reducing the barriers to physical activity participation. Qualified exercise professionals now play a far greater role in effective preparticipation screening and risk stratification and work with a wide range of clientele across the life span including apparently healthy individuals and persons living with chronic medical conditions.

ACKNOWLEDGMENTS

The authors of this chapter are members of the PAR-Q+ Working Group, which is part of the PAR-Q+ Collaboration. The PAR-Q+ Collaboration includes Dr. Shannon S. D. Bredin, Dr. Jamie Burr, Kim Buxton, Dr. Sarah Charlesworth, Dr. Phil Chilibeck, Dr. Neil Eves, Dr. Heather Foulds, Dr. Norman Gledhill, Dr. Jack Goodman, Dr. Veronica Jamnik, Dr. Lee Jones, Dr. Don McKenzie, Dr. Ryan Rhodes, Dr. Michael Riddell, Dr. Roy J. Shephard, Dr. James Stone, Dr. Scott Thomas, and Dr. Darren E. R. Warburton. We would like to acknowledge the generous funding support from the Public Health Agency of Canada, the BC Ministry of Health, and GE Healthcare.

REFERENCES

ACSM & AHA. (1998). American College of Sports Medicine Position Stand and American Heart Association. Recommendations for cardiovascular screening, staffing, and emergency policies at health/fitness facilities. *Medicine and Science in Sports and Exercise*, *30*(6), 1009–1018.

Adams, O. P. (2013). The impact of brief high-intensity exercise on blood glucose levels. *Diabetes, Metabolic Syndrome and Obesity: Targets and Therapy*, 6, 113–122.

AGREE Collaboration. (2001). *Appraisal of Guidelines for Research and Evaluation (AGREE) instrument*. Retrieved from http://www.agreecollaboration.org

AGREE Collaboration. (2003). Development and validation of an international appraisal instrument for assessing the quality of clinical practice guidelines: The AGREE project. *Quality & Safety in Health Care*, *12*(1), 18–23.

Albert, C. M., Mittleman, M. A., Chae, C. U., Lee, I. M., Hennekens, C. H., & Manson, J. E. (2000). Triggering of sudden death from cardiac causes by vigorous exertion. *The New England Journal of Medicine*, *343*(19), 1355–1361.

American College of Sports Medicine (ACSM). (2006). *ACSM's guidelines for exercise testing and prescription* (7th ed.). Baltimore, MD: Lippincott Williams & Wilkins.

American College of Sports Medicine. (2013). *ACSM's guidelines for exercise testing and prescription* (9th ed.). Baltimore: Lippincott Williams & Wilkins.

Bailey, I. (Producer). (2010). *How to get breast-cancer survivors exercising? Video games*. Retrieved from http://www.theglobeandmail.com/life/health-and-fitness/how-to-get-breast-cancer-survivors-exercising-video-games/article597012/

Bailey, D. A., Shephard, R. J., Mirwald, R. L., & McBride, G. A. (1974). A current view of Canadian cardiorespiratory fitness. *Canadian Medical Association Journal*, *111*(1), 25–30.

Balady, G. J., Chaitman, B., Driscoll, D., Foster, C., Froelicher, E., Gordon, N., et al. (1998). Recommendations for cardiovascular screening, staffing, and emergency policies at health/fitness facilities. *Circulation*, *97*(22), 2283–2293.

Balady, G. J., Williams, M. A., Ades, P. A., Bittner, V., Comoss, P., Foody, J. M., et al. (2007). Core components of cardiac rehabilitation/secondary prevention programs: 2007 update: A scientific statement from the American Heart Association Exercise, Cardiac

Rehabilitation, and Prevention Committee, the Council on Clinical Cardiology; the Councils on Cardiovascular Nursing, Epidemiology and Prevention, and Nutrition, Physical Activity, and Metabolism; and the American Association of Cardiovascular and Pulmonary Rehabilitation. *Circulation*, *115*(20), 2675–2682.

Biswas, A., Oh, P. I., Faulkner, G. E., Bajaj, R. R., Silver, M. A., Mitchell, M. S., et al. (2015). Sedentary time and its association with risk for disease incidence, mortality, and hospitalization in adults: A systematic review and meta-analysis. *Annals of Internal Medicine*, *162*(2), 123–132.

Bredin, S. S., Gledhill, N., Jamnik, V. K., & Warburton, D. E. R. (2013). PAR-Q+ and ePARmed-X+: New risk stratification and physical activity clearance strategy for physicians and patients alike. *Canadian Family Physician Médecin de Famille Canadien*, *59*(3), 273–277.

Bredin, S. S. D., Gledhill, N., Jamnik, V., & Warburton, D. E. R. (2015). The PAR-Q+ 12 and ePARmed-X+: As easy as 1, 2, 3. *Health & Fitness Journal of Canada*, *2*(2), 3–10.

Bredin, S. S. D., Jamnik, V., Gledhill, N., & Warburton, D. E. R. (2013). Effective Pre-Participation Screening and Risk Stratification. In D. E. R. Warburton (Ed.), *Health-related exercise Prescription for the qualified exercise professional* (3rd ed., pp. 1–30). Vancouver, WA: Health & Fitness Society of BC.

Bredin, S. S., & Warburton, D. E. R. (2013). Physical activity line: Effective knowledge translation of evidence-based best practice in the real-world setting. *Canadian Family Physician Médecin de Famille Canadien*, *59*(9), 967–968.

Bredin, S. S. D., Warburton, D. E. R., & Lang, D. J. (2013). The health benefits and challenges of exercise training in persons living with schizophrenia: A pilot study. *Brain Sciences*, *3*(2), 821–848.

Bronstad, E., Rognmo, O., Tjonna, A. E., Dedichen, H. H., Kirkeby-Garstad, I., Haberg, A. K., et al. (2012). High-intensity knee extensor training restores skeletal muscle function in COPD patients. *The European Respiratory Journal*, *40*(5), 1130–1136.

Bull, F. C., Kreuter, M. W., & Scharff, D. P. (1999). Effects of tailored, personalized and general health messages on physical activity. *Patient Education and Counseling*, *36*(2), 181–192.

Carneiro, A. V. (2004). Screening for coronary artery disease in assymptomatic adults is not recommended, so why is it still done? *Revista Portuguesa de Cardiologia*, *23*(12), 1633–1638.

Chisholm, D. M., Collis, M. L., Kulak, L. L., Davenport, W., & Gruber, N. (1975). Physical activity readiness. *British Columbia Medical Journal*, *17*, 375–378.

Chisholm, D. M., Collis, M. L., Kulak, L. L., Davenport, W., Gruber, N., & Stewart, G. (1978). *PAR-Q validation report: The evaluation of the self-administered pre-exercise screening questionnaire for adults*. Victoria, BC: BC Ministry of Health and Health and Welfare Canada.

Corrado, D., Basso, C., Rizzoli, G., Schiavon, M., & Thiene, G. (2003). Does sports activity enhance the risk of sudden death in adolescents and young adults? *Journal of the American College of Cardiology*, *42*(11), 1959–1963.

Corrado, D., Basso, C., Schiavon, M., & Thiene, G. (2006). Does sports activity enhance the risk of sudden cardiac death? *Journal of Cardiovascular Medicine (Hagerstown)*, *7*(4), 228–233.

Dahabreh, I. J., & Paulus, J. K. (2011). Association of episodic physical and sexual activity with triggering of acute cardiac events: Systematic review and meta-analysis. *Journal of the American Medical Association*, *305*(12), 1225–1233.

Eickhoff-Shemek, J. M. (2010). An analysis of 8 negligence lawsuits against personal fitness trainers: 3 major liability exposures revealed. *ACSM's Health & Fitness Journal*, *14*(5), 34–37.

Eickhoff-Shemek, J. M., & Herbert, D. L. (2007). Is licensure in your future? Issues to Consider - Part 1. *ACSM's Health & Fitness Journal*, *11*(5), 35–37.

Eickhoff-Shemek, J. M., & Herbert, D. L. (2008a). Is licensure in your future? Issues to consider - Part 2. *ACSM's Health & Fitness Journal*, *12*(1), 36–38.

Eickhoff-Shemek, J. M., & Herbert, D. L. (2008b). Is licensure in your future? Issues to consider - Part 3. *ACSM's Health & Fitness Journal*, *12*(3), 36–38.

Flesher, M., Woo, P., Chiu, A., Charlebois, A., Warburton, D. E., & Leslie, B. (2011). Self-management and biomedical outcomes of a cooking, and exercise program for patients with chronic kidney disease. *Journal of Renal Nutrition*, *21*(2), 188–195.

Fletcher, G. F., Balady, G. J., Amsterdam, E. A., Chaitman, B., Eckel, R., Fleg, J., et al. (2001). Exercise standards for testing and training: A statement for healthcare professionals from the American Heart Association. *Circulation*, *104*(14), 1694–1740.

Fowler-Brown, A., Pignone, M., Pletcher, M., Tice, J. A., Sutton, S. F., & Lohr, K. N. (2004). Exercise tolerance testing to screen for coronary heart disease: A systematic review for the technical support for the U.S. Preventive Services Task Force. *Annals of Internal Medicine*, *140*(7), W9–W24.

Franklin, B. A. (2014). Preventing exercise-related cardiovascular events: Is a medical examination more urgent for physical activity or inactivity? *Circulation*, *129*(10), 1081–1084.

Franklin, B. A., & Billecke, S. (2012). Putting the benefits and risks of aerobic exercise in perspective. *Current Sports Medicine Reports*, *11*(4), 201–208.

Freyssin, C., Verkindt, C., Prieur, F., Benaich, P., Maunier, S., & Blanc, P. (2012). Cardiac rehabilitation in chronic heart failure: Effect of an 8-week, high-intensity interval training versus continuous training. *Archives of Physical Medicine and Rehabilitation*, *93*(8), 1359–1364.

Fuster, V., Gotto, A. M., Libby, P., Loscalzo, J., & McGill, H. C. (1996). 27th Bethesda conference: Matching the intensity of risk factor management with the hazard for coronary disease events. Task Force 1. Pathogenesis of coronary disease: The biologic role of risk factors. *Journal of the American College of Cardiology*, *27*(5), 964–976.

George, K., Shave, R., Warburton, D., Scharhag, J., & Whyte, G. (2008). Exercise and the heart: Can you have too much of a good thing? *Medicine and Science in Sports and Exercise*, *40*(8), 1390–1392.

Gibbons, R. J., Balady, G. J., Bricker, J. T., Chaitman, B. R., Fletcher, G. F., Froelicher, V. F., et al. (2002). ACC/AHA 2002 guideline update for exercise testing: Summary article. A report of the American College of Cardiology/American Heart Association Task Force on Practice Guidelines (Committee to update the 1997 exercise testing guidelines). *Journal of the American College of Cardiology*, *40*(8), 1531–1540.

Gjellesvik, T. I., Brurok, B., Hoff, J., Torhaug, T., & Helgerud, J. (2012). Effect of high aerobic intensity interval treadmill walking in people with chronic stroke: A pilot study with one year follow-up. *Topics in Stroke Rehabilitation*, *19*(4), 353–360.

Gledhill, N. (2002). *The revised PAR-Q*. York University.

Gledhill, N., & Jamnik, V. K. (1992). Development and validation of a fitness screening protocol for firefighter applicants. *Canadian Journal of Sport Sciences = Journal Canadien des Sciences du Sport*, *17*(3), 199–206.

Gledhill, N., & Jamnik, V. K. (2003). *Canadian physical activity, fitness and lifestyle approach* (3rd ed.). Ottawa: Canadian Society for Exercise Physiology.

Goodman, J. M., Thomas, S. G., & Burr, J. (2011). Evidence-based risk assessment and recommendations for physical activity and exercise testing. *Applied Physiology, Nutrition and Metabolism*, *36*(S1), S14–S32.

Hamm, L. F., Sanderson, B. K., Ades, P. A., Berra, K., Kaminsky, L. A., Roitman, J. L., et al. A. (2011). Core competencies for cardiac rehabilitation/secondary prevention professionals: 2010 update: Position statement of the American Association of Cardiovascular and Pulmonary Rehabilitation. *Journal of Cardiopulmonary Rehabilitation and Prevention*, *31*(1), 2–10.

Herbert, D. L. (1987). Is there a legal mandate duty to screen exercise participants prior to exercise? *Exercise Standard and Malpractice Reporter*, *1*(1), 10–12.

Herbert, D. L. (1988a). Are GXTs required for screening all men over 40? *Exercise Standards and Malpractice Reporter*, *2*(2), 18.

Herbert, D. L. (1988b). An examination of four recent cases against fitness instructors. *Exercise Standards and Malpractice Reporter*, *2*(3), 45–47.

Herbert, D. L. (1993). Trainer and coach liable for non-referral of student/athlete to physician. *Exercise Standards and Malpractice Reporter*, *7*(1), 12–13.

Herbert, D. L. (1996). Legal and professional responsibilities of personal training. In S. Roberts (Ed.), *The business of personal training* (pp. 53–64). Champaign, IL: Human Kinetics.

Herbert, D. L. (1999). $320 millon lawsuit filed against health club. *The Exercise Standards and Malpractice Reporter*, *13*(3), 33, 36.

Herbert, D. L., & Eickhoff-Shemek, J. M. (2010). New standards statements legal considerations for the fitness industry. *ACSM's Health & Fitness Journal*, *14*(3), 31–33.

Holleran, C. L., Straube, D. D., Kinnaird, C. R., Leddy, A. L., & Hornby, T. G. (2014). Feasibility and potential efficacy of high-intensity stepping training in variable contexts in subacute and chronic stroke. *Neurorehabilitation and Neural Repair*, *28*(7), 643–651.

Jamnik, V. K., Gledhill, N., & Shephard, R. J. (2007). Revised clearance for participation in physical activity: Greater screening responsibility for qualified university-educated fitness professionals. *Applied Physiology, Nutrition, and Metabolism = Physiologie Appliquée, Nutrition et Métabolisme*, *32*(6), 1191–1197.

Jamnik, V. J., Warburton, D. E. R., Makarski, J., McKenzie, D. C., Shephard, R. J., Stone, J., et al. (2011). Enhancing the effectiveness of clearance for physical activity participation: Background and overall process. *Applied Physiology, Nutrition and Metabolism*, *36*(S1), S3–S13.

La Gerche, A., & Heidbuchel, H. (2014). Can intensive exercise harm the heart? You can get too much of a good thing. *Circulation*, *130*(12), 992–1002.

La Gerche, A., & Prior, D. L. (2007). Exercise—is it possible to have too much of a good thing? *Heart, Lung & Circulation*, *16*(Suppl 3), S102–104.

Maron, B. J., Araujo, C. G., Thompson, P. D., Fletcher, G. F., de Luna, A. B., Fleg, J. L., et al. (2001). Recommendations for preparticipation screening and the assessment of cardiovascular disease in masters athletes: An advisory for healthcare professionals from the working groups of the World Heart Federation, the International Federation of Sports Medicine, and the American Heart Association Committee on Exercise, Cardiac Rehabilitation, and Prevention. *Circulation*, *103*(2), 327–334.

Maron, B. J., & Pelliccia, A. (2006). The heart of trained athletes: Cardiac remodeling and the risks of sports, including sudden death. *Circulation*, *114*(15), 1633–1644.

Mezzani, A., Hamm, L. F., Jones, A. M., McBride, P. E., Moholdt, T., Stone, J. A., et al. (2012). Aerobic exercise intensity assessment and prescription in cardiac rehabilitation: A joint position statement of the European Association for Cardiovascular Prevention and Rehabilitation, the American Association of Cardiovascular and Pulmonary Rehabilitation, and the Canadian Association of Cardiac Rehabilitation. *Journal of Cardiopulmonary Rehabilitation and Prevention*, *32*(6), 327–350.

Mezzani, A., Hamm, L. F., Jones, A. M., McBride, P. E., Moholdt, T., Stone, J. A., et al. (2013). Aerobic exercise intensity assessment and prescription in cardiac rehabilitation: A joint position statement of the European Association for Cardiovascular Prevention and Rehabilitation, the American Association of Cardiovascular and Pulmonary Rehabilitation and the Canadian Association of Cardiac Rehabilitation. *European Journal of Preventive Cardiology*, *20*(3), 442–467.

Mittleman, M. A., Maclure, M., Tofler, G. H., Sherwood, J. B., Goldberg, R. J., & Muller, J. E. (1993). Triggering of acute myocardial infarction by heavy physical exertion. Protection against triggering by regular exertion. Determinants of myocardial infarction onset study investigators. *The New England Journal of Medicine*, *329*(23), 1677–1683.

Mittleman, M. A., & Mostofsky, E. (2011). Physical, psychological and chemical triggers of acute cardiovascular events: Preventive strategies. *Circulation*, *124*(3), 346–354.

Paterson, D. H., & Warburton, D. E. (2010). Physical activity and functional limitations in older adults: A systematic review related to Canada's physical activity guidelines. *The International Journal of Behavioral Nutrition and Physical Activity*, *7*, 38.

Pescatello, L. S., Riebe, D., Arena, R., & American College of Sports Medicine. (2014). *ACSM's guidelines for exercise testing and prescription*. Baltimore, MD: Lippincott Williams & Wilkins.

Reddy, P. R., Reinier, K., Singh, T., Mariani, R., Gunson, K., Jui, J., et al. (2009). Physical activity as a trigger of sudden cardiac arrest: The oregon sudden unexpected death study. *International Journal of Cardiology*, *131*(3), 345–349.

Riebe, D., Franklin, B., Ewing Garber, C., Magal, M., Pescatello, L., Thompson, P. D., et al. (2015, August). Updating the American College of Sports Medicine's recommendations for the exercise pre-participation health screening process. *Medicine and Science in Sports and Exercise*, in Press.

Scheinowitz, M., Dankner, R., Goldbourt, U., & Marom-Klibansky, R. (2008). Preparticipation screening of individuals engaging in noncompetitive physical activity. *Harefuah*, *147*(7), 611–617, 662, 661.

Shephard, R. J. (1988). PAR-Q, Canadian home fitness test and exercise screening alternatives. *Sports Medicine*, *5*(3), 185–195.

Shephard, R. J. (1994). Readiness for physical activity. In C. Corbin & R. Pangrazi (Eds.), *President's council on physical fitness and sports research digest* (Series 1, No. 5). Washington, DC: Department of Health and Human Services.

Shephard, R. J. (2001). Absolute versus relative intensity of physical activity in a dose-response context. *Medicine and Science in Sports and Exercise*, *33*(6 Suppl), S400–S418; discussion S419–420.

Shephard, R. J. (2003). Limits to the measurement of habitual physical activity by questionnaires. *British Journal of Sports Medicine*, *37*(3), 197–206; discussion 206.

Shephard, R. J. (2014). A brief history of exercise and physical activity participation clearance and prescription: 2. Canadian contributions to the development of objective, evidence-based procedures. *Health & Fitness Journal of Canada*, *7*(1), 36–68.

Shephard, R. J. (2015). Qualified fitness and exercise as professionals and exercise prescription: Evolution of the PAR-Q and Canadian Aerobic Fitness Test. *Journal of Physical Activity & Health*, *12*(4), 454–461.

Shephard, R. J., & Johnson, N. (2015). Effects of physical activity upon the liver. *European Journal of Applied Physiology*, *115*(1), 1–46.

Shephard, R. J., Lankenau, B., Pratt, M., Neiman, A., Puska, P., Benaziza, H., et al. (2004). Physical activity policy development: A synopsis of the WHO/CDC consultation, September 29 through October 2, 2002, Atlanta, Georgia. *Public Health Reports*, *119*(3), 346–351.

Shephard, R. J., & Pelzer, A. M. (1966). The working capacity of subjects from an exhibition crowd. *Canadian Medical Association Journal*, *94*(4), 171–174.

Shephard, R. J., Thomas, S., & Weller, I. (1991). The Canadian home fitness test. 1991 update. *Sports Medicine*, *11*(6), 358–366.

Siscovick, D. S., Weiss, N. S., Fletcher, R. H., & Lasky, T. (1984). The incidence of primary cardiac arrest during vigorous exercise. *The New England Journal of Medicine*, *311*(14), 874–877.

Springer, J. B., Eickhoff-Shemek, J. M., & Zuberbuehler, E. J. (2009a). An investigation of pre-activity cardiovascular screening procedures in health/fitness facilities–part I: Is adherence with national standards decreasing? *Preventive Cardiology*, *12*(3), 155–162.

Springer, J. B., Eickhoff-Shemek, J. M., & Zuberbuehler, E. J. (2009b). An investigation of pre-activity cardiovascular screening procedures in health/fitness facilities–part II: Rationale for low adherence with national standards. *Preventive Cardiology*, *12*(4), 176–183.

Stefanelli, F., Meoli, I., Cobuccio, R., Curcio, C., Amore, D., Casazza, D., et al. (2013). High-intensity training and cardiopulmonary exercise testing in patients with chronic obstructive pulmonary disease and non-small-cell lung cancer undergoing lobectomy. *European Journal of Cardio-Thoracic Surgery: Official Journal of the European Association for Cardio-thoracic Surgery*, *44*(4), e260–e265.

Stone, J. A., McCartney, N., Millar, P. J., Tremblay, G., & Warburton, D. E. R. (2007). Risk stratification, exercise testing, exercise prescription, and program safety. In J. A. Stone (Ed.), *Canadian guidelines for cardiac rehabilitation and cardiovascular disease prevention* (3rd ed., pp. 341–385). Winnipeg, MB: Canadian Association of Cardiac Rehabilitation.

Thomas, S. G., Goodman, J. M., & Burr, J. (2011). Evidence-based risk assessment and recommendations for physical activity clearance: Established cardiovascular disease. *Applied Physiology, Nutrition and Metabolism*, *36*(S1), S190–S213.

Thomas, S., Reading, J., & Shephard, R. J. (1992). Revision of the physical activity readiness questionnaire (PAR-Q). *Canadian Journal of Sport Sciences = Journal Canadien des Sciences du Sport*, *17*(4), 338–345.

Thompson, P. D., Arena, R., Riebe, D., & Pescatello, L. S. (2013). ACSM's new preparticipation health screening recommendations from ACSM's guidelines for exercise testing and prescription, ninth edition. *Current Sports Medicine Reports*, *12*(4), 215–217.

Thompson, P. D., Franklin, B. A., Balady, G. J., Blair, S. N., Corrado, D., Estes, N. A., 3rd, et al. (2007). Exercise and acute cardiovascular events placing the risks into perspective: A scientific statement from the American Heart Association Council on Nutrition, Physical Activity, and Metabolism and the Council on Clinical Cardiology. *Circulation*, *115*(17), 2358–2368.

Tremblay, M. S., Warburton, D. E., Janssen, I., Paterson, D. H., Latimer, A. E., Rhodes, R. E., et al. (2011). New Canadian physical activity guidelines. *Applied Physiology, Nutrition, and Metabolism*, *36*(1), 36–46.

Visich, P. S. (2009). The value of graded exercise testing in today's world. *American Journal of Lifestyle Medicine*, *3*(1), 57–62.

Warburton, D. E. R. (2013). The health benefits of physical activity: A brief review. In D. E. R. Warburton (Ed.), *Health-related exercise prescription for the qualified exercise professional* (3rd ed., pp. 1–17). Vancouver, WA: Health & Fitness Society of BC.

Warburton, D. E. R., Bredin, S. S. D., Charlesworth, S., Foulds, H., McKenzie, D. C., & Shephard, R. J. (2011). Evidence-based risk recommendations for best practices in the training of qualified exercise professionals working with clinical populations. *Applied Physiology, Nutrition and Metabolism*, *36*(S1), S232–S265.

Warburton, D. E. R., Bredin, S. S. D., Jamnik, V., & Gledhill, N. (2011). Validation of the PAR-Q+ and ePARmed-X+. *Health & Fitness Journal of Canada*, *4*(2), 38–46.

Warburton, D. E., Charlesworth, S. A., Foulds, H. J., McKenzie, D. C., Shephard, R. J., & Bredin, S. S. (2013). Qualified exercise professionals: Best practice for work with clinical populations. *Canadian Family Physician Médecin de Famille Canadien*, *59*(7), 759–761.

Warburton, D. E., Charlesworth, S., Ivey, A., Nettlefold, L., & Bredin, S. S. (2010). A systematic review of the evidence for Canada's physical activity guidelines for adults. *International Journal of Behavioral Nutrition and Physical Activity*, *7*, 39.

Warburton, D. E., McKenzie, D. C., Haykowsky, M. J., Taylor, A., Shoemaker, P., Ignaszewski, A. P., et al. (2005). Effectiveness of high-intensity interval training for the rehabilitation of patients with coronary artery disease. *The American Journal of Cardiology*, *95*(9), 1080–1084.

Warburton, D. E., Nicol, C., & Bredin, S. S. (2006a). Health benefits of physical activity: The evidence. *Canadian Medical Association Journal*, *174*(6), 801–809.

Warburton, D. E., Nicol, C., & Bredin, S. S. (2006b). Prescribing exercise as preventive therapy. *Canadian Medical Association Journal*, *174*(7), 961–974.

Warburton, D. E. R., Gledhill, N., Jamnik, V. K., Bredin, S. S. D., McKenzie, D. C., Stone, J., et al. (2011a). Evidence-based risk assessment and recommendations for physical activity clearance: Consensus Document 2011. *Applied Physiology, Nutrition and Metabolism*, *36*(S1), S266–S298.

Warburton, D. E. R., Gledhill, N., Jamnik, V. K., Bredin, S. S. D., McKenzie, D. C., Stone, J., et al. (2011b). The physical activity readiness questionnaire for everyone (PAR-Q+) and electronic Physical Activity Readiness Medical Examination (ePARmed-X+): Summary of consensus panel recommendations. *Health & Fitness Journal of Canada*, *4*(2), 26–37.

Warburton, D. E. R., Jamnik, V. K., Bredin, S. S. D., Burr, J., Charlesworth, S., Chilibeck, P., et al. (2011). Executive summary: The 2011 Physical Activity Readiness Questionnaire for Everyone (PAR-Q+) and the Electronic Physical Activity Readiness Medical Examination (ePARmed X+). *Health & Fitness Journal of Canada*, *4*(2), 24–25.

Warburton, D. E. R., Jamnik, V. K., Bredin, S. S. D., & Gledhill, N. (2010). Enhancing the effectiveness of the PAR-Q and PARmed-X screening for physical activity participation. *Journal of Physical Activity and Health*, *7*(Suppl 3), S338–S340.

Warburton, D. E. R., Jamnik, V., Bredin, S. S. D., & Gledhill, N. (2014). The ePARmed-X+ physician clearance follow-up. *Health & Fitness Journal of Canada*, *7*(3), 35–38.

Warburton, D. E. R., Jamnik, V. K., Bredin, S. S. D., & Gledhill, N. (2011). The Physical Activity Readiness Questionnaire for Everyone (PAR-Q+) and electronic Physical

Activity Readiness Medical Examination (ePARmed-X+). *Health & Fitness Journal of Canada, 4*(2), 3–23.

Warburton, D. E. R., Katzmarzyk, P. T., Rhodes, R. E., & Shephard, R. J. (2007). Evidence-informed physical activity guidelines for Canadian adults. *Applied Physiology, Nutrition and Metabolism, 32*(2E), S16–S68.

West Coast Bariatric Surgery (Producer). (2012, June). *West coast bariatric surgery: Our team*. Retrieved from http://www.westcoastbariatricsurgery.com/

Weston, K. S., Wisloff, U., & Coombes, J. S. (2014). High-intensity interval training in patients with lifestyle-induced cardiometabolic disease: A systematic review and meta-analysis. *British Journal of Sports Medicine, 48*(16), 1227–1234.

Whang, W., Manson, J. E., Hu, F. B., Chae, C. U., Rexrode, K. M., Willett, W. C., et al. (2006). Physical exertion, exercise, and sudden cardiac death in women. *Journal of the American Medical Association, 295*(12), 1399–1403.

Whitfield, G. P., Pettee Gabriel, K. K., Rahbar, M. H., & Kohl, H. W., 3rd. (2014). Application of the American Heart Association/American College of Sports Medicine Adult Preparticipation Screening Checklist to a nationally representative sample of US adults aged >=40 years from the National Health and Nutrition Examination Survey 2001 to 2004. *Circulation, 129*(10), 1113–1120.

Williams, M. A. (2001). Exercise testing in cardiac rehabilitation. Exercise prescription and beyond. *Cardiology Clinics, 19*(3), 415–431.

CHAPTER 4

Benefits of Physical Activity on Cognitive Functioning in Older Adults

Danielle M. Wischenka, Carlos Marquez, and Katarina Friberg Felsted

ABSTRACT

As the world becomes more populated and more medically advanced, more people are starting to live longer. There are growing concerns for the health and well-being of an ever-growing population. Aging is accompanied by a series of changes, cognitive decline being one of them. As health becomes more challenging, physical activity may become more cumbersome. However, in many instances, physical activity has been found to prevent and delay cognitive decline. In fact, exercise may prove to be a powerful preventative measure against cognitive impairment in older adults. The aim of this chapter is to explore the evidence base of the effects of physical activity on cognitive decline prevention as well as to review the recommended guidelines for physical activity in this population based on findings in the field.

INTRODUCTION

As humans advance in age, there is a slow, yet progressive, natural decline in cognitive abilities, a concept known as cognitive aging (Deary et al., 2009). Though this decline is a function of aging, it is nonpathological and an experience

http://dx.doi.org/10.1891/0198-8794.36.103

everyone will encounter toward middle age and onward. The literature on cognitive aging is in agreement that decline occurs; however, the process is not fully understood. Dwindling of different neurocognitive domains is fairly dynamic and dependent on demographic, genetic, and environmental factors (Mortensen, et al., 2014). Furthermore, this natural process should not be mistaken for cognitive impairment or dementia, which is typically a product of neurodegenerative processes.

With the advancements in technology and medicine, there are an increasing number of people living many more years, raising concerns that a larger number of people will live with both cognitive and physical ailments (Christensen, Doblhammer, Rau, & Vaupel, 2009). When individuals' cognitive abilities start significantly deviating from what is considered within normal limits for the individual, diagnoses of cognitive impairment and dementia become warranted (Deary et al., 2009). These conditions are usually caused by neurodegenerative, pathological processes that cause deleterious neurocognitive effects associated with different focal areas of the brain. Data from 2010 estimate that there were 35.6 million people in the world living with dementia, with the majority of them residing in low- to middle-income countries (Prince et al., 2013). Prevalence rates are predicted to double every 20 years; by 2050, there will be approximately 115 million people with dementia, with higher rates predicted in other regions such as in South America.

RISK FACTORS OF COGNITIVE DECLINE

Aging is one risk factor, among many others, which contributes to cognitive decline. However, age is typically accompanied by dynamic risk factors that can largely influence one's neurocognitive presentation; for example, cardiovascular disease, poor mental health, lack of physical activity, and poor health behaviors can all affect cognition. Hypertension, hypercholesterolemia, and atherosclerosis are known as vascular risk factors for cognitive decline, as they all can affect the levels of blood supplied to the brain. Furthermore, these factors increase the probability of conditions such as acute ischemic stroke, among others, that can cause cognitive impairment (Deary et al., 2009). Other risk factors that have been implicated for cognitive decline are depression and anxiety, which have been correlated with decline in executive functioning and memory (Diniz et al., 2014; Kaminska, Brodowski, & Karakiewicz, 2015). Furthermore, deficits in neuropsychological domains have also been associated with different diseases, demographic factors, genetic factors, and lack of physical and mental activity in the elderly (Qiu & Fratiglioni, 2015).

PHYSICAL HEALTH AND COGNITIVE FUNCTIONING

Health and wellness are crucial for general well-being in the general population, but they become more crucial components of quality of life as we age. Many researchers highlight the importance of physical health in older adults as it is understood that health affects overall functioning (Fabel & Kempermann, 2008; Hamer & Chida, 2009; Manini & Pahor, 2009). Poor physical health is a leading cause of morbidity and lower quality of life; it can affect mental health and is also a predictor of cognitive functioning in late life (Bherer, Erickson, & Liu-Ambrose, 2013). Independently, aging affects physiological functioning, which, in turn, may limit physical activity and consequently influence other areas of functioning (Manini & Pahor, 2009). In addition, poor physical health in older adults places this population at a higher risk for falls that, in and of itself, is linked to primary as well as secondary causes of cognitive decline (Lautenschlager et al., 2008).

Maintaining physical activity and health in late life serves multiple functions. For example, physical activity engages multiple areas of the brain including frontal systems, the visual cortex, and areas involved in motor activity (Bherer, Erickson, & Liu-Ambrose, 2013). One study investigated the effects of physical activity on cognitive functioning and posited that dancing had a greater positive effect compared to other activities as it recruits and stimulates more neural networks (Verghese et al., 2003). Physical activity can delay neurodegenerative processes and drastic decline in the elderly without neurodegenerative pathology (Salthouse, 2009). Though the literature on the benefits of physical activity is mixed, physical activity does significantly reduce the risk for cardiovascular disease (Salthouse, 2009; Snyder et al., 2014).

Vascular dementia (VaD) occurs after damage to the vasculature induces harm or death to areas of the brain that can be irreversible (Launer et al., 2015). Cardiovascular disease can contribute to existing vascular risk factors and increase the risk for severe cognitive decline (Qiu & Fratiglioni, 2015). In fact, a recent statement released by the American Heart Association (AHA) and the American Stroke Association specified the importance of the contributory burden of vascular risk factors on cognitive impairment and dementia (Snyder et al., 2014).

One of the greatest benefits of physical activity is reducing the vascular burden on the body; in fact, low physical activity, among others, was highlighted as a comorbid condition in the elderly with dementia (Snyder et al., 2014).

Comparatively, those who age with better physical health fare much better than those who age with poorer physical health (Salthouse, 2009). One population-based study investigating physical activity in relation to cognitive impairment found that moderate-to-intense exercise throughout middle and late life reduced the likelihood of mild cognitive impairment (Geda et al., 2010). In general, studies indicate that measures to prevent vascular and cardiovascular risk factors in the earlier stages of life can drastically reduce greater cognitive impairment in late life, physical activity and diet being some of the most effective (Sudeep & Dallas, 2015). Furthermore, leisure activity that is fulfilling and cognitively stimulating can have an additive effect (Geda et al., 2010).

COGNITIVE DECLINE AND DEMENTIA OVERVIEW

Cognitive abilities are rather heterogeneous overall; however, in the aging population, variables of language tend to generally be more preserved than other domains such as memory, executive functioning, and visuospatial abilities (Salthouse, 2009). It is more common to see decreased processing speed and cognitive flexibility in normal cognitive aging (Deary et al., 2009). In addition, memory may be described as sporadically forgetful (e.g., forgetting where one places items) rather than chronic and generally forgetful as in individuals with mild cognitive impairment (MCI) or Alzheimer's dementia (Dickerson et al., 2005). Mood variables also complicate neuropsychological functioning and can resemble symptoms of cognitive impairment, known as pseudodementia. Deficits in attention, processing speed, and executive functioning affect encoding and retention and therefore are not true memory impairments; treating the mood and anxiety symptoms typically ameliorate the cognitive concerns (Kang et al., 2014).

When cognitive decline accelerates to below what is expected in groups of people, given demographic factors, there is concern for further cognitive decline associated with neurodegenerative processes (Langa & Levine, 2014). The initial indicator of this is usually MCI, which is an objective impairment in cognition that does not warrant a diagnosis of dementia (Langa & Levine, 2014). Objective impairments are measured through neuropsychological testing and are typically considered as scores within 1 to 1.5 standard deviations below what is considered average in demographically adjusted normative data in one or more cognitive domains (Albert et al., 2011). Amnestic MCI involves impairment in memory, mixed MCI involves memory and other domains, and nonamnestic MCI does not involve memory. Impairments are not severe enough to cause significant functional decline in activities of daily living; however, there usually is evidence of decline relative to premorbid estimates (Albert et al., 2011).

Once the impairment becomes severe enough and causes significant functional impairment, a diagnosis of dementia is warranted. Dementia, unspecific to pathology, is a neurodegenerative condition defined by the National Institute on Aging and Alzheimer's Association; it causes significant functional decline, is an obvious decline from the premorbid state, relates to significant impairment (two standard deviations below average in a given group) in two or more cognitive domains, and is not due to another general medical condition (McKhann et al., 2011). Recent data indicates that the population of people aged 85 and above is increasing and prevalence rates of dementia within that population are 18%–38% (Gardner, Valcour, & Yaffe, 2013). There are different types of dementia that are based on pathophysiology and patterns of neurocognitive impairment that are demonstrative of the neural networks involved. The most frequently observed types of dementia include Alzheimer's disease (AD)–related dementia, VaD, dementia with Lewy bodies (DLB), and frontotemporal dementia (FTD; Larner, 2014).

FUNCTIONAL IMPAIRMENT IN ADLS AND IADLS

Functional decline in activities of daily living (ADLs) such as difficulties with bathing, dressing, and feeding as well as with instrumental activities with daily living (IADLs) such as shopping, managing finances, and other activities crucial to independent living are typically observed across dementias (Gure, Kabeto, Plassman, Piette, & Langa, 2010). One study in particular made attempts to explore clear-cut differences in functional impairment across dementias and found that there may be higher ADL limitations in those with VaD and dementia due to other etiologies (e.g., Gure et al., 2010). Another study posited that activities requiring more memory and visuospatial abilities were more impaired in AD than in FTD (Park, Harvey, Johnson, & Farias, 2015). However, these conditions are heterogeneous, and differences in functional impairment may be a consequence of other health factors common in aging (Gure et al., 2010). A brief overview of the listed dementias is provided in the following text.

Alzheimer's Dementia

Dementias in general have many common pathophysiological and neuropathological traits. Dementia associated with AD is the most common type of dementia accounting for nearly 60%–70% of all dementia cases (Salthouse, 2009). Alzheimer's pathology is related to neurofibrillary tangles and β-amyloid plaques that develop as we age; there are many theories as to why this occurs but the literature is mixed (McKhann et al., 2011; Weintraub, Wicklund, & Salmon, 2012). The initial changes that occur in Alzheimer's pathology are in the medial temporal lobe structures affecting learning and retention of new information; deficits in problem solving and other areas of executive functioning begin to surface as well (Weintraub et al., 2012). As the disease progresses, language abilities tend to decline, such as object naming, semantic fluency, and semantic knowledge (Weintraub et al., 2012). Declines in visuospatial functioning occur throughout the course of the disease; however, they vary by case.

Vascular Dementia

Diagnosing dementia in general can be complicated; however, diagnosing VaD in particular can be particularly complex (Korczyn, Vakhapova, & Grinberg, 2012). VaD, also known as multi-infarct dementia, is the second-most common type of dementia, following Alzheimer's, and it accounts for up 20% of all dementia cases (Salthouse, 2009). There is currently no consensus on neuropathology in diagnosing VaD although it is understood that pathological changes in the brain occur as a result of vascular diseases such as small vessel disease, lacunar infarct, and ischemic infarct that, among others, have been observed using computed tomography (CT) and magnetic resonance imaging (MRI; Korczyn et al., 2012). Vascular and cardiovascular risk factors such as high blood pressure and atherosclerosis are very amenable to treatment and lifestyle changes such as increasing physical activity and dietary changes and can reduce the chances of vascular changes in the brain (Korczyn et al., 2012; Snyder et al., 2014). Cognitive deficits in VaD tend to vary, though typically one sees disruption in executive features such as attention, problem-solving, and cognitive flexibility (Firbank et al., 2007). Behavioral and emotional changes have also been observed. Given that vascular changes in the brain widely vary, cognitive impairments tend to be diverse (Korczyn et al., 2012).

Dementia With Lewy Bodies

DLB makes up 10%–20% of the cases of dementia, making it the third-most frequently observed dementia (Salthouse, 2009). Lewy bodies are abnormal protein material found in nerve cells in patients with Parkinson's disease; however, DLB is its own subset along the spectrum of dementia (Oda, Yamamoto, & Maeda, 2009). There are cortical and brain stem Lewy bodies and four subtypes of DLB: neocortical type, limbic type, brain stem type, and cerebral type (Oda et al., 2009). Patterns of impairment are comparable to those seen in patients with AD; however, visual hallucinations and visuospatial deficits are fairly prominent in DLB (Oda et al., 2009). The neuropsychological hallmark of DLB is the waxing and waning of cognitive abilities; mild motor symptoms such as parkinsonism features can also be present (Oda et al., 2009). Though memory can still be impaired, the deficits are not as pronounced as in AD. Diagnosis of DLB is usually confirmed posthumously during autopsy when Lewy bodies can be detected.

Frontotemporal Dementia

FTD is a condition that mostly affects frontal and temporal structure and accounts for about 5% of all dementia cases (Hutchinson & Mathias, 2007; Salthouse, 2009). FTD involves two patterns of neurodegeneration that affect language-based abilities and behavior (Weintraub et al., 2012). Executive dysfunction is a distinguishing feature of FTD in that it tends to cause disinhibition, deficits in problem-solving, and overall personality changes that are obvious, relative to the person; this is more common in the behavioral variant, given the frontal neural structures involved (Harciarek & Cosentino, 2013). In the syndrome primarily affecting language, problems are with expressive language, typically due to word-finding difficulties. As the disease progresses, semantic language declines, as does the fund of vocabulary knowledge; problems with reading and writing may also be present (Harciarek & Cosentino, 2013). Memory stays relatively intact compared to AD.

Dementias are complex syndromes that vary from person to person, and many share similar symptomology. Specific details and etiology of these dementias are outside of the scope of this chapter. In general, dementia is a heterogeneous condition affecting many people around the world and given the rate at which the elderly population is growing, it will be an issue warranting more preventative and public health efforts.

THEORIES OF EXERCISE AND COGNITIVE BENEFITS

Several hypotheses have been explored as potential explanations for the link between exercise and cognitive benefits. A systematic review by Fratiglioni and colleagues cited three major hypotheses related to physical activity and cognitive health (2004). The cognitive reserve hypothesis assumes that physical activity and exercise improve nonneural components of the brain, which results in increased perfusion of the brain, leading to larger cognitive reserve. In turn, this cognitive reserve can be used in the case of degenerative diseases such as AD (van Uffelen, Paw, Hopman-Rock, & van Mechelen, 2008). The vascular hypothesis posits that exercise reduces the risk of cardiovascular disease, a contributory factor to vascular burden, which is strongly associated with VaD and dementia in general (Langa & Levine, 2014). Finally, the stress hypothesis emphasizes the benefits of exercise as a stress reducer, as stress increases susceptibility to dementia twofold (van Uffelen et al., 2008). The aforementioned hypotheses attempt to explain the relationship between the general construct of exercise and benefit to cognitive functioning. The aerobic fitness hypothesis implies that potential benefits in cognition are experienced as a result of aerobic exercise (van Uffelen et al., 2008). Studies have suggested that increased aerobic fitness is associated with morphologic changes in the human brain (Colcombe et al., 2006). However, other researchers have reported that improved aerobic fitness cannot be directly attributed to the effects on cognition (Angevaren, Aufdemkampe, Verhaar, Aleman, & Vanhees, 2008; Etnier, Nowell, Landers, & Sibley, 2006). These hypotheses underscore the potential mechanisms underlying the effect of exercise on cognition based on physical and mental processes. The lack of knowledge about the exact mechanisms responsible for changes in cognitive function may explain the different results highlighted throughout the literature (van Uffelen et al., 2008).

EVIDENCE OF PHYSICAL ACTIVITY AND COGNITIVE OUTCOMES

Regular exercise has been noted to have potential benefits for cognitive functioning in animal and human studies. Regular exercise is not precisely defined but is connoted as aerobic exercise that is at least 20–30 minutes per session in which heart rate increases and oxygen is needed so that cardiovascular fitness results. In particular, this implies exercise that sufficiently elevates heart rate to approximately 60% of the maximum, noting that greater than 60% may not be attainable for much of this population (Ahlskog, Geda, Gradd-Radford, & Petersen, 2011). Literature suggests that exercise may have a more direct and favorable effect on brain neuroplasticity and resilience to brain aging and neurodegeneration. It is argued that the benefits of exercise include improved cognition and forestalling of later life cognitive decline. Physical fitness training has also been reported to improve cognitive function in the elderly (Heyn, Abreu, & Ottenbacher, 2004). The noted exercise benefits in the elderly include executive control processes of cognition such as selective attention, planning, inhibition, and working memory (Baker et al., 2010). These benefits may be more pronounced in older women than in older men (Colcombe & Kramer, 2003). In the Canadian Study of Health and Aging, physical activity was found to reduce the risks of cognitive impairment and AD (Laurin, Verreault, Lindsay, MacPherson, & Rockwood, 2001). A 2009 study suggested that adults who routinely engage in physical activity or regular exercise in midlife experienced a significantly lower risk of dementia years later (Hamer & Chida, 2009). Several studies have consistently demonstrated that physical activity is associated with a decreased risk of cognitive decline and dementia in older adults (Laurin et al., 2001; Lytle, Vander, Pandav, Dodge, & Ganguli, 2004; Rockwood & Middleton, 2007). Ahlskog and colleagues have cautioned that these findings may be interpreted as reversed causality, such that individuals with preclinical neurodegenerative disease might be disinclined to exercise (2011). However, the evidence of positive effects for both AD and VaD as related to physical activity has been observed consistently (Aarsland, Sardahaee, Anderssen, Ballard, & Alzheimer's Society Systematic Review group, 2010; Hamer & Chida, 2009), thus demonstrating that baseline physical activity is not associated with prior cognitive decline (Buchman et al., 2009) and that low physical activity is harmful to cognitive health rather than vice versa (Angevaren et al., 2008).

Numerous clinical investigations of physical activity's effects on cognitive outcomes have demonstrated preventative effects in normal populations as well as patients with mild cognitive impairment (Angevaren et al., 2008). A meta-analysis in 2010 by Smith and colleagues of 29 randomized controlled trials (RCTs) documented cognitive benefits from sustained exercise in adults without dementia, noting modest improvements in memory, attention, processing speed, and executive functions. A 2008 review by van Uffelen and colleagues explored the effects of various exercise programs on neuropsychological outcomes in both cognitively healthy and impaired subjects. Town and Lewis reported that physical activity increases the availability of cognitive nutrients, endogenous antioxidants, and other neurotrophic factors (1996). Exercise in healthy subjects resulted in benefits on various measures of cognition including memory, information processing, and executive function. These subjects made use of aerobic exercise, strength exercise, flexibility training, and various combinations of these exercises. Subjects with cognitive decline made observable improvements in general cognitive function and executive functions. Effective interventions for subjects with cognitive decline included aerobic exercise and combination strength exercise and flexibility or balance exercise (Baum, Jarjoura, Polen, Faur, & Rutecki, 2003; van de Winckel, Feys, De Weerdt, & Dom, 2004).

Several studies (Ahlskog et al., 2011; Baker et al., 2010; Lautenschlager et al., 2008; van de Winckel et al., 2004) have focused on the cognitive outcomes of exercise in individuals with dementia. A study conducted by Lautenschlager and colleagues demonstrated that subjects with "memory problems" had demonstrable cognitive benefits when engaged in a moderate-intensity exercise regimen for 6 months as opposed to a sedentary routine; these benefits lasted at 12 and 18 months (2008). A review by Van Uffelen and colleagues revealed that different kinds of exercise may benefit cognitive function regardless of baseline cognitive functioning (2008).

Baker and colleagues (2010) showed significant sex-specific improvement in executive control processes for older adult women (the effect size proved over twice as large as the men's), who were considered high risk for cognitive impairment. Exercise seems to specifically improve areas of the brain where executive processing and memory function reside, which incidentally are the most vulnerable with increasing age (Colcombe & Kramer, 2003; Daniels, Toth, & Jacoby, 2006). These processes are disproportionately vulnerable in those patients who are in preclinical stages of AD. A related study, the Canadian Study of Health and Aging (Middleton, Kirkland, & Rockwood, 2008) indicated that women who participated in "heavy to moderate exercise" lowered their risk for cognitive decline, but there was no such association for men between physical activity and risk. One potential reason for this is the lower fitness, higher body fat, and higher cortisol levels that women showed at baseline (Baker et al., 2010). Jedrziewski, Lee, and Trojanowski (2007) also posit that lower correlations between cognitive function and physical activity for men may simply be due to smaller sample sizes in those studies.

Interestingly, Liu-Ambrose and Donaldson address the effect of resistance training on cognitive function in older adult men (2009). Both moderate- and high-intensity resistance exercise significantly increased cognitive performance in older adult men. As little as 3–6 months of moderate aerobic exercise has been shown to significantly improve executive control in older adults of both sexes by Erickson and Kramer (2009). These changes are seen in older adults with and without dementia, indicating improvement across baseline levels. The Intervention Project on Cerebrovascular Diseases and Dementia in the Community of Ebersberg, Bavaria (INVADE) study by Etgen et al. showed that the protective nature of moderate or high physical activity remained in place at a 2-year follow-up (2010).

Numerous noncognitive nonvascular benefits from exercise are proposed for an aging population, which include reduction of osteoporosis and fracture risk, frailty (Rizzoli et al., 2009; Rockwood, 2004), and mental health benefits of combating depression and anxiety (Conn, 2010; Dunn & Jewell, 2010). Physical activity in the older adult population is also associated with lower incidence of diabetes and optimized blood pressure values (Vogel et al., 2009). Other benefits include improved behavioral management in seniors with dementia (Teri et al., 2003) and a decreased risk of falls (Allan, Ballard, Rowan, & Kenny, 2009), as well as reduced mortality risk in the general population due to long-term fitness (Kokkinos, Sheriff, & Kheirbek, 2011). It would be remiss not to mention adverse effects of exercise such as orthopedic injuries, increased fall risk, and provocation of acute coronary syndromes (Ahlskog et al., 2011). It is therefore important to emphasize that providers should assist patients in selecting the appropriate exercise program for their capabilities and cardiopulmonary status.

PHYSICAL ACTIVITY RECOMMENDATIONS FOR OLDER ADULTS WITH COGNITIVE IMPAIRMENTS

Physical activity has recently been considered a primary behavioral preventive strategy against cognitive decline (Liu-Ambrose & Donaldson, 2009). In considering physical activity recommendations for an older adult population, it is imperative to consider several unique factors within the context of this population in order to feasibly adapt such recommendations. These factors include possible chronic medical conditions, low fitness levels, functional limitations, and/or safety concerns (Manini & Pahor, 2009; Nelson et al., 2007). The U.S.

Department of Health and Human Services advises that older adults with chronic medical conditions seek to understand if and how their conditions affect their ability to do regular physical activity safely (2008). Ahlskog and colleagues stress that the choice of exercise routines must match the patient's capabilities (2011). For example, impaired walking should not limit individuals from exercise; rather, such individuals should engage in sitting exercises such as rowing machines and exercise bicycles. They also note that a patient's interest must be considered lest he or she abandon attempts to engage in physical fitness (Ahlskog et al., 2011).

Maintaining an engaged, active lifestyle has benefits for cognitive functioning across the adult life span (Jopp & Herzog, 2007). And it is never too late: Exercise is associated with decreased risk of subsequent cognitive impairment for individuals who are already in their 80th year of life (Flicker et al., 2005). Exercise is a simple and practical strategy, available at little or no cost and offering many other benefits. Yet, older adults have the lowest rates of physical activity and, perhaps not unrelated, the highest health-care costs (Rice & Fineman, 2004; Troiano et al., 2008).

Physical activity in older adults is linked to preventing, delaying, and slowing cognitive decline (Jedrziewski et al., 2007). While cause and effect may not have been sufficiently demonstrated in exercise interventions regarding cognitive decline, there are several emerging themes in this space (Jedrziewski et al., 2007). The connection between physical activity and cognitive function is inarguable.

With regard to suggested intensity, Rockwood and Middleton report that in longitudinal studies, the risk of "dementia, cognitive impairment, cognitive decline, and Alzheimer's disease is lower" among those who participate in high levels versus those with low levels of physical activity (2007). And according to Colcombe and Kramer, cognitive function is positively affected by a session of at least 30 minutes (2003).

Ahlskog and colleagues suggest that exercise be utilized by all people regardless of their medical comorbidities that limit their ability to exercise fully; however, they caution that major cardiopulmonary disease or other major organ failure may thwart this (2011). It is therefore recommended that individuals suffering from the aforementioned conditions seek advice from their primary care provider in order to assess their ability and capacity to exercise. It is important that such individuals continue to engage in regular physical activity, which is ultimately of large benefit for their health (U.S. Department of Health and Human Services, 2008). It is also acknowledged that sometimes it may be required to withdraw from regular physical activity for a period of time due to illness or injury. In this occurrence, physical activity may be resumed at a lower level and progressively increased to the level prior to the sustained injury or illness

(Elsawy & Higgins, 2010). Consideration of adjustment of physical activity based on body weight is also a necessary component to successful physical activity in elderly adults. Primary care physicians must guide older adults in choosing exercises that will keep them free of injury. In conjunction with appropriate diet, some older adults may require greater amounts of physical activity than the minimum recommendation in order to maintain health and weight (Elsawy & Higgins, 2010). Buchman and colleagues recommend that older individuals who may not be able to engage in formal exercise due to underlying health concerns can still gain benefits from a more active lifestyle by increasing the spectrum of their routine activities (2012).

It is noted that older individuals may decrease their nonexercise activities when they increase their exercise activity (Garland et al., 2011). However, it is recommended that individuals maintain both of these levels. A study conducted by Buchman and colleagues examined physical activity in a group of over 700 older persons without dementia. They found total daily physical activity to be associated with risk of AD, suggesting that nonexercise physical activity may be an important component in augmenting cognition and forestalling AD (2012).

It is recommended that moderate levels of exercise can serve dually as a preventive measure against age-related cognitive decline and brain deterioration as well as a treatment to recover some cognitive deficits already present in older adults (Erickson & Kramer, 2009). Because of the diverse range of disease, mobility, and functioning in older adults, a global recommendation is difficult to issue (Manini & Pahor, 2009). Tremblay and colleagues recommend that adults aged 65 years and above accumulate at minimum 150 minutes of moderate- to vigorous-intensity aerobic physical activity per week in intervals of 10 minutes or greater (2011). Elsawy and colleagues note that vigorous-intensity aerobic activity can be performed for a minimum of 20 minutes 3 days per week (2010). Rovio and colleagues (2005) found a correlation between vigorous exercise sessions and a lowered dementia risk; vigorous was defined as lasting for 20 minutes or more, causing both sweating and breathlessness. Positive correlations between cognitive function and physical exercise were also evident in two additional trials (Colcombe et al., 2004; Fabre, Chamari, Mucci, Masse-Biron, & Prefaut, 2002). These interventions lasted 40–45 minutes, three times a week, and 1 hour, two times a week, respectively.

The ACSM and the AHA also recommend that older adults take a multifactorial approach to physical activity by performing a combination of aerobic, strength, and flexibility exercises (Nelson et al., 2007). An activity plan that incorporates the three aforementioned categories of exercise should be detailed along with logistical considerations of the physical activity, such as how it will be performed, at what time, and in what setting (Elsawy & Higgins, 2010). Those with poor mobility should focus on physical activities that enhance balance and prevent falls (Tremblay et al., 2011). Resistance training, with the benefit of strengthening both bones and muscle mass, in particular, is recommended for senior women who are at greater risk of falls and fractures than men (Liu-Ambrose & Donaldson, 2009). Another significant benefit of resistance training to mitigate cognitive decline is its ability to also lower comorbidities in the older adult population (Liu-Ambrose & Donaldson, 2009).

As mentioned previously, resistance training (Liu-Ambrose & Donaldson, 2009) and aerobic exercise (Erickson & Kramer, 2009) are both forms of exercise demonstrated in clinical research to benefit cognitive health. A meta-analysis in 2003 found that programs combining both aerobic and resistance exercises had greater positive benefits on cognition than aerobic-only training (Colcombe & Kramer, 2003). Elsawy and Higgins note that minimum physical activity for achieving important health benefits include a combination of 150 minutes of moderate-intensity aerobic training per week supplemented with muscle-strengthening activities twice per week (2010). It is therefore recommended that both aerobic-based training and resistance training exercise be incorporated as part of a regimen to maintain both physical and brain health (Liu-Ambrose & Donaldson, 2009). It is also recommended that older adults perform at least 2 nonconsecutive days of moderate- to high-intensity resistance training every week (Manini & Pahor, 2009). Examples of aerobic and muscle-strengthening activities provided by the U.S. Department of Health and Human Services includes bicycle riding, dancing, vacuuming, walking, carrying groceries, washing windows or floors, and yard work/gardening (2008). It should be noted that these recommendations include activities that are considered "nonexercise" activities (e.g., vacuuming), which highlights the previously mentioned findings of Buchman et al. (2012).

It is important to note that as the body ages, the cardiovascular system declines in maximal aerobic performance due to a decrease in cardiac output and oxygen uptake at the site of the muscles (Skinner, Tipton, & Vailas, 1982). Safety is therefore a particularly important consideration in the older adult population when designing, undertaking, and committing to a physical activity regimen. To perform physical activities safely and reduce the risk of injuries, the risks of certain exercises should be understood. A person should engage in activities appropriate for his or her current level of fitness. A person should also increase physical activity gradually; this is particularly emphasized for inactive people beginning a workout regimen (U.S. Department of Health and Human Services, 2008). Current ACSM/AHA guidelines indicate moderate-intensity physical activity for older adults for 30 minutes a day, 5 days a week, or high-intensity exercise for 20 minutes a day, 3 days a week. A critical point when incorporating these guidelines is that they can be applied in 10-minute increments throughout the day and be equally effective (Nelson et al., 2007). Erickson and Kramer, after a comprehensive review on aerobic exercise effects on cognition, state that it can be "safely recommended that moderate levels of exercise can serve as both a preventive measure against age-related cognitive and brain deterioration and a treatment to reverse decay and cognitive deficits already present in older adults" (Erickson & Kramer, 2009, p. 4).

CONCLUSION

As a result of a combination of technological and aging advancements, older adults are living longer than ever before. It is thus crucial to find ways to make this longer life span not simply a time of increased comorbidities and poorer quality of life but a time of generativity and health. The leading causes of death for those 65 and above are often referred to as diseases of choice—a phrase that underscores the importance of both lifestyle and screening. A pressing and pervasive health issue in old age is cognitive decline. Cognitive impairment affects the individuals themselves, their families, caregivers, surroundings, community, and society. The effects can be costly, devastating, and result in a deeply declining quality of life. Statistically, identifying a way to delay cognitive decline ultimately means a lower overall incidence. It is thus imperative to seek options for prevention, delay, and slowing of cognitive decline.

It is vital to note that there is no evidence of exercise having a negative impact on cognition. This can rarely be said of other types of intervention, which are often accompanied by undesirable side effects. Nothing indicates that exercise is unsafe, and there is adequate data showing both benefit and buffering in association with cognitive impairment. This is a powerful medicine in an arsenal to equip middle-aged and older adults with the tools to enhance their health in later life. Future research is needed to establish the type, duration, frequency, and intensity of exercises that are most beneficial to the older adult population wishing to combat cognitive decline.

REFERENCES

Aarsland, D., Sardahaee, F. S., Anderssen, S., Ballard, C., & the Alzheimer's Society Systematic Review group. (2010). Is physical activity a potential preventive factor for vascular dementia? A systematic review. *Aging & Mental Health*, *14*(4), 386–395.

Ahlskog, J. E., Geda, Y. E., Graff-Radford, N. R., & Petersen, R. C. (2011). Physical exercise as a preventive or disease-modifying treatment of dementia and brain aging. *Mayo Clinic Proceedings*, *86*(9), 876–884.

Albert, M. S., DeKosky, S. T., Dickson, D., Dubois, B., Feldman, H. H., Fox, N. C., et al. (2011). The diagnosis of mild cognitive impairment due to Alzheimer's disease: Recommendations from the national institute on aging-Alzheimer's association workgroups on diagnostic guidelines for Alzheimer's disease. *Alzheimer's & Dementia*, *7*(3), 270–279.

Allan, L. M., Ballard, C. G., Rowan, E. N., & Kenny, R. A. (2009). Incidence and prediction of falls in dementia: A prospective study in older people. *PLoS One*, *4*(5), e5521.

Angevaren, M., Aufdemkampe, G., Verhaar, H., Aleman, A., & Vanhees, L. (2008). Physical activity and enhanced fitness to improve cognitive function in older people without known cognitive impairment. *Cochrane Database Systematic Reviews*, (2), CD005381.

Baker, L. D., Frank, L. L., Foster-Schubert, K., Green, P. S., Wilkinson, C. W., McTiernan, A., et al. (2010). Effects of aerobic exercise on mild cognitive impairment: A controlled trial. *Archives of Neurology*, *67*(1), 71–79.

Baum, E. E., Jarjoura, D., Polen, A. E., Faur, D., & Rutecki, G. (2003). Effectiveness of a group exercise program in a long-term care facility: A randomized pilot trial. *Journal of the American Medical Directors Association*, *4*(2), 74–80.

Bherer, L., Erickson, K. I., & Liu-Ambrose, T. (2013). A review of the effects of physical activity and exercise on cognitive and brain functions in older adults. *Journal of Aging Research*, *2013*(2013), 1–8.

Buchman, A. S., Boyle, P. A., Wilson, R. S., Fleischman, D. A., Leurgans, S., & Bennet, A. B. (2009). Association between late-life social activity and motor decline in older adults. *Archives of Internal Medicine*, *168*, 1139–1146.

Buchman, A. S., Boyle, P. A., Yu, L., Shah, R. C., Wilson, R. S., & Bennett, D. A. (2012). Total daily physical activity and the risk of AD and cognitive decline in older adults. *Neurology*, *78*(17), 1323–1329. http://dx.doi.org/10.1212/wnl.0b013e3182535d35

Christensen, K., Doblhammer, G., Rau, R., & Vaupel, J. W. (2009). Ageing populations: The challenges ahead. *The Lancet*, *374*(9696), 1196–1208.

Colcombe, S. J., Erickson, K. I., Scalf, P. E., Kim, J. S., Prakash, R., McAuley, E., et al. (2006). Aerobic exercise training increases brain volume in aging humans. *The Journals of Gerontology.Series A, Biological Sciences and Medical Sciences*, *61*(11), 1166–1170. http://dx.doi.org/61/11/1166

Colcombe, S., & Kramer, A. F. (2003). Fitness effects on the cognitive function of older adults: A meta-analytic study. *Psychological Science*, *14*(2), 125–130.

Colcombe, S. J., Kramer, A. F., Erickson, K. I., Scalf, P., McAuley, E., Cohen, N. J., et al. (2004). Cardiovascular fitness, cortical plasticity, and aging. *Proceedings of the National Academy of Sciences of the United States of America*, *101*(9), 3316–3321.

Conn, V. S. (2010). Depressive symptom outcomes of physical activity interventions: Meta-analysis findings. *Annals of Behavioral Medicine*, *39*(2), 128–138.

Daniels, K., Toth, J., & Jacoby, L. (2006). The aging of executive functions. In E. Bialystok & F. I. M. Craik (Eds.), *Lifespan cognition: Mechanisms of change* (pp. 96–111). New York, NY: Oxford University Press.

Deary, I. J., Corley, J., Gow, A. J., Harris, S. E., Houlihan, L. M., Marioni, R. E., et al. (2009). Age-associated cognitive decline. *British Medical Bulletin*, *92*, 135–152. http://dx.doi.org/10.1093/bmb/ldp033

Dickerson, B. C., Salat, D. H., Greve, D. N., Chua, E. F., Rand-Giovannetti, E., Rentz, D. M., et al. (2005). Increased hippocampal activation in mild cognitive impairment compared to normal aging and AD. *Neurology*, *65*, 404–411.

Diniz, B. S., Reynolds, C. F., Begley, A., Dew, M. A., Anderson, S. J., Lotrich, F., et al. (2014). Brain-derived neurotrophic factor levels in late-life depression and comorbid mild cognitive impairment: A longitudinal study. *Journal of Psychiatric Research*, *49*, 96–101.

Dunn, A. L., & Jewell, J. S. (2010). The effect of exercise on mental health. *Current Sports Medicine Reports*, *9*(4), 202–207. http://dx.doi.org/10.1249/jsr.0b013e3181e7d9af

Elsawy, B., & Higgins, K. E. (2010). Physical activity guidelines for older adults. *American Family Physician*, *81*(1), 55–59.

Erickson, K. I., & Kramer, A. F. (2009). Aerobic exercise effects on cognitive and neural plasticity in older adults. *British Journal of Sports Medicine*, *43*(1), 22–24. http://dx.doi.org/10.1136/bjsm.2008.052498

Etgen, T., Sander, D., Huntgeburth, U., Poppert, H., Förstl, H., & Bickel, H. (2010). Physical activity and incident cognitive impairment in elderly persons: The INVADE study. *Archives of Internal Medicine*, *170*(2), 186–193.

Etnier, J. L., Nowell, P. M., Landers, D. M., & Sibley, B. A. (2006). A meta-regression to examine the relationship between aerobic fitness and cognitive performance. *Brain Research Reviews*, *52*(1), 119–130.

Fabel, K., & Kempermann, G. (2008). Physical activity and the regulation of neurogenesis in the adult and aging brain. *Neuromolecular Medicine*, *10*(2), 59–66.

Fabre, C., Chamari, K., Mucci, P., Masse-Biron, J., & Prefaut, C. (2002). Improvement of cognitive function by mental and/or individualized aerobic training in healthy elderly subjects. *International Journal of Sports Medicine*, *23*(6), 415–421. http://dx.doi.org/10.1055/s-2002-33735

Firbank, M. J., Burton, E. J., Barber, R., Stephens, S., Kenny, R. A., Ballard, C., et al. (2007). Medial temporal atrophy rather than white matter hyperintensities predict cognitive decline in stroke survivors. *Neurobiology of Aging*, *28*(11), 1664–1669.

Flicker, L., Almeida, O. P., Acres, J., Le, M. T. Q., Tuohy, R. J., Jamrozik, K., et al. (2005). Predictors of impaired cognitive function in men over the age of 80 years: results from the Health in Men Study. *Age and Ageing*, *34*, 77–80.

Fratiglioni, L., Paillard-Borg, S., & Winblad, B. (2004). An active and socially integrated lifestyle in late life might protect against dementia. *The Lancet Neurology*, *3*(6), 343–353.

Gardner, R. C., Valcour, V., & Yaffe, K. (2013). Dementia in the oldest: A multi-factorial and growing public health issue. *Alzheimer's Research & Therapy*, *5*(4), 27. http://dx.doi.org/10.1186/alzrt181

Garland, T., Schutz, H., Chappell, M. A., Keeney, B. K., Meek, T. H., Copes, L. E., et al. (2011). The biological control of voluntary exercise, spontaneous physical activity and daily energy expenditure in relation to obesity: Human and rodent perspectives. *The Journal of Experimental Biology*, *214*(Pt. 2), 206–229. http://dx.doi.org/10.1242/jeb.048397

Geda, Y. E., Roberts, R. O., Knopman, D. S., Christianson, T. J., Pankratz, V. S., Ivnik, R. J., et al. (2010). Physical exercise, aging, and mild cognitive impairment: A population-based study. *Archives of Neurology*, *67*(1), 80–86.

Gure, T. R., Kabeto, M. U., Plassman, B. L., Piette, J. D., & Langa, K. M. (2010). Differences in functional impairment across subtypes of dementia, *Journal of Gerentology*, *65*, 434–441.

Hamer, M., & Chida, Y. (2009). Physical activity and risk of neurodegenerative disease: A systematic review of prospective evidence. *Psychological Medicine*, *39*(01), 3–11.

Harciarek, M., & Cosentino, S. (2013). Language, executive function and social cognition in the diagnosis of frontotemporal dementia syndromes. *International Review of Psychiatry*, *25*(2), 178–196.

Heyn, P., Abreu, B. C., & Ottenbacher, K. J. (2004). The effects of exercise training on elderly persons with cognitive impairment and dementia: A meta-analysis. *Archives of Physical Medicine and Rehabilitation*, *85*(10), 1694–1704.

Hutchinson, A. D., & Mathias, J. L. (2007). Neuropsychological deficits in frontotemporal dementia and Alzheimer's disease: A meta-analytic review. *Journal of Neurology, Neurosurgery, and Psychiatry*, *78*(9), 917–928. http://dx.doi.org/10.1136/jnnp.2006.100669

Jedrziewski, M. K., Lee, V. M., & Trojanowski, J. Q. (2007). Physical activity and cognitive health. *Alzheimer's & Dementia*, *3*(2), 98–108.

Jopp, D., & Hertzog, C. (2007). Activities, self-referent memory beliefs, and cognitive performance: Evidence for direct and mediated relations. *Psychology and Aging*, *22*(4), 811–825.

Kamińska, M. S., Brodowski, J., & Karakiewicz, B. (2015). Fall risk factors in community-dwelling elderly depending on their physical function, cognitive status and symptoms of depression. *International Journal of Environmental Research and Public Health*, *12*(4), 3406–3416.

Kang, H., Zhao, F., You, L., Giorgetta, C., Sarkhel, S., & Prakash, R. (2014). Pserudo-Dementia: A neuropsychological review. *Annals of Indian Academy of Neurology*, *17*, 147–154.

Kokkinos, P., Sheriff, H., & Kheirbek, R. (2011). Physical inactivity and mortality risk. *Cardiology Research and Practice*, *2011*, 924945. http://dx.doi.org/10.4061/2011/924945

Korczyn, A. D., Vakhapova, V., & Grinberg, L. T. (2012). Vascular dementia. *Journal of the Neurological Sciences*, *322*(1), 2–10.

Langa, K. M., & Levine, D. A. (2014). The diagnosis and management of mild cognitive impairment: A clinical review. *The Journal of the American Medical Association*, *312*(23), 2551–2561.

Larner, A. (2014). *Dementia in clinical practice: A neurological perspective*. London: Springer.

Launer, L. J., Lewis, C. E., Schreiner, P. J., Sidney, S., Battapady, H., Jacobs, D. R., et al. (2015). Vascular factors and multiple measures of early brain health: CARDIA brain MRI study. *PloS One*, *10*(3), 1–13. http://dx.doi.org/10.1371/journal.pone.0122138

Laurin, D., Verreault, R., Lindsay, J., MacPherson, K., & Rockwood, K. (2001). Physical activity and risk of cognitive impairment and dementia in elderly persons. *Archives of Neurology*, *58*(3), 498–504.

Lautenschlager, N. T., Cox, K. L., Flicker, L., Foster, J. K., van Bockxmeer, F. M., Xiao, J., et al. (2008). Effect of physical activity on cognitive function in older adults at risk for Alzheimer disease: A randomized trial. *The Journal of the American Medical Association*, *300*(9), 1027–1037.

Liu-Ambrose, T., & Donaldson, M. G. (2009). Exercise and cognition in older adults: Is there a role for resistance training programmes? *British Journal of Sports Medicine*, *43*(1), 25–27. http://dx.doi.org/10.1136/bjsm.2008.055616

Lytle, M. E., Vander, B. J., Pandav, R. S., Dodge, H. H., & Ganguli, M. (2004). Exercise level and cognitive decline: The MoVIES project. *Alzheimer Disease and Associated Disorders*, *18*, 57–64.

Manini, T. M., & Pahor, M. (2009). Physical activity and maintaining physical function in older adults. *British Journal of Sports Medicine*, *43*(1), 28–31. http://dx.doi.org/10.1136/bjsm.2008.053736

McKhann, G. M., Knopman, D. S., Chertkow, H., Hyman, B. T., Jack, C. R., Kawas, C. H., et al. (2011). The diagnosis of dementia due to Alzheimer's disease: Recommendations from the national institute on aging-Alzheimer's association workgroups on diagnostic guidelines for alzheimer's disease. *Alzheimer's & Dementia*, *7*(3), 263–269.

Middleton, L., Kirkland, S., & Rockwood, K. (2008). Prevention of CIND by physical activity: Different impact on VCI-ND compared with MCI. *Journal of the Neurological Sciences*, *269*(1), 80–84.

Mortensen, E. L., Flensborg-Madsen, T., Molbo, D., Fagerlund, B., Christensen, U., Lund, R., et al. (2014). The relationship between cognitive ability and demographic factors in late midlife. *Journal of Aging Health*, *26*, 37–53.

Nelson, M. E., Rejeski, W. J., Blair, S. N., Duncan, P. W., Judge, J. O., King, A. C., et al. (2007). Physical activity and public health in older adults: Recommendation from the american college of sports medicine and the american heart association. *Circulation*, *116*(9), 1094.

Oda, H., Yamamoto, Y., & Maeda, K. (2009). Neuropsychological profile of dementia with lewy bodies. *Psychogeriatrics*, *9*(2), 85–90.

Park, L. Q., Harvey, D., Johnson, J., & Farias, S. T. (2015). Deficits in everyday function differ in AD and FTD. *Alzheimer's Disease Associated Disorders*. http://dx.doi.org/10.1097/wad.0000000000000081

Prince, M., Bryce, R., Albanese, E., Wimo, A., Ribeiro, W., & Ferri, C. P. (2013). The global prevalence of dementia: A systematic review and metaanalysis. *Alzheimer's & Dementia*, *9*(1), 63–75. e2.

Qiu, C., & Fratiglioni, L. (2015). A major role for cardiovascular burden in age-related cognitive decline. *Nature Reviews Cardiology*,*12*(5), 267–277.

Rice, D. P., & Fineman, N. (2004). Economic implications of increased longevity in the united states. *Annu.Rev.Public Health*, *25*, 457–473.

Rizzoli, R., Bruyère, O., Cannata-Andia, J. B., Devogelaer, J., Lyritis, G., Ringe, J., et al. (2009). Management of osteoporosis in the elderly. *Current Medical Research and Opinion*, *25*(10), 2373–2387.

Rockwood, K., Howlett, S. E., MacKnight, C., Beattie, B. L., Bergman, H., Hebert, R., et al. (2004). Prevalence, attributes, and outcomes of fitness and frailty in community-dwelling older adults: Report from the Canadian study of health and aging. *The Journals of Gerontology. Series A, Biological Sciences and Medical Sciences*, *59*(12), 1310–1317. http://dx.doi.org/59/12/1310

Rockwood, K., & Middleton, L. (2007). Physical activity and the maintenance of cognitive function. *Alzheimer's & Dementia*, 3(2), S38–S44.

Rovio, S., Kåreholt, I., Helkala, E., Viitanen, M., Winblad, B., Tuomilehto, J., et al. (2005). Leisure-time physical activity at midlife and the risk of dementia and Alzheimer's disease. *The Lancet Neurology*, 4(11), 705–711.

Salthouse, T. (2009). *Major issues in cognitive aging.* New York, NY: Oxford University Press. http://dx.doi.org/10.1093/acprof:oso/9780195372151.001.0001

Skinner, J., Tipton, C., & Vailas, A. (1982). In A. Viidik (Ed.), *Lectures on gerontology* (Vol. 1B ed., pp. 407–439). London: Academic Press.

Smith, P. J., Blumenthal, J. A., Hoffman, B. M., Cooper, H., Strauman, T. A., Welsh-Bohmer, K., et al. (2010). Aerobic exercise and neurocognitive performance: A meta-analytic review of randomized controlled trials. *Psychosomatic Medicine*, *72*(3), 239–252. http://dx.doi.org/10.1097/psy.0b013e3181d14633

Snyder, H. M., Corriveau, R. A., Craft, S., Faber, J. E., Greenberg, S. M., Knopman, D., et al. (2014). Vascular contributions to cognitive impairment and dementia including Alzheimer's disease. *Alzheimer's & Dementia*, *11*(6), 710–717.

Sudeep, S. G., & Dallas, P. S. (2015). Lifestyles and cognitive health: what older individuals can do to optimize cognitive outcomes. *Journal of the American Medical Association*, *314*, 774–775.

Teri, L., Gibbons, L. E., McCurry, S. M., Logsdon, R. G., Buchner, D. M., Barlow, W. E., et al. (2003). Exercise plus behavioral management in patients with aAlzheimer disease: A randomized controlled trial. *The Journal of the American Medical Association*, *290*(15), 2015–2022.

Town, G. I., & Lewis, S. A. (1996). Predictors of impaired cognitive function in men over the age of 80 years: Results from the Health in Men Study. *Thorax*, *51*, 1010–1016.

Tremblay, M. S., Warburton, D. E., Janssen, I., Paterson, D. H., Latimer, A. E., Rhodes, R. E., et al. (2011). New Canadian physical activity guidelines. *Applied Physiology, Nutrition, and Metabolism*, *36*(1), 36–46.

Troiano, R. P., Berrigan, D., Dodd, K. W., Mâsse, L. C., Tilert, T., & McDowell, M. (2008). Physical activity in the united states measured by accelerometer. *Medicine and Science in Sports and Exercise*, *40*(1), 181–188.

U.S. Department of Health and Human Services. (2008). *Physical activity guidelines advisory committee report*. Washington, DC: U.S. Department of Health and Human Services, 2008.

Van de Winckel, A., Feys, H., De Weerdt, W., & Dom, R. (2004). Cognitive and behavioural effects of music-based exercises in patients with dementia. *Clinical Rehabilitation*, *18*(3), 253–260.

Van Uffelen, J. G., Chin A Paw, M. J., Hopman-Rock, M., & van Mechelen, W. (2008). The effects of exercise on cognition in older adults with and without cognitive decline: A systematic review. *Clinical Journal of Sport Medicine: Official Journal of the Canadian Academy of Sport Medicine*, *18*(6), 486–500. http://dx.doi.org/10.1097/jsm.0b013e3181845f0b

Verghese, J., Lipton, R. B., Katz, M. J., Hall, C. B., Derby, C. A., Kuslansky, G., et al. (2003). Leisure activities and the risk of dementia in the elderly. *New England Journal of Medicine*, *348*(25), 2508–2516.

Vogel, T., Brechat, P., Leprêtre, P., Kaltenbach, G., Berthel, M., & Lonsdorfer, J. (2009). Health benefits of physical activity in older patients: A review. *International Journal of Clinical Practice*, *63*(2), 303–320.

Weintraub, S., Wicklund, A. H., & Salmon, D. P. (2012). The neuropsychological profile of Alzheimer disease. *Cold Spring Harbor Perspectives in Medicine*, *2*(4), a006171. http://dx.doi.org/10.1101/cshperspect.a006171

CHAPTER 5

Aerobic Exercise for Older Adults

Dale Avers

ABSTRACT

Older adults move less, making them prone to deconditioning and a host of other consequences including stiffness, weakness, cardiovascular changes, decreased balance, cognitive disorders, insomnia, mood changes, and adverse effects on appetite, to name a few. Because the benefits of aerobic exercise and physical activity are so powerful and pervasive in reversing the consequences of inactivity, the Centers for Disease Control and Prevention (CDC) have established guidelines for all adults of 150 minutes of moderate-intensity physical activity comprising aerobic and strengthening activity. Yet, the majority of older adults do not engage in *any* aerobic activity (CDC, 2013). Aerobic exercise is so important for health and chronic disease management that its prescription is a core competency for most health-care providers. This chapter reviews the effects of aging on aerobic capacity, the benefits of aerobic exercise across many common chronic diseases, and an evidence-based exercise prescription based on appropriate screening for a variety of conditions common to older adults.

BENEFITS OF AEROBIC EXERCISE

It is well known that participation in a regular exercise program is an effective way to reduce and/or prevent functional decline and the burdens of many chronic diseases associated with aging (Taylor, 2014). Aerobic or endurance training can

http://dx.doi.org/10.1891/0198-8794.36.123

help to maintain various aspects of heart and lung function and cardiac output. Aerobic activity enables the body to burn calories, a function referred to as a metabolic equivalent (MET). Aerobic activity is defined as any activity that uses large muscle groups, can be maintained continuously, and is rhythmic in nature (American College of Sports Medicine [ACSM], 2010). Examples of aerobic activities include swimming, running, walking, skiing, aerobic dance, and biking.

Broadly, the three categories of exercise are aerobic training, resistance training, and flexibility training. The benefits of exercise are listed in Table 5.1, which include reducing the burden of chronic diseases seen so frequently in older adults, improving quality of life and well-being, and maintaining function and independence. This chapter highlights the use of aerobic exercise for the maintenance of health and management of chronic disease. The specific and compelling benefits of aerobic/endurance exercise are listed in Table 5.2.

DESCRIPTION OF AEROBIC EXERCISE

For aerobic exercise to be effective, a training effect must occur. A training effect is when the total training load exceeds loads encountered during daily life and when adaptations occur that promote cardiovascular fitness (Pescatello, Arena, Riebe, & Thompson, 2014). Aerobic exercise below a certain level, such as light activities, is unlikely to achieve health-related changes (Taylor, 2014). The ACSM and the Centers for Disease Control and Prevention (CDC) together recommend 150 minutes per

TABLE 5.1
Benefits of Exercise

Reduce the risk of premature death
Reduce the risk of developing and/or dying from heart disease
Reduce high blood pressure or the risk of developing high blood pressure
Reduce high cholesterol or the risk of developing high cholesterol
Reduce the risk of developing colon cancer and breast cancer
Reduce the risk of developing diabetes
Reduce or maintain body weight or body fat
Build and maintain healthy muscles, bones, and joints
Reduce depression and anxiety
Improve psychological well-being
Enhance work, recreation, and sport performance

Source: Pescatello, Arena, Riebe, and Thompson (2014).

TABLE 5.2
Benefits of Aerobic Exercise

Increased maximal oxygen consumption (VO_2max)
Improvement in cardiovascular/cardiorespiratory function (heart and lungs)
Increased maximal cardiac output (amount of blood pumped every minute)
Increased maximal stroke volume (amount of blood pumped with each beat)
Increased blood volume and ability to carry oxygen
Reduced workload on the heart (myocardial oxygen consumption) for any given submaximal exercise intensity
Increased blood supply to muscles and ability to use oxygen
Lower heart rate and blood pressure at any level of submaximal exercise
Increased threshold for lactic acid accumulation
Lowered resting systolic and diastolic blood pressure in people with high blood pressure
Increased HDL cholesterol (the good cholesterol)
Decreased blood triglycerides
Reduced body fat and improved weight control
Improved glucose tolerance and reduced insulin resistance

Note: HDL = high-density lipoprotein.
Source: Gostic (2005).

week of moderate-intensity aerobic activity (i.e., brisk walking) *or* 75 minutes per week of vigorous-intensity aerobic activity. For greater health benefits, older adults should increase their activity to 300 minutes per week of moderate-intensity aerobic activity or 150 minutes of vigorous-intensity aerobic activity (CDC, 2013). This volume of exercise should occur for at least 10 minutes at a time.

MEASURES OF AEROBIC EXERCISE INTENSITY

Intensity of exercise is measured in terms of METs, which indicates how much energy is burned during exercise and physical activities (Table 5.3). METs are used to standardize energy expenditure, which differs from calorie counts, which is dependent on body weight. One MET equals 3.5 mLO_2/kg of body weight per minute, which is what the human body requires at rest. The more effort an activity requires, the higher the MET value. This value is the same for most people, regardless of fitness level. Variations may occur with gender, age, and body

TABLE 5.3
Aerobic Intensity

Activity	RPE (1–10)
Light-intensity activities are defined as 1.1 MET to 2.9 METs.	3–4
Moderate-intensity activities are defined as 3.0 to 5.9 METs.	5–6
Walking at 3.0 mph requires 3.3 METs of energy expenditure and is therefore considered a moderate-intensity activity.	
Vigorous-intensity activities are defined as 6.0 METs or more.	7–8
Running at 10 minutes per mile (6.0 mph) is a 10 MET activity and is therefore classified as vigorous intensity.	8–10

Note: MET = metabolic equivalent; mph = miles per hour; RPE = rate of perceived exertion.
Source: Pescatello et al. (2014).

composition. However, because maximal aerobic capacity declines with age, the relative exercise intensity level (maximum oxygen consumption [VO_2 max]) will be higher for older adults for the same MET level. Even so, physically active older adults may have aerobic capacities comparable to or greater than sedentary younger adults (Pescatello et al., 2014).

Cardiorespiratory fitness is related to the ability to use large muscles in a dynamic way at moderate-to-high intensities for prolonged periods. VO_2 max is the accepted criterion measure of cardiorespiratory fitness. The exercise guidelines by the CDC and ACSM mentioned in the previous section are based on MET levels. Five hundred to 1,000 MET minutes of activity per week is equal to 150 minutes of moderate-intensity activity per week (3.3 METs for 150 minutes per week). A MET level of 6.0 is equivalent to 75 minutes of vigorous activity per week (Office of Disease Prevention and Health Promotion, 2015). Based on these guidelines using MET level as the basis for the recommendations, 1 minute of vigorous-intensity activity is equal to 2 minutes of moderate-intensity activity.

When the energy requirement for an activity exceeds a person's aerobic capacity, the individual can no longer perform that activity. Thus, the ability to maintain a high aerobic capacity is directly related to an older adult's functional independence. Morey et al. established the optimal cut point of a peak VO_2 of ~18 mL/kg/min, which differentiates low versus high function in a group of community-dwelling adults aged 65–90 years (Morey, Pieper, & Cornoni-Huntley, 1998). A healthy 50-year-old man should have a capacity of at least 9.2 METS, a healthy 50-year-old woman should be able to achieve 8.2 METs or higher. METs for common exercise modes and activities are listed in Table 5.4.

TABLE 5.4
Metabolic Equivalents for Aerobic Exercise Modes and Activities

Moderate Activity (3.0–6.0 METs)	Vigorous Activity (>6.0 METs)
Walking at a moderate or brisk pace of 3 to 4.5 mph (20–12.33 min/mile) on a level surface inside or outside such as • Walking to class, work, or the store • Walking for pleasure • Walking the dog • Walking as a break from work Walking downstairs or down a hill Using crutches Hiking	Racewalking and aerobic walking—5 mph or faster (<12 min/mile) Jogging or running Walking and climbing briskly up a hill Backpacking Mountain climbing
Bicyclying 5–9 mph, level terrain, or with few hills Stationary cycling—using moderate effort	Bicycling more than 10 mph or bicycling on steep uphill terrain Stationary bicycling—using vigorous effort
Aerobic dancing—high impact Water aerobics	Aerobic dancing—high impact Step aerobics Water jogging Teaching an aerobic dance class
Calisthenics—light Yoga Gymnastics General home exercises, light or moderate effort, getting up and down from the floor Using a stair-climber machine at a light-to-moderate pace Using a rowing machine with moderate effort	Calisthenics—push-ups, pull-ups, vigorous effort Karate, judo, tae kwon do, jujitsu Jumping rope Performing jumping jacks Using a stair-climber at a fast pace Using a rowing machine—with vigorous effort Using an arm cycling machine—with vigorous effort
Ballroom dancing Line dancing Square dancing Folk dancing Modern dancing, disco Ballet	Professional ballroom dancing—energetically Square dancing—energetically Folk dancing—energetically Clogging

(Continued)

TABLE 5.4
MET Equivalent for Aerobic Exercise Modes and Activities (Continued)

Moderate Activity (3.0–6.0 METs)	Vigorous Activity (>6.0 METs)
Table tennis—competitive Tennis—doubles	Tennis—singles
Golf—wheeling or carrying clubs	
Playing Frisbee Badminton	Handball—general or team Racquetball Squash
Swimming—recreational Treading water—slowly, moderate effort Diving—springboard or platform Aquatic aerobics Waterskiing Snorkeling Surfing, board or body	Swimming, steady-paced laps Synchronized swimming Treading water—fast, vigorous effort Water jogging Water polo Water basketball Scuba diving
Canoeing or rowing a boat at less than 4 mph Rafting—whitewater Sailing—recreational or competition Paddle boating Kayaking—on a lake, calm water	Canoeing or rowing—4 or more mph Kayaking in whitewater rapids
Fishing while walking along a riverbank or while wading in a stream—wearing waders	
Gardening or yard work; raking the lawn bagging grass or leaves, digging, hoeing, light shoveling (less than 10 lb per min), or weeding while standing or bending Planting trees, trimming shrubs and trees, hauling branches, stacking wood Pushing a power mower or tiller	Gardening and yard work: heavy or rapid shoveling (more than 10 lb per minute), digging ditches or carrying heavy loads Felling trees, carrying large logs, swinging an ax, hand-splitting logs, or climbing and trimming trees Pushing a nonmotorized lawn mower
Shoveling light snow	Shoveling heavy snow

(Continued)

TABLE 5.4
MET Equivalent for Aerobic Exercise Modes and Activities (Continued)

Moderate Activity (3.0–6.0 METs)	Vigorous Activity (>6.0 METs)
Moderate housework: scrubbing the floor or bathtub while on hands and knees, hanging laundry on a clothesline, sweeping an outdoor area, cleaning out the garage, washing windows, moving light furniture, packing or unpacking boxes, walking and putting household items away, carrying out heavy bags or trash or recyclables (e.g., glass, newspapers, and plastics), or carrying water or firewood	Heavy housework: moving or pushing heavy furniture (75 lb or more), carrying household items weighing 25 lb or more up a flight of stairs Standing, walking, or walking down a flight of stairs while carrying objects weighing 50 lb or more
Actively playing with children—walking, running, or climbing while playing with children Walking while carrying a child weighing less than 50 lb Walking while pushing or pulling a child in a stroller or an adult in a wheelchair Carrying a child weighing less than 25 lb up a flight of stairs Child care: handling uncooperative young children (e.g., chasing, dressing, lifting into car seat) or handling several young children at one time Bathing and dressing an adult	Vigorously playing with children—running longer distances or playing strenuous games with children Racewalking or jogging while pushing a stroller designed for sport use Carrying an adult or child weighing 25 lb or more up a flight of stairs Standing or walking while carrying an adult or a child weighing >50 lb

Note: lb = pound; MET = metabolic equivalent; min = minute; mph = miles per hour.
Source: Centers for Disease Control and Prevention (2014).

The rate of perceived exertion (RPE; Russell, 1997) is a subjective measure of effortful exertion (Borg, 1998). The RPE correlates numerical descriptors with heart rate and exercise intensity on a scale of 6–20 with 6 equating to a heart rate of 60 and so on. The RPE has been validated for older adults and is particularly useful for those who may have a blunted heart rate response, such as when taking β-blockers. A rate of 11–15 on the Borg RPE corresponds to a percentage of 60%–80% VO_2 max. The original and modified RPE scale that uses anchors of 1–10

TABLE 5.5
Rate of Perceived Exertion

Modified Scale	Original Scale	Percent Effort	Perceived Workload
	6	20%	
	7	30%	Very, very light
	8	40%	
1	9	50%	Very light
2	10	55%	
3	11	60%	Fairly light
	12	65%	
4	13	70%	Moderately hard
	14	75%	
5	15	80%	Hard
6	16	85%	
7	17	90%	Very hard
8	18	95%	
9	19	100%	Very, very hard
10	20	Exhausted	

Source: Avers and Brown (2009).

is illustrated in Table 5.5. Working at an intensity of 5–6 on the modified RPE scale is recommended for a training effect (Pescatello et al., 2014). It is important to be aware that self-perception of RPE among older adults who have not been physically active may be exaggerated, so minimal activity might be perceived as hard effort (high intensity). Musculoskeletal factors that can give the perception of hard effort without a concurrent increase in physiological response include leg fatigue related to inadequate strength, joint pain, and obesity (Hulens, Vansant, Claessens, Lysens, & Muls, 2003; Sutbeyaz, Sezer, Koseoglu, Ibrahimoglu, & Tekin, 2007). If musculoskeletal problems persist in limiting the ability to perform aerobic activity, physical therapy interventions may be indicated.

EFFECTS OF AGING ON AEROBIC CAPACITY

The aging process affects all systems, but of particular importance to aerobic activity is how aging affects the cardiovascular system. In the vessels, arterial walls become stiff and thickened due to collagen deposition, elastin loss, and hypertrophy of the smooth muscle cells (Wan & Wong, 2014). These changes make the blood pressure higher and the heart work harder, which may lead to hypertrophy of the heart muscle. Most older adults have a moderate increase in blood pressure. The baroreceptors, receptors that monitor blood pressure and make changes to maintain blood pressure during rest and activity, become less sensitive with age. The reduced sensitivity of baroreceptors may cause orthostatic hypotension.

The heart's pacemaker system, the sinoatrial (SA) node loses some of its cells with age, which may result in a slightly lower heart rate. The heart's left ventricle may fill more slowly because of a slight increase in the size of the heart and it has less contractility. Heart changes and disease cause arrhythmias such as atrial fibrillation. Lipofuscin, an aging pigment, can be deposited in the heart wall, and the heart muscle cells may degenerate slightly. The heart's valves may thicken and become stiffer, which may result in a heart murmur (Montero, Roberts, & Vinet, 2014).

VO_2 max is the most frequent indicator of overall cardiovascular function and maximum capacity. Consistent findings indicate that VO_2 max decreases approximately 5%–15% per decade beginning at 25–30 years of age (Fletcher et al., 1996). This decline in VO_2 max is attributed to age-related reductions in both maximal cardiac output and maximal arteriovenous oxygen (a-v O_2) difference. Maximal heart rate decreases about 6–10 beats per minute per decade and is responsible for much of the age-associated decrease in maximal cardiac output. The reduction in stroke volume during maximal exercise also contributes to the decline in cardiac output.

The blood in an aging person thickens as a result of less fluid, so blood volume decreases. There is a slower response to blood loss and anemia because red blood cells are not produced as quickly (MedlinePlus, 2015). Neutrophils decrease in number and therefore have less ability to fight off bacteria, reducing the ability to fight off infection. Decreases in vascular capacity and local blood flow regulation, along with a decline in muscle oxidative capacity contribute to the overall reduction in maximal a-v O_2 difference with age. Coupled with poor oxygen delivery mechanisms, mitochrondrial alterations also lead to a reduction in maximum capacity to utilize oxygen at the level of the skeletal muscle (Petrella, 2000).

All of these changes in combination result in decreased VO_2 at a minimum rate of 8%–10% per decade in healthy men and women (Fleg & Lakatta, 1988), which may accelerate to 20%–25% per decade in those aged 70 or above (Fleg et al., 2005). While fitness level can keep the aerobic capacity at a higher level than that for unfit individuals, the decline is the same across all individuals.

Fortunately, even in the face of all these changes, older adults can adapt to a program of regular aerobic training as well as younger people (American College of Sports Medicine et al., 2009). Older adults can achieve the same 10%–30% increase in VO_2 max in response to aerobic/endurance exercise training as younger adults. The magnitude of these adaptations in VO_2 max is a function of training intensity; low-intensity training elicits only marginal changes. The increase in VO_2 max in older adults is a result of improvements in both maximum cardiac output and a-v O_2 difference.

AEROBIC EXERCISE TESTING AND PRESCRIPTION

Preparticipation Health Screening

The purpose of preparticipation health screening is to determine eligibility for participation in exercise and physical activity. The goal of preparticipation health screening is identification of individuals not known to be at risk, discernment of those with medical contraindications for certain types of exercise, recognition of individuals with clinically significant disease(s) or conditions, and detection of individuals who should undergo a medical evaluation and/or exercise testing before beginning an exercise program (Fletcher et al., 2013; Pescatello et al., 2014).

The revised ACSM 2014 preexercise evaluation recommendations reduce the emphasis on the need for medical evaluation prior to initiating a progressive exercise regimen for healthy, asymptomatic individuals to reduce a barrier to initiating a physical activity and exercise program *except* for those individuals at high risk (Pescatello et al., 2014). However, the ACSM recommendations emphasize the identification of clients or classification of participants with known disease, because these individuals are at the greatest risk for an exercise-related cardiac event. The ACSM risk stratification for exercise testing is described in Table 5.6.

All older individuals wishing to initiate a physical activity program should complete a self-report medical history or health risk appraisal questionnaire called a preparticipation health screening. Preparticipation health screening may include cost-effective self-assessments such as the Physical Activity Readiness Questionnaire (PAR-Q; Thomas, Reading, & Shephard, 1992), the exercise and screening test (Exercise Assessment and Screening for You [EASY]; Ory & Resnick, 2008), or the modified AHA/ACSM Health/Fitness Facility Preparticipation Screening Questionnaire (Balady et al., 1998). The PAR-Q asks questions that focus mostly on symptoms that might suggest angina pectoris but that have not been validated on adults above 65. The questionnaire of the Wisconsin Affiliate of the American Heart Association, the AHA/ACSM

TABLE 5.6
New ACSM Recommendations for Exercise Testing Prior to Exercise-Diagnosed Cardiovascular Disease

Unstable or new or possible symptoms of cardiovascular disease
Diabetes mellitus and at least one of the following:
Age > 35 years OR
Type 2 diabetes mellitus > 10-year duration OR
Type 1 diabetes mellitus > 15-year duration OR
Hypercholesterolemia (total cholesterol ≥ 240 mg/L) OR
Hypertension (systolic blood pressure ≥140 or diastolic ≥ 90 mmHg) OR
Smoking OR
Family history of CAD in first-degree relative <60 years OR
Presence of microvascular disease OR
Peripheral artery disease OR
Autonomic neuropathy
End-stage renal disease
Patients with symptomatic or diagnosed pulmonary disease including COPD, asthma, interstitial lung disease, or cystic fibrosis

Note: ACSM = American College of Sports Medicine; CAD = coronary artery disease; COPD = chronic obstructive pulmonary disease.
Source: Pescatello et al. (2014).

Health/Fitness Facility Preparticipation Screening Questionnaire, is slightly more complex than the PAR-Q and uses history, symptoms, and risk factors to determine appropriateness either to participate in an exercise program or to contact their physician or appropriate health-care provider (physician-provider) before participation. The EASY test, an online tool, was more recently developed to screen readiness to exercise and to help individuals follow up on any medical problems that need to be addressed (e.g., new onset of dizziness); it helps the individual match an appropriate exercise program with the underlying medical problems (e.g., exercises that are good to do when one has arthritis; Resnick et al., 2008).

The need for follow-up is determined by the individual's answers to any question in the tools mentioned in the preceding text. Individuals at moderate risk with two or more cardiovascular risk factors listed in Table 5.7 should consult with a health-care provider prior to initiating a physical activity program of a vigorous intensity. However, the majority of these individuals can begin a light- to medium-intensity exercise program such as walking without consulting with their health-care provider. Routine exercise testing is recommended only for individuals at high risk including those diagnosed with cardiovascular disease (CVD), symptoms suggestive of new or changing CVD, diabetes mellitus and additional CVD risk factors, end-stage renal disease, and specified lung disease as listed in Table 5.7 (Pescatello et al., 2014).

TABLE 5.7

Cardiovascular Risk Factors and Defining Criteria

Risk Factor	Defining Criteria
Age	Men ≥ 45 years; women ≥ 55 years
Family history	Myocardia infarction, coronary revascularization, or sudden death before 55 years in father or other male first-degree relative or before 65 years in mother or other female first-degree relative
Cigarette smoking	Current cigarette smoker or those who quit within the previous 6 months or exposure to environmental tobacco smoke
Sedentary lifestyle	Not participating in at least 30 min of moderate-intensity physical activity (40% to <60% VO_2R) on at least 3 days of the week for at least 3 months
Obesity	Body mass index ≥ 30 *or* waist girth > 102 cm (40 in.) for men and >88 cm (35 in.) for women
Hypertension	Systolic blood pressure ≥ 140 mmHg and/or diastolic ≥ 90 mmHg, confirmed by measurements on at least two separate occasions, or on antihypertensive medication
Dyslipidemia	LDL cholesterol ≥ 130 or HDL cholesterol < 40 or on lipid-lowering medication. If total serum cholesterol is all that is available, use ≥200
Prediabetes	Impaired fasting glucose = fasting plasma glucose ≥100 and ≤125 or impaired glucose tolerance = 2 h values in oral glucose tolerance test ≥140 and ≤199 confirmed by measurements on at least two separate occasions
Negative Risk Factors	
HDL cholesterol	≥60

Note: h = hour; HDL = high-density lipoprotein; LDL = low-density lipoprotein; in. = inch.

Source: American College of Sports Medicine (2010); Pescatello et al. (2014).

Individuals With Impaired Aerobic Capacity

For those individuals with known impaired aerobic capacity, performing a careful history and systems review is important. The history should include risk factors for CVD, presence of symptoms such as shortness of breath at rest or with mild exertion, pain or discomfort (or other angina equivalent) in the chest, neck, jaw, arms, or other areas that may result from cardiac ischemia, orthopnea, paroxysmal nocturnal dyspnea, bilateral ankle edema, palpitations, tachycardia, intermittent leg claudication, known heart murmur, and undue fatigue with usual activities (LaPier, 2012). Positive information may, at a minimum, inform the exercise prescription and lead the exercise professional to revise the program to best meet the needs of the participant. A general rule of thumb is to start low and slow, gradually building the program's intensity based on the participant's response. (Fitness program: 5 steps to get started—Mayo Clinic.)

A systems review should then be conducted that will include, at a minimum, physiological baseline measures of blood pressure, heart rate and rhythm, edema, and respiration rate. Screening for integrity of the musculoskeletal, neurological, and integumentary systems will also yield useful information. Table 5.8 lists recommended history items and system review tests. While it is beyond the scope of this chapter to provide detailed interpretation of each question and test, it is assumed the reader recognizes when a question or test is not normal and its implications.

Clinical Measures of Aerobic Impairment

In the presence of aerobic impairments, it is useful to obtain cardiovascular and pulmonary response to functional activity. Obtaining baseline measures of the patient's physiological measures such as heart rate, blood pressure, respiratory rate, and oxygen saturation will yield useful information about the individual's response to activity. Normal and abnormal responses to exercise are listed in Table 5.9. Describing the parameters of graded exercise testing is outside the scope of this chapter; however, it is common to perform submaximal tests such as the 6-minute walk test to ascertain an individual's physiological response to exercise before designing the exercise prescription, described in the following text.

Timed Walk Tests

The 6-minute and 2-minute walk tests are modifications of Cooper's original 12-minute walk test. Walk tests are inexpensive, efficient, require minimal equipment, and can be done anywhere. Walk tests can be used on a wide variety of patients and settings and have norms for many chronic diseases. The 6-minute

TABLE 5.8

History and Systems Review for the Individual With Impaired Aerobic Capacity

Chart Review and/or Oral History	Clinical Findings
	Other significant medical problems
	Current medications
	Risk factors for heart disease
	Lifestyle history (smoking, physical activity, etc.)
	Laboratory data (cholesterol, blood glucose)
	Electrocardiogram
	Pulmonary function tests
	Arterial blood gases
	Diagnostic tests
	Occupational history
	Presence of dizziness or excessive fatigue
Systems Review	Vital signs (heart rate, rhythm, blood pressure, respiration)
	Heart sounds
	Pulmonary auscultation
	BMI, waist circumference
	Range of motion and strength evaluation
	Sensation
	Skin integrity and peripheral circulation (pedal pulses)
	Chest excursion
	Edema
	Oxygen saturation

Note: BMI = body mass index.

walk test is a valid and reliable indicator of aerobic fitness. The average distance walked in a 6-minute walk test of 400 meters correlates to the average distance of a trip or errand in the community and so serves as a useful goal (Shumway-Cook et al., 2002). Assistive devices may be used, but the individual must be able to walk independently. Distance and physiological responses are the main outcomes of walk tests.

TABLE 5.9
Normal and Abnormal Responses to Exercise

Measure	Normal Response	Abnormal Response
Heart rate	60–100 bpm Increases proportionately to the metabolic demand (10 bpm per MET)	Inadequate increase or a sudden drop, which may be attributed to β-blockers, sinus node dysfunction, or chronotropic incompetence and may be an indication to stop exercise (Fletcher et al., 2013; Guccione, Wong, & Avers, 2012; LaPier, 2012). Excessive increase of 120–150 bpm: Use precaution in initiating an exercise program, consult with a physician-provider
Heart rate recovery	Rapid fall within 30 seconds after exercise, followed by a slower return to preexercise level	Slower recovery can be prognostic of cardiovascular disease or poor fitness (Dimkpa, 2009)
Systolic blood pressure (SBP) (reflecting cardiac output)	100–140 mmHg: Increase in proportion to the metabolic demand (pronounced in women as opposed to men). Average rise during a progressive exercise test is about 10 mmHg/MET (Fletcher et al., 2013) After maximum exercise, SBP declines, reaching preexercise levels or lower within 6 min. It can remain lower than preexercise levels for several hours	Inadequate rise of <20–30 mmHg (Exercise Assessment and Screening for You; Fletcher et al., 2013) >200 mmHg: contraindication to exercise, refer to physician-provider (LaPier, 2012)

(*Continued*)

TABLE 5.9
Normal and Abnormal Responses to Exercise *(Continued)*

Measure	Normal Response	Abnormal Response
Diastolic blood pressure (reflecting peripheral resistance)	70–90 mmHg	Increases are prognostic of cardiac disease (Akhras & Jackson, 1991) >115 mmHg: contraindicated to continue exercise, refer to physician-provider (LaPier, 2012)
Respiratory rate	Increases with mild- to moderate-intensity aerobic exercise, then plateaus as exercise intensity continues to increase	Abnormally high response may indicate coronary heart disease (Robbins et al., 1999)
Oxygen saturation	≥90%	Declines indicate heart failure, lung disease 86%–89%: Consider adding supplemental 0_2 and may be an indication to stop exercise. ≤85%: Add or increase supplemental 0_2; contraindication for continuing exercise/activity; refer to physician-provider if remains <90%

Note: bpm = beats per minute; MET = metabolic equivalent; min = minute.

Directions for Walk Tests

Prior to the test, a standard distance of at least 20 feet is mapped. Vital signs are recorded prior to the test. The individual is instructed to walk as far as possible for up to 6 minutes without sitting. The individual is allowed to stop but not allowed to lean or to sit. If sitting or leaning is necessary, the test is terminated at that point and the distance walked to that moment is the result of the test, with the time recorded in addition to the distance. Vital signs are recorded immediately at the end of the test with continuous monitoring until the vital signs return to baseline. It is useful to record how long it took the vital signs to return to baseline. Additionally, the RPE should be recorded. Normative distances for healthy older adults are listed in Table 5.10.

The 2-minute walk test was designed as a modification of the 6-minute walk test for individuals with amputations who could not walk a full 6 minutes (Brooks, Parsons, Hunter, Devlin, & Walker, 2001). The individual walks for 2 minutes and the distance recorded is the result of the test. However, there are no norms for the 2-minute walk test to the degree there are for the 6-minute walk test, and since 2 minutes is a far shorter time than what is required of the average errand in the community, this may have limited usefulness. The 6-minute walk test can still be used for individuals who cannot walk 6 minutes (Guccione, Wong, & Avers, 2012).

The 400-meter walk test is similar to the 6-minute walk test, but it defines a distance to walk (400 meters) versus a length of time. Some have suggested that knowing the distance to walk makes it easier for individuals to pace themselves and therefore achieve a greater effort (Simonsick, Montgomery, Newman, Bauer, & Harris, 2001). Similar to the other walk tests, vital signs are recorded

TABLE 5.10

Normative Values for 6-Minute Walk Test (Rikli & Jones, 1998) and 400-Meter Walk Test

6-Minute Walk Test			400-Meter Walk Test
Age	Men	Women	
60–69	572 m	538 m	
70–79	527 m	471 m	
80–89	417 m	392 m	
			>5 min 30 s is indicative of functional limitations
			Mean time to complete 400 meters is 5 min 11s (Simonsick et al., 2001)

Note: m = meter; min = minute; s = second.

prior to and immediately after the test and the RPE is recorded immediately after. The result is the time it took to complete the 400 meters. Normative results for healthy older adults are listed in Table 5.10. Interestingly, normative scores for the 400 meter walk test are very close to 6 minutes.

Exercise Prescription

Once the health-care provider has evaluated the individual, it is time to design an appropriate aerobic program to match the individuals' abilities. The exercise prescription for healthy older adults does not differ appreciably from that for younger adults. As indicated previously, the exercise recommendation for aerobic exercise is 150 minutes of moderate-intensity exercise per week or 75 minutes of vigorous-intensity exercise per week. The CDC recommends supplementing aerobic exercise with strengthening exercise on at least 2 days per week (CDC, 2015).

Setting Participant Goals and Identifying Barriers and Motivators

The first step in designing an exercise prescription, following screening and testing, is to be clear about the individual's goals. Common goals may be to lose weight, to feel better, to keep up with the grandkids, to lower blood pressure or cholesterol, and so forth. With each of these goals, encouraging regular physical activity and reducing time spent in sedentary activities as part of a healthy lifestyle will yield the most benefits. Addressing real or perceived barriers at the time of eliciting goals can also be beneficial.

Barriers and Motivators

Barriers to sustaining an exercise program differ from those for young people, who cite time as the most significant barrier to exercise, whereas older adults cite poor health as the leading barrier to both physical activity and exercise, as shown

TABLE 5.11

Barriers to Exercise for Older People

Health concerns
Pain
Fear of injury
Safety concerns of physical environment
Accessibility to exercise facility, park or footpath
Lack of counseling from physician-provider
Inadequate knowledge of health benefits of moderate exercise
Lack of social support

Source: Schutzer and Graves (2004).

in Table 5.11 (Schutzer & Graves, 2004). Fear of injury is also a real concern as is a lack of knowledge about how physical activity and exercise can improve chronic health conditions. Thus, counseling by a health professional knowledgeable about the health benefits of physical activity and exercise may be helpful.

Several studies have cited the importance and benefits of the physician-provider's advice and counseling in starting and continuing a physical activity and exercise program in later years (Balde, Figureras, Hawking, & Miller, 2003; CDC, 2012; Weiss, Wolfson, Yaffe, Shrier, & Puts, 2012). Effective counseling can be as simple as writing the CDC's recommended guidelines on a prescription pad (Swinburn, Walter, Arroll, Tilyard, & Russell, 1998).

Pedometers are known to promote exercise adherence and a higher intensity of exercise (Bravata et al., 2007; Mansi, Milosavljevic, Baxter, Tumilty, & Hendrick, 2014; Snyder, Colvin, & Gammack, 2011). One study found that in a group of postmenopausal women (age 45–75 years), 2,800 steps per session met 50% of the minimum exercise recommendation, 5,500 steps per session met 100% of the minimum exercise recommendation, and 6,500 steps per exercise session met 150% of the minimum exercise recommendation (Jordan, Jurca, Locke, Church, & Blair, 2005).

To promote and maintain health, the CDC's recommendations for aerobic exercise are a good place to start, that is, 150 minutes per week of moderate-intensity physical activity on 3–5 days a week, in 30-minute sessions. It is recommended that if participating in aerobic exercise 5 days per week, the individual should include a variety of exercise modes such as walking and swimming or cycling to place different impact-stresses on the body and to utilize different muscle groups. It is also recommended to incorporate strengthening and flexibility into the exercise program.

Because there is a positive dose–response relationship of health benefits that results from increasing exercise intensity, continuous challenge is important. Considering the physical stress theory (Mueller & Maluf, 2002), exercise must be beyond the threshold that maintains fitness. In other words, the body must be challenged sufficiently to incur health benefits. Therefore, it will be necessary to progressively increase the intensity throughout the program, when the perceived exercise effort drops below 5 on a 1–10 scale if more than maintenance is desired.

Exercise Duration and Progression

The duration of any single exercise session should be 30 minutes on 5 or more days per week for a total of 150 minutes *or* vigorous-intensity aerobic exercise done for at least 20–25 minutes 3 or more days per week. To promote or maintain weight loss, 50–60 minutes per day to total 300 minutes of moderate or 150 minutes vigorous daily exercise is recommended (Pescatello et al., 2014). However, as little as 10 minutes of intermittent exercise to accumulate the minimum-duration recommendations is effective. At least 3,000–4,000 steps a day of moderate- to vigorous-intensity walking is another way of looking at duration and intensity.

The rate of progression of the aerobic program is dependent on the level of fitness, exercise tolerance, health status, and individual goals. In the beginning, increasing the minutes of an exercise session is recommended. An increase of 5–10 minutes every 1–2 weeks over the first 4–5 weeks is reasonable for the average adult (Mazzeo et al., 1998). Once the duration has reached 60 minutes in a session or has reached the time available for exercise, intensity should be increased and duration reduced. A good rule of thumb is an activity intensity that allows conversation while breathing rapidly.

Aerobic Exercise Options

The types of exercise that are rhythmic and involve large muscle groups and thus considered aerobic are listed in Table 5.12. Specificity of training is key

TABLE 5.12
Types of Aerobic Exercise

Exercise Group	Description	Recommended for	Examples
A	Endurance activities requiring minimal skill or physical fitness to perform	All adults	Walking, leisurely cycling, aquarobics, slow dancing
B	Vigorous-intensity endurance activities requiring minimal skill	Adults with regular exercise program and/ or at least average physical fitness	Jogging, running, rowing, aerobics, spinning, elliptical exercise, stepping exercise, fast dancing, boxing
C	Endurance activities requiring skill to perform	Adults with acquired skill and/or at least average physical fitness levels	Swimming, cross-country skiing, skating, rowing
D	Recreational sports	Adults with a regular exercise program and at least average physical fitness	Racquet sports, basketball, soccer, downhill skiing, hiking, team sports

Source: Pescatello et al. (2014).

with respect to the individual's goals and functional demands. Exercises of Type A are recommended for all older adults, as they require little skill and are easily adapted to all levels of fitness. Type B exercises are best suited for those who exercise regularly and Type C exercises require skill to perform, and therefore safety can be a concern. Type D exercises are considered recreational and should supplement other types of aerobic exercise rather than be the only type of aerobic exercise done.

Each exercise has its advantages and disadvantages. Walking comes close to the "perfect" exercise as it is safe, low impact, is easily progressed in both duration and intensity, and is ideal for beginning an exercise program. Jogging has the same advantages as walking but may cause joint and muscle discomfort, so it is not recommended for those just beginning an exercise program. Good shoes are recommended for both walking and jogging. Swimming and aquarobics is generally less effective for weight loss compared to walking or jogging and does not reduce the risk of bone loss since it does not involve impact. However, for those very overweight, swimming may be preferred because the water will help support the body weight and reduce the pressure on joints. Risk of injury can be low in swimming and aquarobics. Aquarobics can involve a social aspect that can promote adherence. Outdoor cycling, although putting less stress on joints, can have safety concerns and requires equipment. Riding a stationary bicycle and spinning classes can alleviate the safety concerns. Other aerobic exercises require some degree of skill and should be attempted when some minimal level of exercise tolerance has been achieved with a walking, cycling, or swimming program. Regardless of the type of aerobic exercise chosen, the best exercise is the one the individual is most likely to do. Therefore, convenience and individual preference may be the most important considerations. Fitness level will also dictate what activity is considered aerobic. Any activity, such as gardening or even pushing a grocery cart, that increases heart rate for 10 minutes can be considered aerobic and will have beneficial effects.

EXERCISE PRESCRIPTION FOR SELECTED CHRONIC DISEASES

Arthritis and Obesity

Even though aerobic exercise such as walking or group exercise classes can reduce pain and self-reported physical function in individuals with body mass index ≥ 30, one of the reasons most often cited for not exercising is painful symptoms (Stubbs, Hurley, & Smith, 2015). However, the effect of aerobic exercise on weight loss in individuals with painful osteoarthritis is less known (Khoja,

Susko, Josbeno, Piva, & Fitzgerald, 2014). Individuals may have difficulty sustaining, in the presence of painful osteoarthritis, the 50–60 minutes/session that is required to lose weight. The addition of specific dietary interventions can help facilitate weight loss (Miller et al., 2013). Varying the mode of aerobic exercise from weight bearing (walking) to less-impact modes such as cycling or swimming within a week's session may be a helpful adaption. Additionally, supportive braces, good shoes that absorb impact, and strengthening exercises may be of benefit to help sustain the program. Every feasible mechanism to help the individual sustain an exercise program to promote weight loss will have the additional benefit of significantly reducing musculoskeletal symptoms (Messier, Gutekunst, Davis, & DeVita, 2005).

Diabetes Mellitus

Physical activity and exercise have beneficial effects on both glucose metabolism and insulin sensitivity (Fletcher et al., 2013). An aerobic exercise program of 150 minutes per week and weight reduction of 7% led to a 58% reduction in the incidence of Type 2 diabetes mellitus as compared with a control group, over 2.8 years of follow-up (Knowler et al., 2002).

Aerobic exercise and resistive exercise appear equivalent in their reduction of glycosylated hemoglobin (Yang, Scott, Mao, Tang, & Farmer, 2014). Aerobic exercise also reduced adipose tissue and promoted weight loss. Therefore, promoting aerobic exercise for individuals with diabetes is important. However, there are some concerns that should be addressed when prescribing aerobic exercise. Diabetic retinopathy may pose safety concerns, and therefore indoor exercise may be a better place to start. Foot care and appropriate footwear is critical. Silica gel or midsoles as well as socks of polyester or polyester–cotton blend to prevent blisters and keep the feet dry are recommended (Castaneda, 2003). Careful monitoring of blood glucose before, during, and after exercise to avoid hypoglycemic events is critical, especially as better glycemic control is achieved through exercise. Adjustment in the timing of exercise in relation to medication use and meals as well as food composition may be required (Zinker, 1999).

Cardiac Disease, Hypertension

The benefits of a regular, aerobic program are well known for individuals with cardiac disease and hypertension. Exercise training lowers resting blood pressure in normotensive and hypertensive individuals and in patients with and without CVD. The ACSM guidelines for beginning an aerobic exercise program described earlier with special attention to monitoring the physiological response before, during, and after exercise should provide a safe and effective framework to begin the program.

Heart Failure

Heart failure (HF) can be left or right sided. Dyspnea is the hallmark symptom of HF, although roughly two-thirds of individuals are also limited by leg fatigue during exercise (Norberg, Boman, & Lofgren, 2010). Leg fatigue may be due to the heart's inability to supply adequate blood and oxygen to the working muscles. While chronic HF patients were traditionally counseled to rest and avoid exercise to delay disease progression and to promote diuresis induced by bed rest, it is now known that most HF patients who exercise can markedly improve their functional status and quality of life (McMurray et al., 2012).

Exercise training leads to reduced peripheral vasoconstriction, improved endothelial function, and enhanced endothelial repair, which address the symptom of edema. Regular exercise also addresses muscle wasting and improves peak VO_2 (De Maeyer, Beckers, Vrints, & Conraads, 2013). In a large randomized controlled trial (RCT), exercise lowered the relative risk of mortality over a period of 30 months by 11%, in spite of only 30% of patients reaching a targeted 120 minutes of training per week, and it was safe (O'Connor et al., 2009; Smart & Marwick, 2004). In a further analysis, Keteyian and colleagues found that every 6% increase in VO_2 peak was associated with a 7% lower risk of mortality. Furthermore, moderate exercise volumes of 3 to <5 METs were associated with risk reduction exceeding 30% (Keteyian et al., 2012).

While characteristics of exercise programs vary, a gradual approach is recommended (Piepoli et al., 2011). Long warm-ups are important to promote vasodilation before the demands of exertion. A protocol of at least 10 minutes of stretching, slow walking, or other exercise can increase blood flow to muscles without raising the pulse above 40%–50% of maximum heart rate (Keteyian, 2011).

Interval training with 2 to 4 minutes of exercise followed by 1–3 minutes of rest for up to 38 minutes of exercise led to improvements in aerobic capacity in individuals with left ventricular ejection fraction of 29% and was determined to be safe (Rognmo et al., 2012; Wisloff et al., 2007). These studies indicate the feasibility of interval programs that allow patients to progress gradually until they can sustain continuous exercise for 30–40 minutes. Because one of the goals of exercise is to improve function, exercise intensities up to 90% of VO_2 peak and as low as 40% VO_2 peak have been investigated and found safe and effective (De Maeyer et al., 2013).

Aerobic exercise in the form of cycling, walking, and so forth, is recommended as baseline activity. Stationary cycling at very low workloads with continuous monitoring of heart rate, rhythm, and blood pressure is the most preferred mode of exercise for individuals with HF because of its reproducible power output and low injury rate (De Maeyer et al., 2013; Myers, 2008). Recommended training intensity using RPE 11–13 on the Borg scale of 6–20 (i.e., perceived exertion ranging between "light" and "somewhat hard") is equivalent to a training range (Carvalho, Bocchi, & Guimaraes, 2009). Exercise frequency and duration should be individually determined based on exercise tolerance and may range from as little as 5 minutes to a full 30 minutes for 3–5 sessions per week. Swimming is not appropriate for individuals with HF because of the increases in heart rate, hydrostatically induced volume loading of the thorax and heart, and higher mean pulmonary artery and capillary pressures (Meyer, 2006; Meyer & Leblanc, 2008).

Specific strategies recommended by ACSM for individuals with HF include (Meyers, 1997):

- Close monitoring for signs of decompensation, rapid changes in weight or blood pressure, worse-than usual dyspnea or angina on exertion, or increases in dysrhythmias
- Prolonged warm-up and cool-down sessions
- Low-intensity/long-duration sessions
- Interval training
- Perceived exertion and dyspnea scales take precedence over heart rate and workload targets
- Electrocardiogram (ECG) monitoring for persons with a history of ventricular tachycardia, cardiac arrest (sudden death), or exertional hypotension

Osteoporosis

Low-impact exercise, such as the kind seen with some forms of aerobic exercise can benefit individuals with osteoporosis. For example, a meta-analysis demonstrated that bone density improved at the hip in women who regularly walked (Kelley, 1998). Another study demonstrated the effectiveness of weight-bearing activity, such as walking, on the spine. Modes of aerobic exercise such as elliptical training machines, low-impact aerobics, stair-step machines, and walking may be particularly beneficial.

Peripheral Artery Disease

Much evidence exists that demonstrates the effectiveness of a graduated walking program on the symptoms of peripheral artery disease (PAD). Following the standard recommendations for beginning an exercise program of 3–5 days per week progressing to a total of 30–60 minutes will achieve health benefits and symptom improvement of PAD. Intensity and duration should be monitored by symptoms. Walking into leg pain to a level of 3–4 out of 5 (severe pain) is recommended. Stopping exercise for a short rest when pain reaches a 4 and then beginning again until 30 minutes is reached will increase duration. Ideally, exercise durations should be at least 5 minutes without stopping to rest (Cleveland Clinic, 2015).

Pulmonary Diseases

Individuals with increased airway resistance (chronic bronchitis and asthma), abnormalities of gas exchange (emphysema, pulmonary fibrosis, chronic obstructive pulmonary disease [COPD]), and other lung disease may particularly benefit from aerobic exercise through improving pulmonary blood flow and peripheral muscle conditioning, cardiovascular reconditioning, desensitization to dyspnea, and improved ventilatory efficiency (Maltais et al., 2014). For example, physical conditioning of leg muscles through exercise training reduces lactate production and decreases ventilatory burden. In turn, a lower ventilatory burden allows the patient to breathe more slowly during exercise, thereby reduction dynamic hyperinflation. These effects reduce exertional dyspnea, even without a change in forced expiratory volume (FEV; Spruit et al., 2013).

The general principles of exercise training in individuals with chronic pulmonary disease are no different from those for healthy individuals. The aims are to condition the muscles of ambulation and improve cardiorespiratory fitness to allow an increase in physical activity that is associated with a reduction in breathlessness and fatigue (Spruit et al., 2013). A high level of intensity of continuous exercise (>60% maximal work rate) for 20–60 minutes per session maximizes physiologic benefits. Walking and biking are optimal exercise modalities, if tolerated (Jenkins, Hill, & Cecins, 2010).

Management to minimize symptoms during exercise can include breathing techniques, supplemental oxygen when arterial oxygen tension falls below 88%, and emphasis on interval sessions of 5–10 minutes with adequate rest until the individual builds up tolerance to a full 30-minute session (Lacasse, Goldstein, Lasserson, & Martin, 2006; Nonoyama, Brooks, Lacasse, Guyatt, & Goldstein, 2007).

Pulmonary rehabilitation is a nonpharmacologic therapy, comprehensive and multidisciplinary in its approach that includes patient-centered interventions that include exercise training, self-management education, and psychosocial support. It is usually provided in an outpatient hospital-based program for 6–12 weeks (Nici, Lareau, & ZuWallack, 2010). A recent Cochrane systematic review investigated the effects of pulmonary rehabilitation or respiratory rehabilitation on COPD (McCarthy et al., 2015). The results of 65 RCTs demonstrated moderately large effects for the improvement of dyspnea and fatigue, improvement in emotional function, and enhancement of an individual's control over his or her condition.

Alzheimer's Disease

Aerobic exercise training is increasingly suggested as a therapeutic intervention for Alzheimer's disease (AD) because of its potential effect on cognition (Erickson & Kramer, 2009). While the exact mechanism is unclear, aerobic exercise may positively affect cerebral structure and function, improve neuronal survivability and function, increase cerebral vascularization and neuroendocrine response to stress, decrease neuroinflammation, and reduce certain waste products that are by-products of AD (Fang, 2011). Low cardiovascular fitness has been linked to a greater loss of gray matter and cognitive decline in cognitively nonimpaired individuals (Angevaren, Aufdemkampe, Verhaar, Aleman, & Vanhees, 2008; Erickson et al., 2010). Additionally, cognitive improvement is reported after aerobic exercise training (Buchman, Wilson, & Bennett, 2008), and there is some evidence that participation in an aerobics program improves psychological and behavior symptoms in persons with AD (Hogan, 2005). While no exercise prescription exists for those with AD, incorporating the CDC and ACSM recommendations of 150 minutes per week of moderate intense exercise is a goal. Involving the caregiver as a partner in the aerobic program may improve adherence for the individual with Alzheimers and may help reduce the stress of caregiving. Participating in familiar modes of exercise, such as walking may also improve adherence.

SUMMARY

Aerobic exercise has widespread beneficial effects for older adults, positively affecting all body systems and effectively managing symptoms from many chronic diseases. Aerobic exercise costs little to implement, is readily accessible, and can enhance quality of life. It may be said that aerobic exercise is essential to an older person's well-being for an investment of as little as 30 minutes 5 days a week.

REFERENCES

Akhras, F., & Jackson, G. (1991). Raised exercise diastolic blood pressure as indicator of ischaemic left ventricular dysfunction. *Lancet, 337*(8746), 899–900.

American College of Sports Medicine, Chodzko-Zajko, W. J., Proctor, D. N., Fiatarone Singh, M. A., Minson, C. T., Nigg, C. R., et al. (2009). American College of Sports Medicine position stand. Exercise and physical activity for older adults. *Medicine and Science in Sports and Exercise, 41*(7), 1510–1530.

American College of Sports Medicine. (Ed.). (2010). *ACSM's guidelines for exercise testing and prescription* (8th ed.). Baltimore, MD: American College of Sports Medicine.

Angevaren, M., Aufdemkampe, G., Verhaar, H. J., Aleman, A., & Vanhees, L. (2008). Physical activity and enhanced fitness to improve cognitive function in older people without known cognitive impairment. *Cochrane Database of Systematic Reviews (Online)*, (3), CD005381.

Avers, D., & Brown, M. (2009). White paper: Strength training for the older adult. *Journal of Geriatric Physical Therapy, 32*(4), 148–152.

Balady, G. J., Chaitman, B., Driscoll, D., Foster, C., Froelicher, E., Gordon, N., et al. (1998). AHA/ACSM joint statement: Recommendations for cardiovascular screening, staffing and emergency polices at health/fitness facilities. *Medicine & Science in Sports & Exercise, 30*(6), 2283–2293.

Balde, A., Figureras, J., Hawking, D., & Miller, J. (2003). Physician advice to the elderly about physical activity. *Journal of the Aging and Physical Activity, 11*, 90–97.

Borg, G. (1998). *Borg's perceived exertion and pain scales*. Champaign, IL: Human Kinetics.

Bravata, D. M., Smith-Spangler, C., Sundaram, V., Gienger, A. L., Lin, N., Lewis, R., et al. (2007). Using pedometers to increase physical activity and improve health: A systematic review. *The Journal of the American Medical Association, 298*(19), 2296–2304.

Brooks, D., Parsons, J., Hunter, J., Devlin, M., & Walker, J. (2001). The 2-minute walk test as a measure of functional improvement in persons with lower limb amputation. *Archives of Physical Medicine and Rehabilitation, 82*(10), 1478–1483.

Buchman, A. S., Wilson, R. S., & Bennett, D. A. (2008). Total daily activity is associated with cognition in older persons. *The American Journal of Geriatric Psychiatry: Official Journal of the American Association for Geriatric Psychiatry, 16*(8), 697–701.

Carvalho, V. O., Bocchi, E. A., & Guimaraes, G. V. (2009). The Borg scale as an important tool of self-monitoring and self-regulation of exercise prescription in heart failure patients during hydrotherapy. A randomized blinded controlled trial. *Circulation Journal: Official Journal of the Japanese Circulation Society, 73*(10), 1871–1876.

Castaneda, C. (2003). Diabetes control with physical activity and exercise. *Nutrition in Clinical Care*, 6(2), 89–96.

Centers for Disease Control and Prevention. (2012). *Trends in adults receiving a recommendation for exercise and physical activity from a physician or other health care provider.* Retrieved from http://www.cdc.gov/nchs/data/databriefs/db86.htm

Centers for Disease Control and Prevention (2013). Adult participation in aerobic and muscle-strengthening physical activities - United States, 2011. *MMWR. Morbidity and Mortality Weekly Report, 62*(17), 326–330.

Centers for Disease Control and Prevention. (2014). *Physical activity intensity*. Retrieved from http://www.cdc.gov/nccdphp/dnpa/physical/pdf/PA_Intensity_table_2_1.pdf

Centers for Disease Control and Prevention. (2015). *Physical activity recommendations for older adults*. Retrieved from http://www.cdc.gov/physicalactivity/everyone/guidelines/olderadults.html

Cleveland Clinic. (2015). *Peripheral Arterial Disease (PAD) & exercise*. Retrieved from http://my.clevelandclinic.org/services/heart/disorders/pad/padexercise

De Maeyer, C., Beckers, P., Vrints, C. J., & Conraads, V. M. (2013). Exercise training in chronic heart failure. *Therapeutic Advances in Chronic Disease, 4*(3), 105–117.

Dimkpa, U. (2009). Post-exercise heart rate recovery: An index of cardiovascular fitness. *Journal of Exercise Physiology, 12*(1), 10–22. Retrieved from https://www.asep.org/asep/asep/Dimpka%2012(1)10-22.doc

Erickson, K. I., & Kramer, A. F. (2009). Aerobic exercise effects on cognitive and neural plasticity in older adults. *British Journal of Sports Medicine, 43*(1), 22–24.

Erickson, K. I., Raji, C. A., Lopez, O. L., Becker, J. T., Rosano, C., Newman, A. B., et al. (2010). Physical activity predicts gray matter volume in late adulthood: The cardiovascular health study. *Neurology, 75*(16), 1415–1422. http://dx.doi.org/10.1212/wnl.0b013e3181f88359

Exercise Assessment and Screening for You (EASY) Screening Group. (2007). *Exercise and screening for you tool 2007*. Retrieved from http://www.easyforyou.info/index.asp

Fang, Y. (2011). Guiding research and practice: A conceptual model for aerobic exercise training in Alzheimer's disease. *American Journal of Alzheimer's Disease and Other Dementias, 26*(3), 184–194.

Mayo Clinic. *Fitness programs: 5 steps to get started - Mayo Clinic*. Retrieved from http://www.mayoclinic.org/healthy-lifestyle/fitness/in-depth/fitness/art-20048269

Fleg, J. L., & Lakatta, E. G. (1988). Role of muscle loss in the age-associated reduction in VO2 max. *Journal of Applied Physiology (Bethesda, Md.: 1985), 65*(3), 1147–1151.

Fleg, J. L., Morrell, C. H., Bos, A. G., Brant, L. J., Talbot, L. A., Wright, J. G., et al. (2005). Accelerated longitudinal decline of aerobic capacity in healthy older adults. *Circulation, 112*(5), 674–682.

Fletcher, G. F., Ades, P. A., Kligfield, P., Arena, R., Balady, G. J., Bittner, V. A., et al. (2013). Exercise standards for testing and training: A scientific statement from the American Heart Association. *Circulation, 128*(8), 873–934.

Fletcher, G. F., Balady, G., Blair, S. N., Blumenthal, J., Caspersen, C., Chaitman, B., et al. (1996). Statement on exercise: Benefits and recommendations for physical activity programs for all Americans. A statement for health professionals by the Committee on Exercise and Cardiac Rehabilitation of the Council on Clinical Cardiology, American Heart Association. *Circulation, 94*(4), 857–862.

Gostic, C. L. (2005). The crucial role of exercise and physical activity in weight management and functional improvement for seniors. *Clinics in Geriatric Medicine, 21*(4), 747–756.

Guccione, A., Wong, R., & Avers, D. (2012). *Geriatric Physical Therapy* (3rd ed.). St Louis, MO: Elseiver.

Hogan, M. (2005). Physical and cognitive activity and exercise for older adults: A review. *International Journal of Aging & Human Development, 60*(2), 95–126.

Hulens, M., Vansant, G., Claessens, A. L., Lysens, R., & Muls, E. (2003). Predictors of 6-minute walk test results in lean, obese and morbidly obese women. *Scandinavian Journal of Medicine & Science in Sports, 13*(2), 98–105.

Jenkins, S., Hill, K., & Cecins, N. M. (2010). State of the art: How to set up a pulmonary rehabilitation program. *Respirology (Carlton, Vic.), 15*(8), 1157–1173.

Jordan, A. N., Jurca, G. M., Locke, C. T., Church, T. S., & Blair, S. N. (2005). Pedometer indices for weekly physical activity recommendations in postmenopausal women. *Medicine and Science in Sports and Exercise, 37*(9), 1627–1632.

Kelley, G. A. (1998). Aerobic exercise and bone density at the hip in postmenopausal women: A meta-analysis. *Preventive Medicine, 27*(6), 798–807.

Keteyian, S. J. (2011). Exercise training in congestive heart failure: Risks and benefits. *Progress in Cardiovascular Diseases, 53*(6), 419–428.

Keteyian, S. J., Leifer, E. S., Houston-Miller, N., Kraus, W. E., Brawner, C. A., O'Connor, C. M., et al. (2012). Relation between volume of exercise and clinical outcomes in patients with heart failure. *Journal of the American College of Cardiology, 60*(19), 1899–1905.

Khoja, S. S., Susko, A. M., Josbeno, D. A., Piva, S. R., & Fitzgerald, G. K. (2014). Comparing physical activity programs for managing osteoarthritis in overweight or obese patients. *Journal of Comparative Effectiveness Research, 3*(3), 283–299.

Knowler, W. C., Barrett-Connor, E., Fowler, S. E., Hamman, R. F., Lachin, J. M., Walker, E. A., et al. (2002). Reduction in the incidence of type 2 diabetes with lifestyle intervention or metformin. *The New England Journal of Medicine, 346*(6), 393–403.

Lacasse, Y., Goldstein, R., Lasserson, T. J., & Martin, S. (2006). Pulmonary rehabilitation for chronic obstructive pulmonary disease. *The Cochrane Database of Systematic Reviews,* (4), CD003793.

LaPier, T. (2012). Impaired aerobic capacity/endurance. In A. Gucionne, R. Wong, & D. Avers (Eds.), *Geriatric Physical Therapy* (2nd ed., p. 229). St. Louis, MO: Elseiver.

Maltais, F., Decramer, M., Casaburi, R., Barreiro, E., Burelle, Y., Debigare, R., et al. (2014). An official American Thoracic Society/European Respiratory Society statement: Update on limb muscle dysfunction in chronic obstructive pulmonary disease. *American Journal of Respiratory and Critical Care Medicine, 189*(9), e15–e62.

Mansi, S., Milosavljevic, S., Baxter, G. D., Tumilty, S., & Hendrick, P. (2014). A systematic review of studies using pedometers as an intervention for musculoskeletal diseases. *BMC Musculoskeletal Disorders, 15*, 231.

Mazzeo, R. S., Cavanagh, P., Evans, W. J., Fiatarone, M. A., Hagberg, J., McAuley, E., et al. (1998). ACSM position stand: Exercise and physical activity for older adults. *Medicine & Science in Sports & Exercise, 30*(6), 992–1008.

McCarthy, B., Casey, D., Devane, D., Murphy, K., Murphy, E., & Lacasse, Y. (2015). Pulmonary rehabilitation for chronic obstructive pulmonary disease. *The Cochrane Database of Systematic Reviews, 2*, CD003793.

McMurray, J. J., Adamopoulos, S., Anker, S. D., Auricchio, A., Bohm, M., Dickstein, K., et al. (2012). ESC guidelines for the diagnosis and treatment of acute and chronic heart failure 2012: The task force for the diagnosis and treatment of acute and chronic heart failure 2012 of the European Society of Cardiology. Developed in collaboration with the Heart Failure Association (HFA) of the ESC. *European Heart Journal, 33*(14), 1787–1847.

MedlinePlus. (2015). *Aging changes in the heart and blood vessels*. Retrieved from http://www.nlm.nih.gov/medlineplus/ency/article/004006.htm

Messier, S. P., Gutekunst, D. J., Davis, C., & DeVita, P. (2005). Weight loss reduces knee-joint loads in overweight and obese older adults with knee osteoarthritis. *Arthritis Rheum, 52*(7), 2026–2032.

Meyer, K. (2006). Left ventricular dysfunction and chronic heart failure: Should aqua therapy and swimming be allowed? *British Journal of Sports Medicine, 40*(10), 817–818.

Meyer, K., & Leblanc, M. C. (2008). Aquatic therapies in patients with compromised left ventricular function and heart failure. *Clinical and Investigative Medicine, 31*(2), E90–E97.

Meyers, J. N. (1997). Congestive heart failure. In American College of Sports Medicine (Ed.), *Exercise management for persons with chronic diseases and disabilities* (p. 48). Champaign, IL: Human Kinetics.

Miller, C. T., Fraser, S. F., Levinger, I., Straznicky, N. E., Dixon, J. B., Reynolds, J., et al. (2013). The effects of exercise training in addition to energy restriction on functional capacities and body composition in obese adults during weight loss: A systematic review. *PloS One, 8*(11), e81692.

Montero, D., Roberts, C. K., & Vinet, A. (2014). Effect of aerobic exercise training on arterial stiffness in obese populations: A systematic review and meta-analysis. *Sports Medicine (Auckland, N.Z.), 44*(6), 833–843.

Morey, M. C., Pieper, C. F., & Cornoni-Huntley, J. (1998). Physical fitness and functional limitations in community-dwelling older adults. *Medicine and Science in Sports and Exercise, 30*(5), 715–723.

Mueller, M. J., & Maluf, K. S. (2002). Tissue adaptation to physical stress: A proposed "Physical Stress Theory" to guide physical therapist practice, education, and research. *Physical Therapy, 82*(4), 383–403.

Myers, J. (2008). Principles of exercise prescription for patients with chronic heart failure. *Heart Failure Reviews, 13*(1), 61–68.

Nici, L., Lareau, S., & ZuWallack, R. (2010). Pulmonary rehabilitation in the treatment of chronic obstructive pulmonary disease. *American Family Physician, 82*(6), 655–660.

Nonoyama, M. L., Brooks, D., Lacasse, Y., Guyatt, G. H., & Goldstein, R. S. (2007). Oxygen therapy during exercise training in chronic obstructive pulmonary disease. *The Cochrane Database of Systematic Reviews*, (2), CD005372.

Norberg, E. B., Boman, K., & Lofgren, B. (2010). Impact of fatigue on everyday life among older people with chronic heart failure. *Australian Occupational Therapy Journal, 57*(1), 34–41.

O'Connor, C. M., Whellan, D. J., Lee, K. L., Keteyian, S. J., Cooper, L. S., Ellis, S. J., et al. (2009). Efficacy and safety of exercise training in patients with chronic heart failure: HF-ACTION randomized controlled trial. *The Journal of the American Medical Association, 301*(14), 1439–1450.

Office of Disease Prevention and Health Promotion. (2015). *Appendix 1: Translating scientific evidence about total amount and intensity of physical activity into guidelines.* Retrieved from http://health.gov/PAGUIDELINES/guidelines/appendix1.aspx

Ory, M. G., & Resnick, B. (2008). *Exercise and screening for you.* Retrieved from http://www.easyforyou.info/downloads/EASYScreeningToolHardCopyFINAL040308.pdf

Pescatello, L. S., Arena, R., Riebe, D., & Thompson, P. D. (Eds.). (2014). *ACSM's guidelines for exercise testing and prescription* (9th ed.). Baltimore, MD: Wolters Kluwer Lippincott, Williams & Wilkins.

Petrella, R. J. (2000). Moderate aerobic exercise to increase fitness in older adults. *Clinical Journal of Sports Medicine, 10*(4), 307–378.

Piepoli, M. F., Conraads, V., Corra, U., Dickstein, K., Francis, D. P., Jaarsma, T., et al. (2011). Exercise training in heart failure: From theory to practice. A consensus document of the Heart Failure Association and the European Association for cardiovascular prevention and rehabilitation. *European Journal of Heart Failure, 13*(4), 347–357.

Resnick, B., Ory, M. G., Hora, K., Rogers, M. E., Page, P., Bolin, J. N., et al. (2008). A proposal for a new screening paradigm and tool called Exercise Assessment and Screening for You (EASY). *Journal of Aging and Physical Activity, 16*(2), 215–233.

Rikli, R. E., & Jones, C. J. (1998). The reliability and validity of a 6-minute walk test as a measure of physical endurance in older adults. *Journal of Aging & Physical Activity, 6*, 3630–375.

Robbins, M., Francis, G., Pashkow, F. J., Snader, C. E., Hoercher, K., Young, J. B., et al. (1999). Ventilatory and heart rate responses to exercise: Better predictors of heart failure mortality than peak oxygen consumption. *Circulation, 100*(24), 2411–2417.

Rognmo, O., Moholdt, T., Bakken, H., Hole, T., Molstad, P., Myhr, N. E., et al. (2012). Cardiovascular risk of high- versus moderate-intensity aerobic exercise in coronary heart disease patients. *Circulation, 126*(12), 1436–1440.

Russell, W. D. (1997). On the current status of Rated Perceived Exertion. *Perceptual Motor Skills, 84*(3 Pt. 1), 799–808.

Schutzer, K. A., & Graves, B. S. (2004). Barriers and motivations to exercise in older adults. *Preventive Medicine, 39*(5), 1056–1061.

Shumway-Cook, A., Patla, A. E., Stewart, A., Ferrucci, L., Ciol, M. A., & Guralnik, J. M. (2002). Environmental demands associated with community mobility in older adults with and without mobility disabilities. *Physical Therapy, 82*(7), 670–681.

Simonsick, E. M., Montgomery, P. S., Newman, A. B., Bauer, D. C., & Harris, T. (2001). Measuring fitness in healthy older adults: The health ABC long distance corridor walk. *Journal of the American Geriatrics Society, 49*(11), 1544–1548.

Smart, N., & Marwick, T. H. (2004). Exercise training for patients with heart failure: A systematic review of factors that improve mortality and morbidity. *The American Journal of Medicine, 116*(10), 693–706.

Snyder, A., Colvin, B., & Gammack, J. K. (2011). Pedometer use increases daily steps and functional status in older adults. *Journal of the American Medical Directors Association, 12*(8), 590–594.

Spruit, M. A., Singh, S. J., Garvey, C., ZuWallack, R., Nici, L., Rochester, C., et al. (2013). An official American Thoracic Society/European Respiratory Society statement: Key concepts and advances in pulmonary rehabilitation. *American Journal of Respiratory and Critical Care Medicine, 188*(8), e13–e64.

Stubbs, B., Hurley, M., & Smith, T. (2015). What are the factors that influence physical activity participation in adults with knee and hip osteoarthritis? A systematic review of physical activity correlates. *Clinical Rehabilitation, 29*(1), 80–94.

Sutbeyaz, S. T., Sezer, N., Koseoglu, B. F., Ibrahimoglu, F., & Tekin, D. (2007). Influence of knee osteoarthritis on exercise capacity and quality of life in obese adults. *Obesity (Silver Spring, Md.), 15*(8), 2071–2076.

Swinburn, B. A., Walter, L. G., Arroll, B., Tilyard, M. W., & Russell, D. G. (1998). The green prescription study: A randomized controlled trial of written exercise advice provided by general practitioners. *American Journal of Public Health, 88*(2), 288–291.

Taylor, D. (2014). Physical activity is medicine for older adults. *Postgraduate Medical Journal, 90*, 26–32.

Thomas, S., Reading, J., & Shephard, R. J. (1992). Revision of the Physical Activity Readiness Questionnaire (PAR-Q). *Canadian Journal of Sport Sciences, 17*(4), 338–345.

Wan, M., & Wong, R. Y. (2014). Benefits of exercise in the elderly. *Canadian Geriatrics Society Journal of CME, 4*, 5–8.

Weiss, D., Wolfson, C., Yaffe, M., Shrier, I., & Puts, M. (2012). Physician counseling of older adults about physical activity: The importance of context. *American Journal of Health Promotion, 27*(2), 71–74.

Wisloff, U., Stoylen, A., Loennechen, J. P., Bruvold, M., Rognmo, O., Haram, P. M., et al. (2007). Superior cardiovascular effect of aerobic interval training versus moderate continuous training in heart failure patients: A randomized study. *Circulation, 115*(24), 3086–3094.

Yang, Z., Scott, C. A., Mao, C., Tang, J., & Farmer, A. J. (2014). Resistance exercise versus aerobic exercise for type 2 diabetes: A systematic review and meta-analysis. *Sports Medicine (Auckland, N.Z.), 44*(4), 487–499.

Zinker, B. A. (1999). Nutrition and exercise in individuals with diabetes. *Clinics in Sports Medicine, 18*(3), 585–606, vii–viii.

CHAPTER 6

Exercise for Osteoarthritis of the Hip and Knee

Tracey E. Howe

ABSTRACT

Osteoarthritis (OA) is the most common form of arthritis and is a painful, chronically disabling joint disease that often significantly compromises function and independence. With the generalized rise in the age of the global population, the number of people suffering from musculoskeletal disorders throughout the world will increase dramatically over the coming decades. International clinical guidelines recommend exercise for the treatment of OA. Given the current and predicted future global burden of OA of the hip and knee, the aim of this chapter is to summarize the evidence from recent systematic reviews published in English on the effectiveness of land- and water-based exercise programs for people with OA of the hip and knee. The primary outcomes considered, based on the recommendations of the Outcome Measures in Rheumatology (OMERACT) conference OMERACT III, are pain and function. Recent systematic reviews have examined the effectiveness of exercise on pain and function compared with controls: land- versus water-based exercise, individual versus group exercise, and exercise prior to surgery for people with OA of the hip, the knee, and lower limb (hip and knee combined). Generally, most forms of exercise have been demonstrated to have significant positive effects on pain and function at the end of the exercise program, but unless participants continue the program, the sustainability of these

http://dx.doi.org/10.1891/0198-8794.36.155

effects in the longer term are questionable. However, exercise appears to be a safe intervention, with few adverse effects reported. A number of considerations relating to the design and reporting of primary research in this area are discussed.

INTRODUCTION

Osteoarthritis (OA) is the most common form of arthritis and is a painful, chronically disabling joint disease that often significantly compromises function and independence. OA can present in the spine and hands, but the most frequently affected joints are the main load-bearing joints, the hips and knees. Approximately one in four people may develop symptomatic hip OA in their lifetime (Murphy et al., 2010); the lifetime prevalence for hip OA is estimated to be 25.3% but it is much higher for knee OA, 44.7% (Murphy et al., 2008). The global age-standardized point prevalence for hip and knee OA in 2010 was 3.8% (95% uncertainty interval 3.6 to 4.1) and was higher in females peaking at age 50 years (March et al., 2014).

The symptoms of OA include pain, joint stiffness, muscle weakness and atrophy, altered proprioception, and limitations in functional activities and social participation. Joint malalignment may be present in progressive disease states and this can result in bone-on-bone joint pain. Hip and knee OA accounts for about 10.5% of the total disability burden in terms of years lived, with disabilities for all musculoskeletal diseases combined.

With the generalized rise in the age of the global population, the number of people suffering from musculoskeletal disorders throughout the world will increase dramatically over the coming decades. For example in the United States, the number of adults with arthritis is projected to increase from 47.8 million in 2005 to 67 million in 2030 (Hootman & Helmick, 2006). This will result in an exponential increase in the global burden of disability from OA hip and knee; therefore, finding cost-effective and safe treatment to minimize the symptoms for people with OA hip and knee is imperative.

Traditionally, treatment of OA involves pharmacological interventions such as paracetamol/acetaminophen, nonsteroidal anti-inflammatory drugs, and intra-articular steroids. Nonpharmacological interventions include exercise, education, weight reduction, appliances, heat and cold therapy, transcutaneous electrical nerve stimulation, pulsed electromagnetic field, and laser and galvanic stimulation; joint replacement is the most common surgical intervention.

THE ROLE OF PHYSICAL ACTIVITY AND EXERCISE

It is well documented that regular moderate-intensity physical activity—such as walking, cycling, or participating in sports—has been shown to have significant benefits for general health of populations, such as reducing the risk of cardiovascular diseases, diabetes, colon and breast cancer, and depression; decreasing the risk of a hip or vertebral fracture; and helping control weight. Indeed, global recommendations on physical activity for health for adults are participation in moderate physical activity, for example, walking, cycling, and household chores for at least 30 minutes per session, five times per week, or vigorous activity for at least 25 minutes per session, three times per week (World Health Organization [WHO], 2010a). It can be postulated then that participation in regular physical activity may be sufficient to protect against the development of OA or relieve symptoms of OA hip and knee. However, it has been reported that only 27.8% of individuals with arthritis engage in physical activity to a level that is sufficient to experience these benefits (Hootman, Macera, Ham, Helmick, & Sniezek, 2003). The terms *physical activity* and *exercise* are often used interchangeably. Physical activity in daily life can be categorized into occupational, sports, conditioning, household, or other activities. Exercise is a subset of physical activity that is planned, structured, and repetitive and has the objective of improvement or maintenance of physical fitness or a desired therapeutic effect (Caspersen, Powell, & Christenson, 1985). Exercise has been demonstrated to be effective in a number of groups, for example, improving balance in older people (Howe, Rochester, Neil, Skelton, & Ballinger, 2011) and preventing and managing osteoporosis in postmenopausal women (Howe et al., 2011).

International clinical guidelines such as Osteoarthritis Research Society International guidelines for the nonsurgical management of knee OA (McAlindon et al., 2014; Roddy et al., 2006) recommend exercise as a low-cost safe intervention with few reported adverse effects. The aim of therapeutic exercise programs is to relieve the symptoms of OA of the hip or knee including pain, joint stiffness, muscle weakness, and subsequent reduction in function. Therapeutic exercise programs for OA hip and knee frequently include land- or water-based exercise designed to improve muscle strength, range of movement in the joint, or aerobic capacity, or combinations of these. These exercise programs are typically designed and supervised by health professionals but may also be undertaken at home as part of self-management strategies.

Outcome measurement in clinical studies requires the use of valid, reliable, and responsive measurement procedures that adequately capture important aspects of the condition. In 1997, participants at the OMERACT III conference agreed (≥90%) on a core set of four domains for outcome measurement in future Phase III clinical studies of hip, knee, and hand OA. The four domains identified were pain, physical function, patient global assessment, and, for studies of at least 1 year, joint imaging (Bellamy et al., 1997). This has been further confirmed by Paskins, Sanders, and Hassell (2014) in their systematic review comparing patient experiences of the OA consultation with general practitioner (GP) attitudes and beliefs about OA. The authors found that pain management and fear of disability were consultation priorities for patients. Patients seem keen to explore nonpharmacological interventions, whereas GPs reported frustration and lack of knowledge about issues to do with lifestyle changes.

Functioning and disability, according to the International Classification of Functioning, Disability and Health (ICF; WHO, 2010b), are viewed as a complex interaction between the health condition of the individual and the contextual factors of the environment as well as personal factors. The ICF focuses on impact, creating a foundation and a common framework allowing all conditions to be compared using a common metric—the impact on the functioning of the individual "in his or her world."

Recognizing the global burden of OA of the hip and knee, this chapter summarizes the evidence from recent systematic reviews on the effectiveness of exercise programs for OA of the hip and knee on pain and function.

Exercise and Osteoarthritis of the Hip

Three systematic reviews have examined the effects of exercise on OA of the hip (Fransen, McConnell, Hernandez-Molina, & Reichenbach, 2014; Hernández-Molina, Reichenbach, Zhang, Lavalley, & Felson, 2008; Romeo, Parazza, Boschi, Nava, & Vanti, 2013).

A recently updated Cochrane review, search updated to February 2013 (Fransen et al., 2014) included 10 studies (549 participants), 7 of which were judged as having a low risk of bias. The studies included participants with mostly mild-to-moderate symptomatic hip OA, alone or with knee OA. Except for one study where participants enrolled in a tai chi program, all other participants underwent land-based exercise programs consisting of traditional muscle strengthening, functional training, and aerobic fitness programs, supervised either individually or as part of a group. Participants in the control groups did not exercise. Meta-analysis of high-quality evidence from nine studies (549 participants) demonstrated that exercise reduced pain (standardized mean difference [SMD] −0.38, 95% CI −0.55 to −0.20) equivalent to 8 points on a scale 0–100 (95% CI 4 to 11 points; number needed to treat for an additional beneficial outcome [NNTB] = 6). Physical function also improved (SMD −0.38, 95% CI −0.54 to −0.05) equivalent to 7 points on a 0–100 scale (95% CI 1 to 12 points; NNTB = 6). Only three small studies (183 participants) evaluated quality of life and they demonstrated no benefit from exercise for participants' quality of life (SMD −0.07, 95% CI −0.23 to −0.36).

These findings are consistent with a previous high-quality meta-analysis of nine studies (1,234 participants) comparing exercise programs of durations longer than 4 weeks with control (Hernández-Molina et al., 2008). Results indicate beneficial effect of exercise on pain with an effect size (ES) of −0.38 (95% CI −0.68 to −0.08; $p = 0.01$), but there was high heterogeneity ($I^2 = 75\%$) among studies. The heterogeneity was caused by one trial consisting of an exercise intervention that was not administered in person. When the authors removed this study leaving eight studies (493 participants) with a similar exercise strategy (specialized hands-on exercise training, all of which included at least some element of muscle strengthening), exercise demonstrated a benefit on pain with an ES of −0.46 (95% CI −0.64 to −0.28; $p < 0.0001$).

In contrast, a descriptive review involving 10 Studies, 2 of which involved manual therapy (Romeo et al., 2013), concluded that at mid- and long-term follow-up land-based exercises showed insufficient evidence of effectiveness with respect to pain and quality of life, but positive results were found for physical function. The authors also concluded that water-based exercises significantly reduced fall risk when combined with functional exercises. They stated that programs containing progressive and gradual exposure to difficult activities, education, and exercises promoted better outcomes, higher adherence to home program, and increased amount of physical activity, especially walking.

Exercise and Osteoarthritis of the Knee

Eight reviews examined studies investigating the effects of exercise on OA of the knee (Devos-Comby, Cronan, & Roesch, 2006; Focht, 2006; Fransen et al., 2015; Jansen, Viechtbauer, Lenssen, Hendriks, & de Bie, 2011; Juhl, Christensen, Roos, Zhang, & Lund, 2014; Petrella, 2000; Roddy, Zhang, & Doherty, 2005; Tanaka, Ozawa, Kito, & Moriyama, 2013).

A recently updated Cochrane review (Fransen et al., 2015), search updated to May 2013, undertook meta-analysis of data immediately after completion of exercise programs, compared with controls. They defined exercise as any land-based nonperioperative therapeutic exercise regimen aimed at relieving the symptoms of OA, regardless of content, duration, frequency, or intensity. High-quality evidence from 44 studies (3,537 participants) indicated that pain was reduced (SMD −0.49, 95% CI −0.39 to −0.59), equivalent to 12 points (95% CI 10 to 15 points) on a scale of 0–100 points. Moderate-quality evidence from 44 studies (3,913 participants) showed that exercise improved physical function (SMD −0.52, 95% CI −0.39 to −0.64), equivalent to 10 points (95% CI 8 to 13 points) on a scale of 0–100 points. Furthermore, high-quality evidence from 13 studies (1,073 participants) revealed that exercise improved quality of life (SMD 0.28, 95% CI 0.15 to 0.40) equivalent to 4 points (95% CI 2 to 5 points) on a scale of 0–100 points.

Encouragingly, Fransen et al. (2015) reported a sustained treatment effect at 2–6 months after intervention. Evidence from 12 studies (1,468 participants) indicated reduction in pain (SMD −0.24, 95% CI −0.35 to −0.14), equivalent to

6 (3–9) points on a scale of 0–100 points. Ten studies (1,279 participants) indicated sustainability of effect on physical function (SMD −0.15, 95% CI −0.26 to −0.04), equivalent to improvement of 3 (1–5) points on a scale of 0–100-points. This confirmed the large significant ES (SMD −0.94, 95% CI −1.31 to −0.57) of exercise on knee pain reported by Tanaka et al. (2013) based on eight studies (unclear number of participants).

In a review comparing exercise with control in 12 studies (808 participants), Devos-Comby et al. (2006) concluded that exercise had only a small-to-moderate effect on physical outcomes as assessed by self-report and direct measures with ES = 0.29 (95% CI 0.23 to 0.36); a small positive effect was seen on direct measures of impairment in 11 studies (740 participants) with a mean ES = 0.15 (95% CI 0.08 to 0.23). This is supported by the findings of two descriptive reviews (Focht, 2006; Petrella, 2000). Focht (2006) reported significant differences in pain between exercise and control interventions with small (0.25) to large (2.75) ESs based on 18 studies (2,320 participants). Petrella (2000) found small-to-moderate beneficial effects of exercise treatment for pain, small beneficial effects on disability, and moderate-to-great beneficial effects were observed according to patient global assessment of effect.

In a review of 12 studies (unknown number of participants) comparing three types of exercise interventions, Jansen et al. (2011) reported that the ES on pain for strength training was ES = 0.38 (95% CI 0.23 to 0.54), for exercise, it was ES = 0.34 (95% CI 0.19 to 0.49), and the ES on pain for exercise plus manual mobilization was ES = 0.69 (95% CI 0.42 to 0.96). Furthermore, each intervention also improved physical function significantly. However, metaregression indicated that exercise plus manual mobilizations improved pain significantly more than exercise alone ($p = 0.03$). Subgroup analyses by Tanaka et al. (2013) showed a larger effect for non-weight-bearing strengthening exercise (SMD −1.42, 95% CI −2.09 to −0.75) compared with weight-bearing strengthening exercise (SMD −0.70, 95% CI −1.05 to −0.35) and aerobic exercise (SMD −0.45, 95% CI −0.77 to −0.13).

Juhl et al. (2014) examined the effects of different types of exercise programs on pain in 47 studies (4,028 participants). Positive effects on pain relief were found for aerobic, resistance, and performance exercise (SMD 0.67, 0.62, and 0.48, respectively; $p = 0.733$). Single-type exercise programs were more efficacious than programs that included different exercise types (SMD 0.61 versus 0.16; $p < 0.001$). The effect of aerobic exercise on pain relief increased with an increased number of supervised sessions (slope 0.022, 95% CI 0.002 to 0.043). More pain reduction occurred with quadriceps-specific exercise than with general lower limb exercise (SMD 0.85 versus 0.39; $p = 0.005$) and when supervised exercise was performed at least three times a week (SMD 0.68 versus 0.41; $p = 0.017$). No impact of intensity, duration of individual sessions, or patient characteristics was found. Similar results were found by Roddy et al. (2005) in

13 studies. Pooled ESs for pain were 0.52 for aerobic walking and 0.39 for quadriceps strengthening, and for self-reported disability, ES was 0.46 for aerobic walking and 0.32 for quadriceps strengthening.

Exercise for Osteoarthritis of the Lower Limb

Ten reviews included studies involving participants with OA of either their hip or knee (Bartels et al., 2007; Brosseau et al., 2004; Daly Iversen, 2010; Pelland et al., 2004; Pisters et al., 2007; Tiffreau et al., 2007; Uthman et al., 2014; van Baar, Assendelft, Dekker, Oostendorp, & Bijlsma, 1999; Waller et al., 2014; Wallis & Taylor, 2011)

Uthman et al. (2014) in an analysis of 60 studies (44 knee, 2 hip, 14 mixed with 2,118 participants) reported that for pain relief, several types of exercise programs were significantly more effective than control. These included (a) strengthening, (b) flexibility plus strengthening, (c) flexibility plus strengthening plus aerobic, (d) aquatic strengthening, and (e) aquatic strengthening plus flexibility. Furthermore, a combined intervention of strengthening, flexibility, and aerobic exercise was also significantly more effective than the no-exercise control for improving limitation in function (SMD –0.63, 95% credible interval –1.16 to –0.10).

ESs from 11 studies, 10 on the knee and 1 on the hip (van Baar et al., 1999) indicated small-to-moderate beneficial effects of exercise therapy on pain, small beneficial effects on both disability outcome measures, and moderate-to-great beneficial effects according to the patient's global assessment of effect. However, only two studies had an acceptable validity score as well as sufficient power and another two studies had an acceptable validity score, but low power.

In a best-evidence synthesis of 11 studies (5 high and 6 low quality; Pisters et al., 2007), strong evidence was found for no long-term effectiveness on pain and self-reported physical function, moderate evidence for long-term effectiveness on patient global assessment of effectiveness, and conflicting evidence for observed physical function. For exercise programs with additional booster sessions, moderate evidence was found for long-term effectiveness on pain, self-reported physical function, and observed physical function.

This is further confirmed by descriptive reviews of 12 studies (1,363 participants; Brosseau et al., 2004) and 18 studies (1 hip, 6 hip and knee, 11 knee; Daly Iversen, 2010) that indicated that various forms of aerobic exercise, such as a walking program, jogging in water, yoga, and tai chi can have statistically significant effects on pain, joint tenderness, functional status, and respiratory capacity for patients with OA.

A review of 22 studies (2,325 participants) concluded that strengthening exercises alone have some effects on improving pain and functional outcomes (Pelland et al., 2004). However, in order to maximize their effectiveness, it is necessary to combine them with a more complete exercise program including range of motion (ROM), stretching, functional balance, and aerobic exercises.

Individual Versus Group Exercise

The effectiveness of individual or collective group exercise programs for knee or hip OA was examined in 29 studies (21 knee, 1 hip, and 7 knee and hip) (Tiffreau et al., 2007). The authors reported that the benefit of individual and group exercise programs is low-to-moderate for pain, strength, and ability to walk, and that there is no evidence of the superiority of one modality over the other. However, they observed that effectiveness is not maintained over time if the exercise program is not continued.

Aquatic Versus Land-Based Exercise

The effects of aquatic based exercise were examined by Waller et al. (2014). They included 11 studies (6 knee and hip, 3 knee only, 1 hip only, and 1 any lower limb OA in a total of 1,092 participants). Effects directly after intervention revealed a small but significant effect from aquatic exercise on pain (SMD 0.26, 95% CI 0.11 to 0.41), stiffness (SMD 0.20, 95% CI 0.03 to 0.36), self-reported and objectively measured physical functioning (SMD 0.30, 95% CI 0.18 to 0.43; and SMD 0.22, 95% CI 0.07 to 0.38, respectively), physical functioning at activity level (SMD 0.22, 95% CI 0.01 to 0.42), ROM (SMD 0.56, 95% CI 0.14 to 0.99), and quality of life (SMD 0.24, 95% CI 0.04 to 0.45). Only two studies examined effects at 3- and 6-month follow–up, but the effects had been lost at both follow-up measurement points.

An earlier meta-analysis comparing aquatic with land-based exercise at the end of treatment for combined knee and hip OA revealed that there was a small-to-moderate effect on function (SMD 0.26, 95% CI 0.11 to 0.42) and a small-to-moderate effect on quality of life (SMD 0.32, 95% CI 0.03 to 0.61). A minor effect of a 3% absolute reduction (0.6 fewer points on a 0–20 scale) and 6.6% relative reduction from baseline was found for pain. There was no evidence of effect on walking ability or stiffness immediately after the end of treatment (Bartels et al., 2007). From the one trial including participants with hip OA alone, which compared aquatic exercise with land-based exercise, no evidence of effect on pain, function, or quality of life was observed. However, for the one study including participants with knee OA, there was a large effect on pain (SMD 0.86, 95% CI 0.25 to 1.47; 22% relative percent improvement), immediately after the treatment program but no evidence of effect on stiffness or walking ability.

Positive effects of exercise programs involving aquatic strengthening and aquatic strengthening plus flexibility on pain were also confirmed by Uthman et al. (2014).

Exercise Prior to Surgery

Only one review (Wallis & Taylor, 2011) has examined the effects of exercise prior to joint replacement surgery. They included 23 studies (1,461 participants) and found moderate-quality evidence that preoperative exercise interventions for knee OA reduced pain prior to knee replacement surgery (SMD 0.43, 95% CI 0.13 to 0.73). Meta-analyses provided evidence of low-to-moderate quality that exercise interventions for hip OA reduced pain (SMD 0.52, 95% CI 0.04 to 1.01) and improved activity (SMD 0.47, 95% CI 0.11 to 0.83) prior to hip replacement surgery. Meta-analyses provided low-quality evidence that exercise with education programs improved activity after hip replacement with reduced time to reach functional milestones during hospital stay, for example (SMD 0.50, 95% CI 0.10 to 0.90), for first-day walking.

Is Exercise Safe?

Adverse events attributed to exercise programs have been reported but these are typically small numbers (Fransen et al., 2014; Fransen et al., 2015; Waller et al., 2014), and were all related to increased pain and specifically in the knee or back (Fransen et al., 2015).

Considerations

There are many common deficiencies in the reports of the primary studies included in the reviews considered in this chapter, many of which are detailed in the extension to the Consolidated Standards of Reporting Trials (CONSORT) statement for randomized controlled trials of nonpharmacological interventions (Boutron et al., 2008). This includes the complexity of the intervention, difficulties of blinding, and the influence of care providers' expertise and volume of care of centers on treatment effect.

Many studies do not include sufficient detail to allow subsequent comparison of the exercise interventions. This information should include the dose of interventions such as duration, frequency, and intensity. Furthermore, many self-management strategies include exercise but also include other interventions such as pain management, weight reduction, education, and generalized physical activity. This makes it difficult to unpack any potential effects of exercise.

Other areas of consideration include level of supervision if any, type of supervisor, environment in which the intervention is delivered, adherence to the intervention, and method by which this is monitored, calculated, and reported. Blinding is also a particular issue for exercise interventions but not impossible, and authors should explain how they attempted to blind participants and therapists. This is of course closely related to sham therapy, again difficult but not impossible to achieve for exercise interventions. This could, for example, include the use of generalized stretching programs and and attention only activities where activities do not have any therapeutic effect but participants receive the same amount of attention as those receiving the proposed therapeutic interventions or usual care.

The choice of appropriate, valid, and reliable outcome measures is an area that should receive attention. The conclusions of a recent systematic review suggest that further good-quality research investigating measurement properties of performance (function) measures including responsiveness and interpretability in people with hip and/or knee OA is needed (Dobson et al., 2012).

Other issues relate to the duration of surveillance. This is often inadequate; typically, data ends on completion of the intervention with no follow-up or at best short-term follow-up data. It has been demonstrated that initial compliance with exercise programs is high because of loyalty to the therapist (Campbell et al., 2001). However, reasons underpinning continued compliance is more complex, involving willingness and ability to accommodate exercises within everyday life, the perceived severity of symptoms, attitudes toward arthritis and comorbidity, and previous experiences of OA. A necessary precondition for continued compliance was the perception that the exercise was effective in ameliorating unpleasant symptoms. A Cochrane review (Jordan, Holden, Mason, & Foster, 2010) concluded that interventions such as supervised or individualized exercise therapy and self-management techniques might enhance exercise adherence for chronic musculoskeletal pain in adults.

Many studies of exercise lack power; the sample size should be adequate to provide a high probability of detecting as significant an ES of a given magnitude if such an effect actually exists. Furthermore, the severity of OA of participants is frequently not quantified by the authors of studies. This could have important implications on the data obtained and conclusions drawn from these studies. Future studies should include this information, as this would allow future reviews to undertake subgroup analysis in which the intervention effect is evaluated in a defined subset of the participants by severity of symptoms. Finally, adverse event reporting is often inadequate; this can mislead by introducing a bias favoring the intervention. The emphasis on treatment benefit, together with lack of information on harmful effects, creates difficulties for people who are trying to make balanced decisions (Cochrane Adverse Effects Methods Group, 2015).

CONCLUSIONS

This chapter has summarized the findings of recent systematic reviews that have examined the effectiveness of exercise on pain and function compared with controls: land- versus water-based exercise, individual versus group exercise, and exercise prior to surgery for people with OA of the hip, the knee, and lower limb (hip and knee combined). Generally, most forms of exercise have been demonstrated to have significant positive effects on pain and function at the end of the exercise program, but unless participants continue the program, the sustainability of these effects in the longer term is questionable. However, exercise appears to be a safe intervention with few adverse effects reported.

There are a number of important considerations relating to the design and reporting of primary research in this area. Future studies are needed to determine the optimum dose of exercise programs (intensity, duration, and frequency) and to determine methods to optimize compliance with the aim of integrating exercise into people's lifestyle. It is important, however, that any further studies should be cognizant of the reporting guidelines of the CONSORT statement.

REFERENCES

Bartels, E. M., Lund, H., Hagen, K. B., Dagfinrud, H., Christensen, R., & Danneskiold-Samsøe, B. (2007). Aquatic exercise for the treatment of knee and hip osteoarthritis. *Cochrane Database of Systematic Reviews*, (4), CD005523. doi:10.1002/14651858.CD005523.pub2

Bellamy, N., Kirwan, J., Boers, M., Brooks, P., Strand, V., Tugwell, P., et al. (1997). Recommendations for a core set of outcome measures for future phase III clinical trials in knee, hip, and hand osteoarthritis. Consensus development at OMERACT III. *The Journal of Rheumatology*, *24*(4), 799–802.

Boutron, I., Moher, D., Altman, D. G., Schulz, K., Ravaud, P., & CONSORT group. (2008). Extending the CONSORT Statement to randomized trials of nonpharmacologic treatment: Explanation and elaboration. *Annals of Internal Medicine*, *148*(4), 295–309.

Brosseau, L., Pelland, L., Wells, G., Macleay, L., Lamothe, C., Michaud, G., et al. (2004). Efficacy of aerobic exercises for osteoarthritis (part II): A meta-analysis. *Physical Therapy Reviews*, *9*(3), 125–145.

Campbell, R., Evans, M., Tucker, M., Quilty, B., Dieppe, P., & Donovan, J. L. (2001). Why don't patients do their exercises? Understanding non-compliance with physiotherapy in patients with osteoarthritis of the knee. *Journal of Epidemiology Community Health*, *55*(2), 132–138. doi:10.1136/jech.55.2.132

Caspersen, C. J., Powell, K. E., & Christenson, G. M. (1985). Physical activity, exercise, and physical fitness: Definitions and distinctions for health-related research. *Public Health Reports*, *100*(2), 126–131.

Cochrane Adverse Effects Methods Group. (2015). *More about us*. Retrieved from http://aemg.cochrane.org/more-about-us

Daly Iversen, M. (2010). Managing hip and knee osteoarthritis with exercise: What is the best prescription? *Therapeutic Advances in Musculoskeletal Disease*, 2(5), 279–290.

Devos-Comby, L., Cronan, T., & Roesch, S. (2006). Do exercise and self-management interventions benefit patients with osteoarthritis of the knee? A metaanalytic review. *The Journal of Rheumatology*, 33, 744–756.

Dobson, F., Hinman, R. S., Hall, M., Terwee, C. B., Roos, E. M., & Bennell, K. L. (2012). Measurement properties of performance-based measures to assess physical function in hip and knee osteoarthritis: A systematic review. *Osteoarthritis Cartilage*, *20*(12), 1548–1562. doi:10.1016/j.joca.2012.08.015

Focht, B. C. (2006). Effectiveness of exercise interventions in reducing pain symptoms among older adults with knee osteoarthritis: A review. *Journal of Aging and Physical Activity*, *14*(2), 212–235.

Fransen, M., McConnell, S., Harmer, A., Van der Esch, M., Simic, M., & Bennell Kim, L. (2015). Exercise for osteoarthritis of the knee. *Cochrane Database of Systematic Reviews*, (1), CD004376. doi:10.1002/14651858.CD004376.pub3

Fransen, M., McConnell, S., Hernandez-Molina, G., & Reichenbach, S. (2014). Exercise for osteoarthritis of the hip. *Cochrane Database of Systematic Reviews*, (4), CD007912. doi:10.1002/14651858.CD007912.pub2

Hernández-Molina, G., Reichenbach, S., Zhang, B., Lavalley, M., & Felson, D. (2008). Effect of therapeutic exercise for hip osteoarthritis pain: Results of a meta-analysis. *Arthritis and Rheumatism*, *59*(9), 1221–1228.

Hootman, J., & Helmick, C. (2006). Projections of US prevalence of arthritis and associated activity limitations. *Arthritis and Rheumatism*, *54*, 226–229.

Hootman, J., Macera, C., Ham, S., Helmick, C., & Sniezek, J. (2003). Physical activity levels among the general US adult population and in adults with and without arthritis. *Arthritis Rheumatism*, *49*, 129–135.

Howe, T. E., Rochester, L., Neil, F., Skelton, D. A., & Ballinger, C. (2011). Exercise for improving balance in older people. *Cochrane Database of Systematic Reviews*, (11), CD004963. doi: 10.1002/14651858.CD004963.pub3

Howe, T. E., Shea, B., Dawson, L. J., Downie, F., Murray, A., Ross, C., et al. (2011). Exercise for preventing and treating osteoporosis in postmenopausal women. *Cochrane Database of Systematic Reviews*, (7), CD000333. doi: 10.1002/14651858.CD000333.pub2

Jansen, M. J., Viechtbauer, W., Lenssen, A. F., Hendriks, E. J. M., & de Bic, R. A. (2011). Strength training alone, exercise therapy alone, and exercise therapy with passive manual mobilization each reduce pain and disability in people with knee osteoarthritis: A systematic review. *Journal of Physiotherapy*, *57*(1), 11–20. doi: http://dx.doi.org/10.1016/S1836-9553(11)70002-9

Jordan, J., Holden, M A., Mason, E., & Foster, N. (2010). Interventions to improve adherence to exercise for chronic musculoskeletal pain in adults. *Cochrane Database of Systematic Reviews*, (1), CD005956. doi:10.1002/14651858.CD005956.pub2

Juhl, C., Christensen, R., Roos, E., Zhang, W., & Lund, H. (2014). Impact of exercise type and dose on pain and disability in knee osteoarthritis: A systematic review and meta-regression analysis of randomized controlled trials. *Arthritis and Rheumatology*, *66*(3), 622–636. doi:10.1002/art.38290

March, L., Smith, E. U., Hoy, D. G., Cross, M. J., Sanchez-Riera, L., Blyth, F., et al. (2014). Burden of disability due to musculoskeletal (MSK) disorders. *Best Practice & Research.Clinical Rheumatology*, *28*(3), 353–366. doi:10.1016/j.berh.2014.08.002

McAlindon, T., Bannuru, R., Sullivan, M., Arden, N., Berenbaum, F., Bierma-Zeinstra, S., et al. (2014). OARSI guidelines for the non-surgical management of knee osteoarthritis. *Osteoarthritis and Cartilage*, *22*(3), 363–388. doi:10.1016/j.joca.2014.01.003

Murphy, L. B., Helmick, C. G., Schwartz, T. A., Renner, J. B., Tudor, G., Koch, G., et al. (2010). One in four people may develop symptomatic hip osteoarthritis in his or her lifetime. *Osteoarthritis and Cartilage*, *18*(11), 1372–1379.

Murphy, L. B., Schwartz, T. A., Helmick, C. G., Renner, J. B., Tudor, G., Koch, G., et al. (2008). Lifetime risk of symptomatic knee osteoarthritis. *Arthritis and Rheumatism*, *59*, 1207–1213.

Paskins, Z., Sanders, T., & Hassell, A. (2014). Comparison of patient experiences of the osteoarthritis consultation with GP attitudes and beliefs to OA: A narrative review. *BMC Family Practice*, *15*, 46.

Pelland, L., Brosseau, L., Wells, G., MacLeay, L., Lambert, J., Lamothe, C., et al. Tugwell, P. (2004). Efficacy of strengthening exercises for osteoarthritis (part 1): A meta-analysis. *Physical Therapy Reviews*, *9*(2), 77–108.

Petrella, R. J. (2000). Is exercise effective treatment for osteoarthritis of the knee? *British Journal of Sports Medicine*, *34*(5), 326–331. doi:10.1136/bjsm.34.5.326

Pisters, M. F., Veenhof, C., Meeteren, N. L., Ostelo, R. W., Bakker, D. H., Schellevis, F. G., & Dekker, J. (2007). Long-term effectiveness of exercise therapy in patients with osteoarthritis of the hip or knee: A systematic review. *Arthritis and Rheumatism*, *57*(7), 1245–1253.

Roddy, E., Zhang, W., & Doherty, M. (2005). Aerobic walking or strengthening exercise for osteoarthritis of the knee: A systematic review. *Annals of the Rheumatic Diseases*, *64*(4), 544–548.

Roddy, E., Zhang, W., Doherty, M., Arden, N. K., Barlow, J., Birrell, F., et al. (2006). Evidence-based clinical guidelines: A new system to better determine true strength of recommendation. *Journal of Evaluation in Clinical Practice*, *12*(3), 347–352.

Romeo, A., Parazza, S., Boschi, M., Nava, T., & Vanti, C. (2013). Manual therapy and therapeutic exercise in the treatment of osteoarthritis of the hip: A systematic review. *Reumatismo*, *65*(2), 63–74. doi:10.4081/reumatismo.2013.63

Tanaka, R., Ozawa, J., Kito, N., & Moriyama, H. (2013). Efficacy of strengthening or aerobic exercise on pain relief in people with knee osteoarthritis: A systematic review and meta-analysis of randomized controlled trials. *Clinical Rehabilitation*, *27*(12), 1059–1071.

Tiffreau, V., Mulleman, D., Coudeyre, E., Lefevre-Colau, M. M., Revel, M., & Rannou, F. (2007). The value of individual or collective group exercise programs for knee or hip osteoarthritis: Elaboration of French clinical practice guidelines. *Annales de Readaptation et de Medecine Physique*, *50*(9), 741–746.

Uthman, O. A., van der Windt, D. A., Jordan, J. L., Dziedzic, K. S., Healey, E. L., Peat, G. M., & Foster, N. E. (2014). Exercise for lower limb osteoarthritis: Systematic review incorporating trial sequential analysis and network meta-analysis. *British Journal of Sports Medicine*, *48*(21), 1579.

van Baar, M., Assendelft, W., Dekker, J., Oostendorp, R., & Bijlsma, J. (1999). Effectiveness of exercise therapy in patients with osteoarthritis of the hip or knee: A systematic review of randomized clinical trials. *Arthritis and Rheumatism*, *42*(7), 1361–1369.

Waller, B., Ogonowska-Slodownik, A., Vitor, M., Lambeck, J., Daly, D., Kujala, U. M., & Heinonen, A. (2014). Effect of therapeutic aquatic exercise on symptoms and function associated with lower limb osteoarthritis: A systematic review with meta-analysis. *Physical Theraphy*, *94*(10), 1383–1395. doi:10.2522/ptj.20130417

Wallis, J. A., & Taylor, N. F. (2011). Pre-operative interventions (non-surgical and non-pharmacological) for patients with hip or knee osteoarthritis awaiting joint replacement surgery--a systematic review and meta-analysis. *Osteoarthritis and Cartilage / OARS, Osteoarthritis Research Society*, *19*(12), 1381–1395. doi:10.1016/j.joca.2011.09.001

World Health Organization. (2010a). *Global recommendations on physical activity for health*. Retrieved from http://apps.who.int/iris/bitstream/10665/44399/1/9789241599979_eng.pdf

World Health Organization. (2010b). *International classification of functioning, disability and health (ICF)*. Retrieved from http://www.who.int/classifications/icf/en/

CHAPTER 7

The Flexibility Debate

Implications for Health and Function as We Age

Liza Stathokostas and Anthony A. Vandervoort

ABSTRACT

Flexibility is the range of motion (ROM) available in a joint or group of joints and can be increased via a flexibility or stretching program. Despite the well-established and long-standing inclusion of stretching programs for fitness routines, there are currently scientific discussions regarding the utility of stretching exercises, which are regularly recommended for overall health and conducted as a part of preexercise protocols to reduce injury and increase performance in athletic-type activities. The implication of this "debate" for the older adult population warrants further discussion, as age-related declines in joint-specific ROM are observed. For the majority of the aging population, ROM status may not be related to fitness activity performance but rather to performance of the activities of daily living. For this reason, the promotion of flexibility in the older adult population is substantial. This chapter reviews the age-related declines of various body parts and how they may relate to function and quality of life as we age. Existing recommendations are based on limited evidence precluding the offering of guidance as to a flexibility intervention related to maintaining or improving functional ROM for older adults.

While ROM decreases with age, older adults do maintain the ability to regain ROM. This chapter summarizes the role of physical activity levels and exercise interventions in the maintenance and training of ROM. The pressing need for high-quality, purposive study of flexibility is warranted in order to establish the magnitude of impact on function.

http://dx.doi.org/10.1891/0198-8794.36.169

INTRODUCTION

Physical fitness standards have been proposed to identify the level of fitness and physical activity needed to remain independent as we age (Rikli & Jones, 2013), and high levels of evidence demonstrate the significant role of exercise training in increasing and maintaining physical fitness across the older adult age range (Paterson & Warburton, 2010). In fact, recently updated international physical activity guidelines are focused on minimum prescriptions of physical fitness components for optimal functional health as well as overall health (Paterson & Warburton, 2010). Whereas the utility of some components of physical fitness (cardiorespiratory fitness and muscle strength and power) are supported by high levels of evidence, one component of physical fitness, flexibility, is not.

The inclusion of flexibility exercise (i.e., stretching) has been a long-standing one in health, fitness, and sport prescriptions. Early recommendations include static stretching as a critical component of warm-up prior to exercise, largely for the purpose of injury prevention. While widespread acceptance of preexercise stretching exists among the general public's consciousness, the past decade has seen a challenge to this long-standing view and the lack of strong evidence (specifically randomized controlled trials [RCTs]) for its support has been identified (Thacker, Gilchrist, Stroup, & Kimsey, 2004). The recommendation for stretching before exercise and as an activity in and of itself is even more pervasive when applied to the older adult population. There is an inordinate amount of emphasis and promotion of the importance of flexibility for older adults, but as in the younger populations, it is unwarranted based on current best evidence (Stathokostas, Little, Vandervoort, & Paterson, 2012). This is not to say that there is no relationship, but rather that one has not yet been demonstrated conclusively. In fact, a lack of evidence recommending stretching routines outside of a rehabilitative context has been identified (Stathokostas et al., 2012).

Simply stated, flexibility is the range of motion (ROM) available in a joint or group of joints; functionally, it can be considered the joint's ability to pass through a given ROM without significant impingement or restriction in performing a given task (American College of Sports Medicine [ASCM], 2014) and can be increased by various methods of stretching (Table 7.1). The ROM of any joint is determined by the distensibility of the joint capsule, muscle viscosity, and the compliance of ligaments and tendons. Two types of connective tissue can affect ROM: fibrous connective tissue (fascia, ligaments, and tendons, consisting primarily of collagen) and elastic connective tissue, many of which undergo changes as a result of immobilization and/or aging. For example, degenerative changes of the intervertebral disc and surrounding structures can lead to alteration of the mechanical properties of the functional spinal unit, with a trend toward spinal stiffening with the increasing degeneration (Galbusera et al., 2014). Flexible,

TABLE 7.1
Various Stretching Techniques

Stretching Technique	Description
Ballistic stretching	Rapid lengthening of the muscle by use of bouncing movements
Dynamic stretching	Gradual progression through movement
Isometric stretching	Static stretching against an immobile force
Passive stretching	Slow sustained muscle lengthening with a partner
Proprioceptive neuromuscular facilitation	Passive muscle lengthening with a partner after an antagonistic muscle contraction
Static stretching	Slow, sustained muscle lengthening held for some duration

pain-free joints are important for well-being, and so the informal observations made of those of advanced age and subjectively reported feelings about "stiffness" by older adults cannot be ignored. However, we need to delineate the primary aging process from the clinical condition of stiffness (the common residual problem of joint immobilization, joint contracture) and investigate whether it is possible to remain "vital and supple" into older age (with/without flexibility training).

AGE-RELATED CHANGES IN FLEXIBILITY WITH AGE

Joint flexibility may decrease across the age span (beginning in mid- to late-20s) (Nonaka et al., 2002; Roach & Miles, 1991; Shields et al., 2010), with the rate of decline dependent on the body part measured, the training status of the sample, and population being studied. For example, a loss of as much as 50% has been observed between young and old in spinal extension (Einkauf, Gohdes, Jensen, & Jewell, 1987) and ankle mobility (Vandervoort et al., 1992). Specific to the older age range, the rate of decline in a generally healthy sample has been shown to be 0.5° per year in males and 0.6° per year in females of upper body flexibility (shoulder abduction) and declines in hip flexion of 0.6° per year in males and 0.7° per year in females (Stathokostas, McDonald, Little, & Paterson, 2013). A 1% decline per year in shoulder abduction ROM of older men and women has been reported in a sample reporting high disability (Bassey, Morgan, Dallosso, & Ebrahim, 1989). Rates of 1.5° per year have been reported for lower back flexion (Einkauf et al., 1987).

Potential critical periods of decline in flexibility across the older adult age range have been identified. James and Parker (James & Parker, 1989) reported decreases in active and passive motion in lower limb joints during the period of 70 to 92 years, with the decline becoming more pronounced during the ninth decade. While not significant, Charkravarty and Webley (Chakravarty & Webley, 1993) reported a greater decline in ROM in a group over the age of 75 years versus an age group 65–74 years, adding support for the trend for an accelerated decline in flexibility in the oldest old. Recently, using piecewise linear regression, an accelerated decline was documented to occur at age of 71 years in both upper and lower body flexibility, as shown in Figures 7.1–7.4 (Stathokostas et al., 2013).

FLEXIBILITY, AGE, AND FUNCTIONAL CAPACITY

The observed declines in flexibility with age are purported to affect normal daily function. It is often mentioned that upper body flexibility is known to be important for activities such as getting dressed and reaching for objects and that lower body flexibility is important for maintaining normal walking patterns and activities involving bending and reaching. These associative statements are most often inferred, and there is surprisingly a paucity of evidence that directly links changes in joint specific flexibility with matched functional outcomes. One of the most thoroughly studied joints is the ankle, with decreased strength

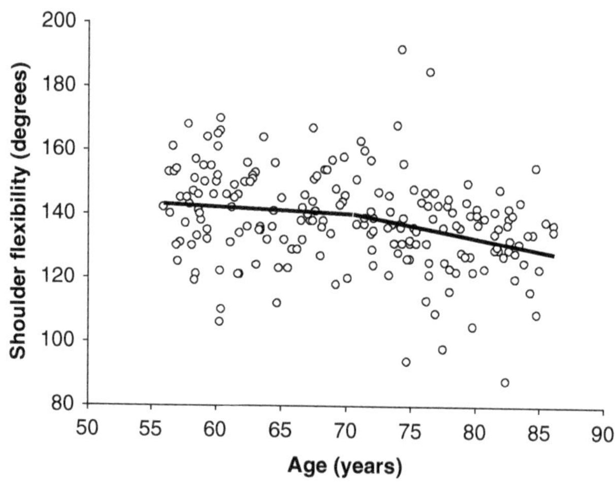

FIGURE 7.1 Age analysis for shoulder flexibility in men. Piecewise linear regression s-segment model shows breaking at age 71 years. Rate of decline prior to age 71 is –0.20° per year and –0.80° per year thereafter (R^2 of fit $R^2 = 0.09$). Reproduced with permission from Stathokostas et al. (2013).

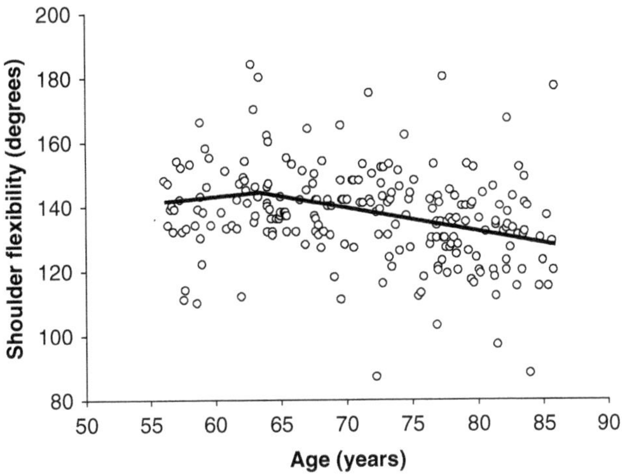

FIGURE 7.2 Age analysis for shoulder flexibility in women. Piecewise linear regression s-segment model shows breaking at age 63 years. Rate of change prior to age 63 is 0.38° per year and –0.74° per year thereafter (R^2 of fit $R^2 = 0.09$). Reproduced with permission from Stathokostas et al. (2013).

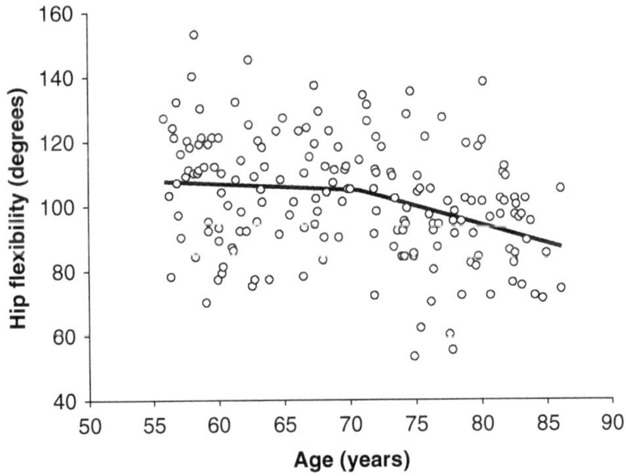

FIGURE 7.3 Age analysis for hip flexion in men. Piecewise linear regression s-segment model shows breaking at age 71 years. The rate of decline prior to 71 years is –0.19° per year and –1.16° per year thereafter (R^2 of fit $R^2 = 0.11$). Reproduced with permission from Stathokostas et al. (2013).

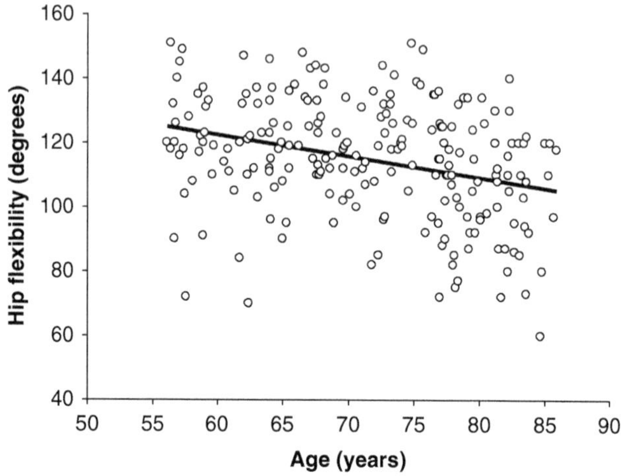

FIGURE 7.4 Age analysis for hip flexion in women. Piecewise linear regression s-segment model shows breaking at age 86 years. The rate of decline prior to 86 years is –0.66° per year and –2.67° per year thereafter (R^2 of fit R^2 = 0.08). Reproduced with permission from Stathokostas et al. (2013).

and flexibility of the muscles around the ankle joint identified as risk factors for falls with age, as shown in Figure 7.5 (Vandervoort, 1999). Tainaka, Takizawa, Katamoto, and Aoki (2009) showed that ankle dorsiflexion ROM was a significant physical fitness factor in predicting 6-year incidence of disability. Shoulder flexibility was also identified as one determinant of independence when comparing a group of independently living older adults versus those in rest or nursing homes. Conversely, there was no association between hip flexion changes with age and self-reported difficulty with stair climbing (Stathokostas et al., 2013). Finally, we compared our results to reference values, indicating that shoulder abduction ROM of 120° and hip flexion values of 30°–50° (for most hip-related functional activities) were considered to be lower end thresholds associated with functional loss (Badley, Wagstaff, & Wood, 1984). Using the "reference" that a value of <120° was related to functional loss, among our community-dwelling, disability-free sample, the probability of the age-related decline in shoulder flexibility falling to below the reference values was very low; less than approximately 10 subjects beyond age 75 years fell below this "functional threshold," and the average for the 85-year-old was close to 130°. For hip flexibility, we were not aware of any similar data to establish a functional threshold. These studies might suggest that the roles of flexibility and function with aging are population dependent and may not be as influential in younger or healthy subgroups of older adults. For example, in a large sample of older adults reporting reduced mobility,

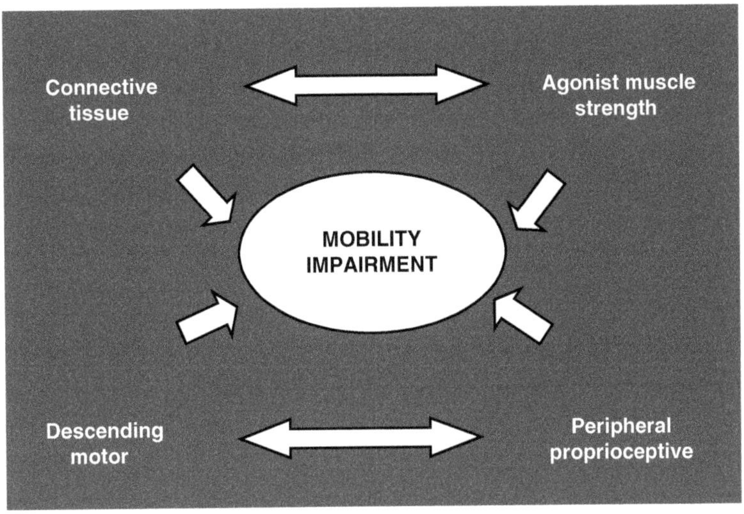

FIGURE 7.5 Key factors in joint mobility. Adapted with permission from Vandervoort (1999).

for activities that involve a high level of physical ability and endurance, such as walking several blocks or getting up from the floor, trunk extensor muscle endurance and knee flexion ROM were important (Bean et al., 2013).

FLEXIBILITY, AGING, AND QUALITY OF LIFE

It has been reported that older adults find personal benefits of physical activity (posed collectively as strength, balance, and flexibility; Franco et al., 2015). In addition, physical function has been shown to be positively associated with perceived quality of life (QOL) in older persons as assessed by the Short Physical Performance Battery (Fusco et al., 2012). However, the direct and independent relationship of flexibility with QOL, well-being, and successful aging has been not been adequately studied. The limited studies in this area indicate that upper and lower body flexibility were not associated with self-rated health and life satisfaction in a sample of independently living, generally healthy older adults (Stathokostas et al., 2013), whereas life satisfaction and social engagement was associated with shoulder ROM in a large sample of older men and women living with a specific arthritis-related disability in that joint (Bassey et al.,1989). Similarly, a study of nonagenarians where almost half the sample reported an orthopedic condition or chronic condition, observed a significant association between upper body flexibility and health-related QOL (Fabre et al., 2007). However, in contrast, proprioception and flexibility (sit and reach) were not correlated with the Short Form-12 (SF-12) in a sample of nursing home residents (Ozcan, Donat, Gelecek, Ozdirenc, & Karadibak, 2005). Low-active older adults increased QOL in a combined strengthening and flexibility intervention (Awick et al., 2015). Spinal ROM in middle- and older-aged adults was associated with QOL (Imagama et al., 2011). While further research is required to understand the role of flexibility in QOL and successful aging, an association is likely related to the presence of a disability or a range of joint motion below some critical threshold.

FLEXIBILITY, PHYSICAL ACTIVITY LEVELS, AND AGING

Although the loss in flexibility with age has been attributable, in part, to decreased activity (i.e., the difference in rate of change in flexibility across joints has been attributed to the degree of use of those joints), the literature describing the influence of physical activity on flexibility and the aging process is limited. The approach of investigating whether "flexibility training" is warranted in older adults by observing whether overall physical activity levels are sufficient to maintain ROM with age is intriguing. It has been established that efforts greater than those provided by activities of daily living or light activities are needed for cardiorespiratory and muscular fitness and functional gains (Paterson & Warburton, 2010). No relationship between self-reported overall physical activity levels and upper or lower body flexibility has been reported (Stathokostas et al., 2013). Similarly, no relationship was observed when physical activity was classified into high and low physical activity categories (Walker, Sue, & Miles-Elkousy, 1984) or when comparing sedentary versus active older adults (Miotto, Chodzko-Zajko, Reich, & Supler, 1999). Bassey et al. (1989) studied the association between shoulder abduction and self-reported customary use of the shoulder and found an association; however, it should be noted that the effect was not significant in women in multiple regression (replaced by effort score), and the effect of customary use was greater in those with a disability. This finding may suggest that a more closely matched flexibility and activity-specific measurement is more reflective of the role of physical activity in the change in flexibility with age.

Further insight is gained when identifying studies of structured, purposeful, repetitive physical activity, that is, exercise. In a small sample of 30 older women, Rikli and Bush (1986) found a significant difference for trunk and shoulder flexibility in active versus nonactive women, where active meant vigorous activity for at least 30 minutes, 3 days per week. This study reported a significant age-by-activity interaction for shoulder flexibility but not for trunk flexion. Voorrips (Voorrips, Lemmink, van Heuvelen, Bult, & van Staveren, 1993), in a sample of 50 women with a mean age of 72 years, reported significantly greater flexion at the hip and spine in women who self-reported high activity levels (several hours per week in aerobic-type exercises). A 5-year longitudinal study by Lan (Lan, Chen, & Lai, 2008) demonstrated that baseline and follow-up thoracolumbar flexibility values were higher in older adults participating in a Chinese conditioning program of repeated motions and postures with ROM warm-up versus a sedentary control group. Further, while both groups showed an age-related decline over the 5 years, the control group had a larger decline in flexibility, supporting a positive role of "physical activity" in attenuating the decline in flexibility with age.

FLEXIBILITY TRAINING AND AGING

While it would appear that overall daily physical activity does not positively influence flexibility in older adults, there may be a role for more structured physical activity. As indicated in the studies in the preceding text, flexibility appears to change with engagement in a general exercise or fitness program. Recently, flexibility has been shown to increase in older adults after interventions involving Pilates (Bullo et al., 2015) and resistance training (Carneiro et al., 2015). However, these studies do not focus solely on the role or individual contribution of flexibility training.

Flexibility training encompasses a planned, deliberate, and regular program of exercises that can progressively increase the useable ROM of a joint or set of joints over a period of time, thereby allowing older adults to optimize their flexibility. In an attempt to establish evidence-based guidelines for the prescription of flexibility exercises, we have previously detailed the literature related to interventions specifically designed for flexibility improvement and observation of resultant functional outcomes (26 studies; Stathokostas et al., 2012). Based on the available literature, the review was not able to provide a consensus on flexibility-training prescription for healthy older adults due to the lack of studies solely involving flexibility training and due to the lack of consistency in the flexibility protocols employed. Furthermore, this review found variation in the value of flexibility training for functional outcomes that may be related to the maintenance of independence in daily activities of older adults. The more influential and high-quality studies of community-dwelling older adults in this review (Table 7.2) showed very comparable effects to the overall outcomes of the 26 studies, namely, variation regarding the value of flexibility training for functional outcomes that may be related to the maintenance of independence in daily activities of older adults. In a subgroup of the very old (≥80 years), frail, and assisted-living populations, there were significant improvements seen in functional reach, sit-to-stand, and 30 meter walk times, but no changes in the physical performance test, and mixed results were observed for flexibility, strength, balance, and timed up-and-go tests. This subgroup was very similar to the rest of the populations in terms of interventions received, although this group had less consistency in the flexibility-related outcome measures. Frequency and duration differences between studies showed no noticeable differences. When different muscle groups were targeted, the flexibility outcomes were expectantly fairly body part specific. Regarding the different flexibility-training methods, active assisted stretching had positive and sometimes significant improvements in several outcome measures as compared to the inactive control group but these were less significant than the improvements seen with the proprioceptive neuromuscular facilitation (PNF) techniques. Weighted flexibility exercises were similar to nonweighted exercises in one study but significantly better than nonweighted exercises in another. One study showed agonist contract–relax PNF to be much more effective than contract–relax PNF and static stretching for both ROM and electromyography activity. The overall results point to PNF stretching being more effective than non-PNF techniques for improving flexibility outcomes but not necessarily functional outcome measures. More recently, a practical protocol of flexibility training for spinal ROMs was proposed and resulted in significant increases in sacral/hip and thoracic ROMs (Battaglia et al., 2014); however, no functional outcomes were related to those changes. Due to the low level of evidence and grade available to formulate a prescription for flexibility training, the current Canadian Physical Activity Guidelines for Older Adults do not include a comment on flexibility (Canadian Society for Exercise Physiology, 2011). However, guidance for the improvement in ROM when needed can be found in the ASCM Position Stand for Exercise and Physical Activity for Older Adults (2009), which also identifies the need for further work in this area.

While flexibility training interventions has been shown to increase flexibility and joint ROM in older adults, future studies should consider the relationship that increased flexibility and joint ROM have with functional outcomes to determine if the increased flexibility is beneficial and worthwhile in terms of maintaining or increasing functional capacity for healthy older adults.

THE ROLE OF FLEXIBILITY IN WARM-UP PRIOR TO AN EXERCISE SESSION

While the lack of evidence precludes informing a concise prescription for flexibility in older adults, much can still be gleaned from resources aimed at young and middle-aged adults. The main goal of a warm-up, as indicated by its name, is to engage in submaximal aerobic activity for the purpose of raising body (and thus muscle) temperature by 1–2°C (Young & Behm, 2002). The rise in muscle temperature results in increased muscle compliance, increased nerve conduction

TABLE 7.2

Flexibility Training Studies Examining the Relationship Between Flexibility and Functional Abilities in Older Adults

Publication Study Type	Objective	Methods	Outcomes	Comments and Conclusions
Bird et al., 2009 Randomized crossover trial Focus: major muscle groups	To determine the effect of community-based resistance-training (RT) vs. flexibility-training (FT) programs on balance and related measures	n = 32 Age: mean 67 yr Males = 18, females = 14 *Pre-post:* 16 wks, 4-wk washout, 16 wks (crossover) *Intervention* Both groups had 3 sessions wk^{-1} for 16 wks, then 4-wk washout, then switch to other group for 16 wks RT: 2–3 sets of 10–12 repetitions FT: 40–45 min with 16–20 stretches; two stretches for each of hamstrings, quadriceps, back, and chest *Assessments* Balance, force plate Timed up and go (UG) 10 times sit to stand Step test Lower limb strength (right and left knee—flexion and extension) with an isokinetic dynamometer	Lower limb strength increased significantly in the RT group, but not in the flexibility group and there was a significant difference between the two groups. Significant improvements were seen in both groups for timed UG, 10 times sit to stand, and step test. Significant improvements in medial–lateral sway *range* were seen in the flexibility group only. Significant decreases in sway *velocity* were seen in both conditions.	Significant improvements in balance performance were achieved with both RT and standing FT programs in healthy untrained older adults. Flexibility program did incorporate some degree of balance training in the nature of the flexibility tasks.

(*Continued*)

TABLE 7.2

Flexibility Training Studies Examining the Relationship Between Flexibility and Functional Abilities in Older Adults (*Continued*)

Publication Study Type	Objective	Methods	Outcomes	Comments and Conclusions
Brown et al., 2000 Randomized controlled trial (RCT) Focus: major muscle groups	To examine effects of low-intensity exercise on factors associated with frailty (gait, flexibility, strength, balance, sensation, response time, coordination) vs. flexibility control group	n = 87 Age: 83 ± 4 yr *Pre-post:* 3 mo *Intervention* EXER: 22 low-intensity strength and flexibility exercise for upper and lower body 3x/wks for total of 36 sessions (~3 mo) HOME: 9 upper and lower body flexibility exercises Conducted at home (self-report), option to participate on site 1·wk^{-1} *Assessments* Strength: physical performance test, isokinetic dynamometer (knee flexors/extensors, ankle flexors/extensors), handheld dynamometer (upper extremities)	*Strength* Significant increases in knee flexor and extensor strength (9% change vs. −1% in control), and shoulder abductors. *Range of motion (ROM)* Flexibility increased in all measurements and in both groups. *Balance* Significant improvements in EXER group for obstacle course, full tandem of Romberg, Berg balance test, and one-limb standing time. No significant changes in control group.	These results suggest that the more comprehensive the exercise intervention, the greater the likely scope of improvement in frailty.

		ROM: goniometry (shoulders, hips, knees, ankles, trunk) Balance: static (Romberg test), dynamic (balance bean, obstacle course, and gait speed), and weight shift (Berg balance test) Gait: pressure-sensitive foot switches Coordination: Purdue peg board Speed of response: red light to green light, stepping on brake and gas pedals Sensation: Semmes-Weinstein monofilaments	*Gait* Significant change in preferred walking cadence in EXER group. *Coordination* Difference between groups was "*almost* significant." *Response time* Unchanged in both groups. Sensation: No apparent differences.	
King et al., 2000 RCT Focus: major muscle groups	To evaluate the effects of two different community-based physical activity regimens—on 1-yr physical performance outcomes, perceived functioning, and well-being in a sample of community-dwelling, sedentary women and men	n = 103 Age: 70 ± 4 yr Males = 36, females = 67 *Pre-post*: 12 mo, 6 mo interim assessment 2 exercise classes/wk and home exercise at least 2·wk^{-1} Classes 1 hr, home exercise built up to 40-min sessions	(values reported separately for men and women for each group) *Functional capacity/endurance* Submax HR: Fit & Firm had significantly greater improvement vs. Stretch & Flex. *Strength and flexibility* Lift-and-reach task: Fit & Firm had significantly greater upper body strength than Stretch & Flex. Sit to stand: No significant results.	Community-based physical activity regimens focusing on moderate-intensity endurance and strengthening exercises or flexibility exercises can be delivered through a combination of formats that result in improvements in important functional and quality-of-life outcomes.

(*Continued*)

TABLE 7.2

Flexibility Training Studies Examining the Relationship Between Flexibility and Functional Abilities in Older Adults (*Continued*)

Publication Study Type	Objective	Methods	Outcomes	Comments and Conclusions
		Experimental group (Fit & Firm) Progressive moderate-intensity endurance and strengthening exercises 5–10 min warm-up, 40–45 min aerobic and strength-training circuit, 5–10 min cooldown; target heart rate 60%–75% HRR Control group (Stretch & Flex) Stretching and flexibility exercises 5–10 min warm-up, 40 min stretching section, 5–10 min relaxation exercises; stretching for neck, shoulders, back, chest, waist, hamstrings, calves, and hands *Assessments* Functional capacity/endurance: Graded treadmill exercise test (GXT) Strength and flexibility: Upper body strength (lift-and-reach task), lower body strength (sit to stand), and flexibility (sit and reach [SR] with Accuflex 1 Sit and Reach box) Self-rated physical performance: a self-efficacy questionnaire	SR: Men assigned to Stretch & Flex had significantly greater increases than men in Fit & Firm. No statistical difference in women, but trend for greater improvement for women in Fit & Firm vs. Stretch & Flex. Women in Fit & Firm had significantly greater increases in flexibility at 12 mo than men. *Self-rated physical performance* Significantly greater increases in walking distance and self-efficacy for heavy lifting in Fit & Firm than in Stretch & Flex. *Perceived functioning and well-being* Only pain scale had significantly greater effects for Stretch & Flex (also statistically significant within group) than Fit & Firm.	

		Perceived functioning and well-being: scales from the Medical Outcomes Study (MOS) including physical functioning, bodily pain, emotional well-being, energy/fatigue, sleep problems, sense of mastery, and self-esteem		
Klein, Stone, Phillips, Gangi, & Hartman, 2002 Prospective two-stage intervention Focus: major muscle groups	To examine the impact of proprioceptive neuromuscular facilitation (PNF) on physical function in an assisted-living population by assessing ROM and isometric strength	$n = 14$ Age: 87 ± 6.5 yr Male = 2, female = 12 Baseline (T1), pre-training (T2, 5 wks), post-training (T3, 10 wks) Pre-training 1 wk^{-1} visit with trainer to increase rapport and interest in participation *Training program* 40–60 min, 2 wk^{-1} Warm-up, cool down, and flexibility (single set 15–20 min, later 2–3 sets) Flexibility: 8 exercises using passive contract–relax PNF technique (6 s isometric contraction, then passive stretch held for 20 s, then 20 s rest). Hamstrings, gluteals, shins, calves, and back	$n = 11$ Statistically significant differences in 6 of 18 variables: Sit to stand decreased significantly from 9.33 to 7.91 s ($p = 0.42$). No change in balance, get up and go, single-leg stand. Ankle flexion ROM decreased (improved) from 26.25° to 20.27° ($p = 0.009$). Shoulder-flexion ROM increased from 163.8 ° to 177.6° (p=0.016). No change in hip flexion, hip extension, ankle extension, functional reach, SR.	PNF flexibility training can improve ROM, isometric strength, and selected physical function tasks in assisted-living older adults. Because the training period was short, 10 wks, the results suggest that continued training might have a greater impact on physical function and the ability to perform routine daily activities.

(*Continued*)

TABLE 7.2

Flexibility Training Studies Examining the Relationship Between Flexibility and Functional Abilities in Older Adults (Continued)

Publication Study Type	Objective	Methods	Outcomes	Comments and Conclusions
		Assessments Isometric strength (dynamometer), flexibility (bubble inclinometer for shoulders, hips, and ankles; SR for spine; functional reach for shoulder) Mobility: get-up-and-go test, sit to stand	Significant increases in strength for hip extension and ankle flexion/extension. No change in hip flexion, shoulder extension, shoulder flexion strength.	
Stanziano, Roos, Perry, Lai, & Signoril, 2009 RCT Focus: major muscle groups	To examine impact of an active assisted (AA) flexibility program on ROM and functional performance variables in older persons living in a residential retirement community (RRC)	n = 17 Age: 88 ± 5.4 yr Experimental group n = 8 90 ± 4.5 yr 1 male, 7 female Control group n = 9 88 ± 6.2 yr 3 male, 6 female *Pre-post:* 8 wks; $2 \cdot wk^{-1}$	n = 13 Flexibility Significant increases in ROM made by experimental group for all measures but left-side BS and right-side SR. Control group showed no change in any flexibility measure but a significant loss in ROM for right-side knee extension.	Eight wks of AA stretching may be an effective intervention for improving ROM, mobility, and functional power for older persons living in an RRC. Data provide clear link between flexibility and functional performance in older persons and support the inclusion of flexibility training in interventions designed to increase independence in older persons.

Experimental group 10 stretches: back scratch (BS; shoulder flexion/abduction), standing thigh (hip hyperextension), side lunge (hip abduction), overhead back (shoulder hyperflexion), overhead side (lateral trunk flexion), cross chest (horizontal shoulder adduction), seated trunk twist (trunk rotation), seated hamstring (trunk/hip flexion), and seated calf (dorsiflexion) 10 repetitions, 4–5 s each Control group Arts and crafts class with limited physical exertion *Assessment* Conducted 1 wk pretraining and posttraining period Flexibility: BS test; modified chair SR test; Supine knee extension (KE) test; modified total body rotation (BR) test	Functionality Experimental group significantly improved CS and MRPT, while control had significant declines. Experimental group significantly improved in AC and the GJST, while control had no change. Experimental group reduced time taken to complete the UG and GS.

(*Continued*)

TABLE 7.2

Flexibility Training Studies Examining the Relationship Between Flexibility and Functional Abilities in Older Adults (*Continued*)

Publication Study Type	Objective	Methods	Outcomes	Comments and Conclusions
		Strength/power: 30-s chair stand (CS); modified ramp power test (MRPT); 30-s arm curl (AC); gallon jug shelf test (GJST) Mobility: 50-foot gait speed test (GS); 8-foot timed UG		
Takeshima et al., 2007 Non-RCT Focus: major muscle groups	To compare the effects of a walking-based aerobic program, a band-based resistance program, a stretching flexibility program, a customized balance program, and a Tai Chi program on functional fitness in a group of community older adults	n = 117 73 ± 6 yr 64 male, 49 female *Pre-post:* 12 wks *Intervention* Supervised 2 days· wk^{-1} (RES, BAL, FLEX, T-CHI) 3 days per wk (AER) AER—outdoor walking RES—progressive elastic band exercises for all major muscle groups BAL—eyes open/closed, exercise on floor, on foam mats FLEX—15 static stretches for upper and lower body (15–20 s each) T-CHI—standardized 24 forms	Improvement in cardiorespiratory fitness (12-min walk) was limited to AER (16%) RES, BAL, AND T-CHI resulted in improvements in upper and lower body strength and balance/agility. RES showed greatest upper body strength improvement (31%). BAL showed greatest lower body strength improvement (40%). Balance/agility were similar across RES, BAL, AND T-CHI (10%).	It is recommended that older adults participate in a well-rounded exercise program vs. single mode. RES, BAL, and TAI CHI cross domains not specifically targeted in their design. AER necessitates aerobic-specific activity to improve cardiorespiratory fitness.

	Assessments Functional fitness 30-s AC test 30-s CS time 3-foot timed UG BS test Chair SR Test 12-min walk test	Functional reach, similar improvements for AER (13%), BAL (16%), RES (15%). No significant changes in either FLEX or control (CON) group on any measure.	With FLEX, lack of improvement suggests that further study is needed to explore the effect of flexibility exercise training in older adults.

Note: PNF = proprioceptive neuromuscular facilitation; HR = heart rate; HRR = heart rate reserve.

velocity, and enzyme cycling (Young & Behm, 2002). While traditionally considered a staple of warm-up, available evidence suggests that static stretching may be detrimental to subsequent strength-, power-, speed, and agility-type performance (Peck, Chomko, Gaz, & Farrell, 2014). In addition, there is now a general consensus that stretching in addition to warm-up does not positively affect the incidence of overuse injuries (Thacker, Gilchrist, Stroup, & Kimsey, 2004). There is evidence that preparticipation stretching reduces the incidence of muscle strains, but there is clearly a need for further work (McHugh & Cosgrove, 2010). Thus, due to equivocal evidence thus far, the current ASCM's guidelines for exercise testing and prescription (ACSM, 2014) recommended the removal of static stretching as part of a warm-up routine for strength and power activities.

Older adults may be less concerned with high-performance benefits from increased flexibility and more focused on being safely active and safely performing activities of daily living. Injury and fall prevention are also common motives for recommending flexibility programs to older adults. The 2011 ACSM position stand (Garber et al., 2011) notes that flexibility training may enhance postural stability and balance when combined with resistance training; however, no consistent link has been shown between regular flexibility exercise and a reduction of musculoskeletal injuries or delayed onset of muscle soreness. In contrast, other exercise modalities, such as Tai Chi Chu'an, involving gait, balance, coordination, functional exercises, and muscle strengthening seem to have the greatest impact on balance in older adults (Hackney & Wolf, 2014). As such, the choice of this modality involving gentle stretching into controlled postures (and challenging other fitness variables) may be a more effective option for injury prevention. In summary, a general whole-body warm-up by gradually increasing the physical activity intensity up to that of the target level of the exercise session followed by dynamic stretching is advisable, with static stretching conducted after the exercise session.

CONCLUSIONS

Definite conclusions in the flexibility debate are premature and await further analyses that are able to discern whether the age-related losses in flexibility impact functional outcomes to an important extent. There is also the question about what degree of loss of ROM might relate to disability. In particular, a more direct matching of specific limb ROM and meaningful functional outcome is needed. Additionally, the specific type of physical activity that may influence the age-related loss needs to be further elucidated. While there is a lack of evidence to recommend stretching routines outside of a rehabilitative context, there is no apparent health or functional risk in including flexibility exercises. As such, in light of increases in functional outcomes achieved by other exercise modes (endurance, aerobic exercise, strengthening exercises), a formal program of stretching exercises can be included as an adjunct to the above, but the current literature would indicate that it would not add much to the overall functional benefits of exercise.

REFERENCES

American College of Sports Medicine. (2014). *ACSM's resource manual for guidelines for exercise testing and prescription* (7th ed.). Baltimore, MD: Lippincott Williams & Wilkins.

American College of Sports Medicine, Chodzko-Zajko, W. J., Proctor, D. N., Fiatarone Singh, M. A., Minson, C. T., Nigg, C. R., et al. (2009). American College of Sports Medicine position stand. Exercise and physical activity for older adults. *Medicine and Science in Sports and Exercise, 41*, 1510–1530. http://dx.doi.org/10.1249/mss.0b013e3181a0c95c

Awick, E. A., Wójcicki, T. R., Olson, E. A., Fanning, J., Chung, H. D., Zuniga, K., et al. (2015). Differential exercise effects on quality of life and health-related quality of life in older adults: A randomized controlled trial. *Quality of Life Research, 24*, 455–462. http://dx.doi.org/10.1007/s11136-014-0762-0

Badley, E. M., Wagstaff, S., & Wood, P. H. N. (1984). Measures of functional ability (disability) in arthritis in relation to impairment of range of joint movement. *Annals of the Rheumatic Diseases*, 43, 563–569.

Bassey, E. J., Morgan, K., Dallosso, H. M., & Ebrahim, S. B. J. (1989). Flexibility of the shoulder joint measured as range of abduction in a large representative sample of men and women over 65 years of age. *European Journal of Applied Physiology and Occupational Physiology, 58*, 353–360.

Battaglia, G., Bellafiore, M., Caramazza, G., Paoli, A., Bianco, A., & Palma, A. (2014). Changes in spinal range of motion after a flexibility training program in elderly women. *Clinical Interventions in Aging, 11*, 653–660. http://dx.doi.org/10.2147/cia.s59518

Bean, J. F., Latham, N. K., Holt, N., Kurlinksi, L., Ni, P., Leveille, S., et al. (2013). Which neuromuscular attributes are most associated with mobility among older primary care patients? *Archives of Physical Medicine and Rehabilitation, 94*, 2381–2388. http://dx.doi.org/10.1016/j.apmr.2013.07.026

Bird, M.L., Hill, K., Ball, M., Williams, A.D. (2009). Effects of resistance- and flexibility-exercise interventions on balance and related measures in older adults. *Journal of Aging and Physical Activity*, 17(4), 444–454.

Brown, M., Sinacore, D. R., Ehsani, A. A., Binder, E. F., Holloszy, J. O., & Kohrt, W. M. (2000). Low- intensity exercise as a modifier of physical frailty in older adults. *Archives of Physical Medicine and Rehabilitation, 81*, 960–965.

Bullo, V., Bergamin, M., Gobbo, S., Sieverdes, J. C., Zaccaria, M., Neunhaeuserer, D., et al. (2015, March 12). The effects of Pilates exercise training on physical fitness and wellbeing in the elderly: A systematic review for future exercise prescription. *Preventative Medicine, 75*, 1–11. pii: S0091-7435(15)00073-0. http://dx.doi.org/10.1016/j.ypmed.2015.03.002

Canadian Society for Exercise Physiology. (2011). *Canadian physical activity guidelines for older: Adults 65 years and older*. Retrieved from http://www.csep.ca/english/view.asp?x=804

Carneiro, N. H., Ribeiro, A. S., Nascimento, M. A., Gobbo, L. A., Schoenfeld, B. J., Achour Júnior, A., et al. (2015, March 15). Effects of different resistance training frequencies on flexibility in older women. *Clinical Interventions in Aging, 10*, 531–538. http://dx.doi.org/10.2147/cia.s77433

Chakravarty, K., & Webley, M. (1993). Shoulder joint movement and its relationship to disability in the elderly. *Journal of Rheumatology*, *20*, 1359–1361.

Einkauf, D. K., Gohdes, M. L., Jensen, G. M., & Jewell, M. J. (1987). Changes in spinal mobility with increasing age in women. *Physical Therapy*, *67*, 370–375.

Fabre, J. M., Wood, R. H., Cherry, K. E., Su, L. J., Cress, M. E., King, C. M., et al. (2007). Age-related deterioration in flexibility is associated with health-related quality of life in nonagenarians. *Journal of Geriatric Physical Therapy*, *30*, 16–22.

Franco, M. R., Tong, A., Howard, K., Sherrington, C., Ferreira, P. H., Pinto, R. Z., et al. (2015, January 13). Older people's perspectives on participation in physical activity: A systematic review and thematic synthesis of qualitative literature. *British Journal of Sports Medicine*, *49*(19), 1268–1276. http://dx.doi.org/10.1136/bjsports-2014-094015

Fusco, O., Ferrini, A., Santoro, M., Lo Monaco, M. R., Gambassi, G., & Cesari, M. (2012). Physical function and perceived quality of life in older persons. *Aging Clinical and Experimental Research*, *24*, 68–73.

Galbusera, F., van Rijsbergen, M., Ito, K., Huyghe, J. M., Brayda-Bruno, M., & Wilke, H. J. (2014). Ageing and degenerative changes of the intervertebral disc and their impact on spinal flexibility. *European Spine Journal, 23*, S324–S332. http://dx.doi.org/10.1007/s00586-014-3203-4

Garber, C. E., Blissmer, B., Deschenes, M. R., Franklin, B. A., Lamonte, M. J., Lee, I. M., et al. (2011). American College of Sports Medicine position stand. Quantity and quality of exercise for developing and maintaining cardiorespiratory, musculoskeletal, and neuromotor fitness in apparently healthy adults: Guidance for prescribing exercise. *Medicine and Science in Sports and Exercise, 43*, 1334–1359. http://dx.doi.org/10.1249/mss.0b013e318213fefb

Hackney, M. E., & Wolf, S. L. (2014). Impact of Tai Chi Chu'an practice on balance and mobility in older adults: An integrative review of 20 years of research. *Journal of Geriatriac Physical Therapy*, *37*, 127–135. http://dx.doi.org/10.1519/jpt.0b013e3182abe784

Imagama, S., Matsuyama, Y., Hasegawa, Y., Sakai, Y., Ito, Z., Ishiguro, N., et al. (2011). Back muscle strength and spinal mobility are predictors of quality of life in middle-aged and elderly males. *European Spine Journal, 20*, 954–961. http://dx.doi.org/10.1007/s00586-010-1606-4

James, B., & Parker, A. W. (1989). Active and passive mobility of lower limb joints in elderly men and women. *American Journal of Physical Medicine and Rehabilitation*, 68, 162–167.

King, A. C., Pruitt, L. A., Phillips, W., Oka, R., Rodenburg, A., & Haskell, W. L. (2000). Comparative effects of two physical activity programs on measured and perceived physical functioning and other health-related quality of life outcomes in older adults. *The Journal of Gerontology. Series A, Biological Sciences and Medical Sciences*, 55, M74–M83.

Klein, D. A., Stone, W. J., Phillips, W. T., Gangi, J., & Hartman, S. (2002). PNF training and physical function in assisted-living older adults. *Journal of Aging and Physical Activity*, *10*, 476–488.

Lan, C., Chen, S., & Lai, J. (2008). Changes of aerobic capacity, fat ratio and flexibility in older TCC practitioners: A five-year follow-up. *The American Journal of Chinese Medicine*, *36*, 1041–1050.

McHugh, M. P., & Cosgrave, C. H. (2010). To stretch or not to stretch: The role of stretching in injury prevention and performance. *Scandinavian Journal of Medicine and Science in Sports*, *20*, 169–181. http://dx.doi.org/10.1111/j.1600-0838.2009.01058.x

Miotto, J. M., Chodzko-Zajko, W. J., Reich, J. L., & Supler, M. M. (1999). Reliability and validity of the fullerton functional fitness test: An independent replication study. *Journal of Aging and Physical Activity, 7*, 339–353.

Nonaka, H., Mita, K., Watakabe, M., Akataki, K., Suzuki, N., Okuwa, T., et al. (2002). Age-related changes in the interactive mobility of the hip and knee joints: A geometrical analysis. *Gait and Posture*, *15*, 236–243.

Ozcan, A., Donat, H., Gelecek, N., Ozdirenc, M., & Karadibak, D. (2005). The relationship between risk factors for falling and the quality of life in older adults. *BMC Public Health, 5*, 90.

Paterson, D. H., & Warburton, D. E. (2010). Physical activity and functional limitations in older adults: a systematic review related to Canada's physical activity guidelines. *Internation Journal of Behaviour Nutrition and Physical Activity*, *7*(1), 38. http.//dx.doi.org/10.1186/1479-5868-7-38

Peck, E., Chomko, G., Gaz, D. V., & Farrell, A. M. (2014). The effects of stretching on performance. *Current Sports Medicine Reports*, *13*, 179–185.

Rikli, R., & Busch, S. (1986). Motor performance of women as a function of age and physical Nactivity level. *Journals of Gerontology*, *41*, 645–649.

Rikli, R. E., & Jones, C. J. (2013). Development and validation of criterion-referenced clinically relevant fitness standards for maintaining physical independence in later years. *Gerontologist*, 53, 255–267. http://dx.doi.org/10.1093/geront/gns071

Roach, K. E., & Miles, T. P. (1991). Normal hip and knee active range of motion: The relationship to age. *Physical Therapy*, *71*, 656–665.

Shields, M., Tremblay, M. S., Laviolette, M., Craig, C. L., Janssen, I., & Gorber, S. C. (2010). Fitness of Canadian adults: Results from the 2007–2009 *Canadian Health Measures Survey Health Reports*, *21*, 21–35.

Stanziano, D. C., Roos, B. A., Perry, A. C., Lai, S., & Signorile, J. F. (2009). The effects of an active- assisted stretching program on functional performance in elderly persons: A pilot study. *Clinical Interventions in Aging*, *4*, 115–120.

Stathokostas, L., Little, R. M., Vandervoort, A. A., & Paterson, D. H. (2012). Flexibility training and functional ability in older adults: A systematic review. *Journal of Aging Research*, 2012, 1–30. http://dx.doi.org/10.1155/2012/306818

Stathokostas, L., McDonald, M. W., Little, R. M., & Paterson, D. H. (2013). Flexibility of older adults aged 55-86 years and the influence of physical activity. *Journal of Aging Research, 2013*, 1–8. http://dx.doi.org/10.1155/2013/743843

Tainaka, K., Takizawa, T., Katamoto, S., & Aoki, J. (2009). Six-year prospective study of physical fitness and incidence of disability among community-dwelling *Japanese elderly women. Geriatrics and Gerontology International, 9*, 21–28. http://dx.doi.org/10.1111/j.1447-0594.2008.00492.x

Takeshima, N., Rogers, N. L., Rogers, M. E., Islam, M. M., Koizumi, D., & Lee, S. (2007). Functional fitness gain varies in older adults depending on exercise mode. *Medicine and Science in Sports and Exercise*, *39*, 2036–2043.

Thacker, S. B., Gilchrist, J., Stroup, D. F., & Kimsey, C. D. (2004). The impact of stretching on sports injury risk: A systematic review of the literature. *Medicine and Science in Sports and Exercise, 36*, 371–378.

Vandervoort, A. A. (1999). Ankle mobility and postural stability. *Physiotherapy Theory Practice*, *15*, 91–103. http://dx.doi.org/10.1080/095939899307793

Vandervoort, A. A., Chesworth, B. M., Cunningham, D. A., Paterson, D. H., Rechnitzer, P. A., & Koval, J. J. (1992). Age and sex effects on mobility of the human ankle. *Journal of Gerontology*, *47*, M17–M21.

Voorrips, L. E., Lemmink, K. A., van Heuvelen, M. J., Bult, P., & van Staveren, W. A. (1993). The physical condition of elderly women differing in habitual physical activity. *Medicine and Science in Sports and Exercise*, *25*, 1152–1157.

Walker, J. M., Sue, D., & Miles-Elkousy, N. (1984). Active mobility of the extremities in older subjects. *Physical Therapy*, *64*, 919–923.

Young, W., & Behm, D. G. (2002). Should static stretching be used during a warm-up for strength and power activities? *Strength and Conditioning Journal*, *24*, 33–37.

CHAPTER 8

Resistance Training

Recommendations for Age-Relevant Benefits

James F. Konopack

ABSTRACT

The physiological changes associated with the aging process include a gradual and progressive reduction in skeletal muscle as well as reductions in bone mineral density and changes in body fatness. These changes both influence and are influenced by changing activity patterns, most particularly decreases in physical activity, and can result in functional limitations as well as poor psychological outcomes. Resistance training can ameliorate and, in some cases, reverse some of the normal losses associated with the aging process. Skeletal muscle in particular generally retains its plasticity throughout the life span, leading to the availability of benefits from resistance training among even the oldest old. The current chapter provides an accessible review of musculoskeletal changes from middle to older adulthood and concludes with several recommendations for ways to maximize the age-relevant benefits of resistance training that are intended to be helpful for a wide audience including researchers, health-care workers, students, and fitness professionals. These recommendations focus on the design of safe and effective resistance training protocols and emphasize psychosocial considerations to maximize participant adherence to and satisfaction with the exercise regimen. Recommendations for additional resources for general audiences are also provided.

http://dx.doi.org/10.1891/0198-8794.36.193

INTRODUCTION

In the field of gerontology and geriatrics, experts are commonly asked—by the general public and colleagues alike—about strategies to optimize physical activity, particularly during older adulthood. Common questions include, "Which modes of physical activity are best for me?" "Is there truly a dose–response relationship between physical activity and health, such that more is always better?" "Are certain types of activity contraindicated for individuals with my health status and limitations?" "Of all of the various types of exercise, which will best help me maintain my health and independence in my advancing years, so I can keep doing the things I love to do—or start doing them again after having stopped?" Being able to cogently respond to questions like these with empirical support is critically important when it comes to maximizing quality of life into older adulthood. This chapter examines the ways in which resistance training optimizes health and function along several dimensions of well-being, making it an indispensable mode of physical activity and a key component of successful aging. It begins with a brief review of the physiological changes to the musculoskeletal system associated with aging and concludes with evidence-based recommendations designed to maximize the age-relevant benefits of resistance training.

AGE-RELATED MUSCLE LOSS

As has been well documented in the research literature, the normal aging process is associated with a gradual decrease in lean body mass, most prevalently in the form of skeletal muscle tissue. In particular, there is a decrease in muscle cell cross-sectional area and a disproportionate loss of Type II (i.e., fast-twitch) muscle fibers compared with Type I (i.e., slow-twitch) fibers, as well as maladaptive changes in muscle quality (Green, 2007, p. 121). This process of age-related, progressive muscle loss is known as *sarcopenia*, a term that first appeared in a paper on the methodological problems associated with determining the nutritional status of older adults in epidemiological research (Rosenberg, 1989). In the average adult, sarcopenia results in a reduction of approximately 40% of one's skeletal muscle mass between roughly the ages of 20 and 70 (Nair, 2005). The good news, however, is that skeletal muscle generally retains its plasticity, thereby remaining responsive to training stimuli throughout the life span.

Aerobic forms of physical activity such as brisk walking, bicycling, and swimming, among others, have been shown in some studies to slow the process of sarcopenia, possibly through the preservation of mitochondrial content within the skeletal muscle (e.g., Broskey et al., 2014). Other studies, however, have found aerobic modes of activity to be less effective in reducing the loss of muscle with aging (e.g., Klitgaard et al., 1990). Indeed, the maximum benefits to muscular strength and size during older adulthood are widely acknowledged to result from a program of progressive resistance training, for which there is a consistent pattern of findings based on substantial data in the literature (Chodzko-Zajko et al., 2009). Physical activities that specifically focus on building and maintaining muscle strength and quality are, therefore, of extreme importance in order to attenuate this process. (See also Chapter 9 on this subject for a more complete discussion of the prevention and management strategies of sarcopenia.)

Encouragingly, the hypertrophic consequences of resistance exercise are not limited to the periods of young and middle adulthood. Indeed, a well-designed program of progressive resistance training is effective for not only slowing the gradual process of sarcopenia but also improving muscle quality and increasing muscle size and strength, even among the oldest old. In a frequently cited landmark study, Fiatarone and colleagues (1994) demonstrated that a progressive resistance training program for frail nursing home residents (*M* age = 87.1 years, 63% female) dramatically reversed the effects of muscular disuse from physical inactivity and aging, with significant gains in muscle strength. Thus, there is no point after which the effects of resistance training diminish; Strength improvements are possible and resistance training is tolerable and effective throughout adulthood. It follows that physical activities focused on increasing strength, even among the physically frail oldest old, can improve functional fitness and the performance of the activities of daily living.

SHIFTS IN BODY COMPOSITION ASSOCIATED WITH AGE

If left unchecked by insufficient physical activity, sarcopenia gradually reduces one's skeletal muscle mass, but fat mass tends to increase with advancing age up to about age 75, after which total body fat decreases and is increasingly redistributed from subcutaneous to central, visceral fat depots. The result is "less fat where it should be and more fat where it should not be, with substantial clinical consequences" (Kirkland, Tchkonia, Pirtskhalava, Han, & Karagiannides, 2002, p. 757). Although total fat mass typically decreases from middle to older adulthood, the simultaneous reduction in muscle mass results in an increase in percent body fat, even with a stable body mass index, as the proportion of fat mass to fat-free mass increases. This phenomenon has been referred to as "sarcopenic obesity" and is a threat to several dimensions of health (Zamboni, Mazzali, Fenton, Rossi, & De Francesco, 2008).

Because of the well-known costs associated with excess body fatness (see Katzmarzyk & Janssen, 2004, for an analysis of the economic as well as public health costs), there is a need to safely control, if not reduce, body fat storage throughout the life span. Aerobic forms of physical activity will, on average, result in higher energy expenditure when measured against resistance exercises of similar length and intensity, but resistance training itself can be a useful tool for controlling body composition with aging. Alexander's (2002) paper on the role of resistance training in weight loss provided evidence that resistance training improves body composition mainly through a resultant increase in the participant's resting metabolic rate (RMR). As RMR is the primary contributor to daily energy expenditure, its increase through resistance training would forestall or reverse undesirable weight gain via metabolic adaptation.

Along this line, prior research has also explored whether the physiologic adaptation to resistance training is preserved or degraded under conditions of reduced calorie intake, which is a commonly used strategy for inducing weight loss but also an undesirable occurrence in frail older adults who could benefit from greater energy intake. In an earlier work, Donnelly et al. (1993) demonstrated that positive muscular adaptations to resistance training are possible even when participants experience controlled calorie restriction. More recently, Jo (2013) found support for the muscle-sparing and muscle-building qualities of resistance training even when exposed to very low calorie diets. In that study, participants who walked plus performed resistance training three times weekly for 12 weeks showed no changes in RMR even in the face of a 1120 kcal/day energy intake, whereas participants who followed identical consumption and walking patterns but did not perform resistance training saw an average of a 350.8 kcal/day drop in RMR (Jo, 2013). Because a loss or gain of 1 pound of body mass requires a shift in energy balance of 3,500 kcal, this 350 kcal/day change to RMR would correspond to a net change in weight of approximately 1 pound per 10 days. While this result is encouraging, however, additional work is needed to substantiate this rate and extent of RMR adaptation and its effects on body weight and composition.

BONE HEALTH AND RESISTANCE TRAINING

With normal aging also comes a concomitant reduction in bone health after middle adulthood. Specifically, the density of minerals within bone decreases for both men and women by age 40 and progresses at an approximate rate of 0.5%–1% per year, though women are likely to experience periods of accelerated bone mineral depletion during and following menopause; a frequent consequence in older adulthood is fracture due to osteoporosis (Demontiero, Vidal, & Duque, 2012; recommended reading for a review of the pathophysiological mechanisms underlying bone loss). Fortunately, as with skeletal muscle, but to a lesser extent, bone retains some of its plasticity with advancing age. Bone mineral density is responsive to exercise training that involves regular stress—typically compression of the bone via a combination of the act of weight-bearing and muscular pressure—though lifetime bone mass reaches its peak sometime between the late teens and late 30s for most people, the exact timing of which varies by sex and across skeletal sites (Berger et al., 2010). Moreover, it should also be noted that the adaptability of bone to regular load-bearing activity may be moderated by age at some skeletal sites (e.g., hip), with greater bone responsivity in early or middle adulthood than in older adulthood in certain populations (Winters-Stone, Leo, & Schwartz, 2012). The combination of osteoporosis, sarcopenia, and obesity has been termed "osteosarcopenic obesity" and comes with a host of negative clinical implications such as increased morbidity and mortality, frailty, impaired function and quality of life, and falls or fractures (Ormsbee et al., 2014). Physical activities such as resistance training are therefore specifically indicated for strengthening bone as well as muscle across the life span, thereby reducing osteoporosis and fracture risk among other clinical outcomes.

PSYCHOLOGICAL CONSIDERATIONS RELATED TO FUNCTIONAL STRENGTH

With the loss of fitness through physical inactivity comes a cluster of risks to psychological health that are, fortunately, amenable to change through physical activity. These psychological outcomes include depression; emotional well-being; cognitive function, particularly executive control function; and health-related quality of life (Lox, Martin Ginis, & Petruzzello, 2014, pp. 283–403). An excellent summary of the psychological benefits of exercise and physical activity among older adults was included in the most recent Position Stand on Exercise and Physical Activity for Older Adults from the American College of Sports Medicine (ACSM; Chodzko Zajko et al., 2009, pp. 1520–1523). Germane to the current chapter was the ACSM's update of their previous position stand to include a section on the psychological benefits of resistance exercise training (Chodzko-Zajko et al., 2009, pp. 1522–1523), which included evidence strongly supporting high-intensity resistance training as an effective tool in treating clinical depression.

RECOMMENDATIONS FOR SUCCESSFUL AGING WITH RESISTANCE TRAINING

The set of recommendations that follows is intended to supplement, rather than replace, the physical activity recommendations for older adults that have been published by leading public health and exercise science organizations in recent years. Authoritative sources specifically addressing resistance training include the joint recommendations on physical activity and public health in older adults from the ACSM and the American Heart Association (Nelson et al., 2007) as well as the ACSM Position Stand on Exercise and Physical Activity for Older Adults (Chodzko-Zajko et al., 2009) and are essential desk references for researchers, clinicians, and fitness professionals working with older adults. It should also be noted that the recommendations issued in the following text pertain to older adults without significant functional limitations. In some ways, this is a difficult proposition, as many older adults have some form of chronic condition or illness, but these recommendations are designed to be practical recommendations suitable to academicians, health-care practitioners, students, and fitness professionals. In instances in which some recommendations designed for healthy older adults may be contraindicated, it is best to explore condition- or disease-specific exercise recommendations (e.g., those with osteoarthritis are directed to the American Geriatrics Society Panel on Exercise and Osteoarthritis, 2001, pp. 815–817). In determining a person's risk stratification and readiness for exercise, the reader is strongly urged to first consult the second chapter of the *ACSM's Guidelines for Exercise Testing and Prescription* (Thompson, 2014, pp. 19–38) and have prospective exercise participants confer with their primary health-care providers as needed.

Participants Should Seek Reliable Instruction

For the most reliable instruction, seek out individuals with certifications from trustworthy fitness organizations, such as the ACSM, which offers various types of health fitness and clinical certifications and is the "gold standard" in fitness certification in the United States, and the American Council on Exercise, which provides a Senior Fitness Specialist certification. Among many other reasons, this is essential for the success of the following recommendations.

Learn and Practice Correct Form

Physical activities such as walking and bicycling require little to no formal instruction in order to perform them safely and effectively throughout one's lifetime, but resistance-training exercises, when improperly executed, can range from counterproductive to dangerous. Injuries in the form of sprains, dislocations, and strains as well as impact injuries from the weights themselves are occasionally observed when participants use incorrect form and may result in the termination of the exercise program, if not a hospital visit (Gray & Finch, 2014). This recommendation, then, is closely coupled with the previous recommendation to seek out reliable instruction on how to perform weighted movements safely and effectively. Fitness experts are encouraged to seek out fellow practitioners to solicit objective feedback on their own resistance training performance.

Select Appropriate Activities

When designing a resistance-training program, exercises should encompass all major muscle groups across approximately 8–10 exercises. Because there is evidence indicating that strength gains may be limited to narrow ranges of joint angles with isometric strength training (Fleck & Kraemer, 2014, p. 13), it is recommended that resistance exercise movements utilize complex, multijoint movements whenever possible unless otherwise contraindicated and are performed to their full range of motion. If participants find this difficult to accomplish with a given weight or training load, reduce the weight or otherwise modify the stimulus until a full range of motion is possible through the desired number of repetitions.

Sample movements include squats, lunges, or leg presses; bench presses, shoulder raises, or push-ups; and upright or seated rows; among many alternatives. For a free and accessible guide to strength-focused activities that can be done at home, see the web resource provided by the Centers for Disease Control and Prevention and listed in the concluding section of this chapter.

Train With Appropriate Frequency

For many older adults, a resistance-training regimen that includes major muscle groups of both the upper and lower body can be well tolerated when performed twice weekly. Several sources recommend a frequency of two *or more* times per week, but two weekly training sessions of the same muscle group can be effective for improving muscle quality in older adults. Additionally, adults of all ages will often experience delayed-onset muscle soreness (DOMS) shortly after undertaking a novel training program, particularly following movements that involve longer eccentric muscle action (i.e., lengthening of the muscle, usually associated with the lowering of the weight; Fleck & Kraemer, 2014, p. 2). DOMS results from the body's natural inflammatory response to minute damage incurred during the exercise stimulus, typically peaks approximately 48 hours after the exercise bout, and can last for 4 days (McCall, 2015, p. 422). For this reason as well as the fact that muscular hypertrophy occurs during the rest *between* rather than *during* training sessions, easing into a new training program in both frequency and intensity is recommended, and frequency of training should not exceed three times per week after the initial few weeks for most individuals.

Perform Resistance Movements With Moderate Intensity in Mind

Intensity of the exercise itself can be thought of as the effort required to perform the movement as a percentage of the maximal effort (i.e., the one-repetition maximum or 1RM; Fleck & Kraemer, 2014, p. 5). Consistent with previous recommendations (Nelson et al., 2007), resistance-training movements should allow for 10–15 repetitions of each movement of such intensity that moderate-to-high effort is required (e.g., 5–8 on a 10-point scale from resting [0] to maximal effort [10]), but not so high that the participant performs the Valsalva maneuver (i.e., holding one's breath with a closed glottis while completing the lift; Fleck & Kraemer, 2014, p. 12). Holding one's breath is difficult to avoid during near-maximal lifts but is strongly discouraged in general, as doing so results in a spike in systolic blood pressure. Controlled exhalation during the concentric, or contractile, phase of movement is recommended instead. Recall that a self-reported intensity of 5–8 on a 10-point scale signifies 50%–80% of one's maximal effort; yet it is sufficient to induce muscular adaptation. Movements should be challenging enough so that they cannot be performed more than 15–20 times, but not so difficult that they cannot be performed at least 6–8 times before failure.

Structure Resistance-Training Programs to Maximize Self-Efficacy

Self-efficacy can be described as an individual's belief in his or her ability to successfully carry out a specific task, and according to Bandura's (1977) seminal work, can be derived from any of four primary sources of information: (a) mastery experiences or personal accomplishments, (b) vicarious experiences or modeling, (c) social persuasion, and (d) the interpretation of physiological or affective states. An increase in self-efficacy for exercise is valuable for a number of reasons, not least of which is its reciprocally causal relationship with exercise adherence (McAuley & Blissmer, 2000). In addition, previous research has shown that individuals' self-efficacy perceptions predict performance on functional fitness tasks, particularly those requiring the use of strength or speed (Konopack et al., 2008).

In working with patients or clients or developing an exercise program, it is possible to structure exercise in ways that will maximize the participants' self-efficacy using the additional recommendations listed in the following text (for more on the theoretical underpinnings of exercise in older adults, see Chapter 11):

- **Start with small performance goals and plan to make gradual, incremental gains.** This is an easily implemented recommendation that targets the most significant source of self-efficacy information (mastery experience through personal accomplishment). The quality of feedback given by instructors, clinicians, or other authority figures to the exercising individual can also influence self-efficacy levels—for better or for worse (e.g., McAuley, Talbot, & Martinez, 1999; Motl, Konopack, Hu, & McAuley, 2006)—and is therefore important to keep in mind. To this end, even the most professional and conscientious fitness specialist with reliable degrees/certifications may be unaware of the determinants of self-efficacy and how it, in turn, contributes to exercise adherence, perceived exertion, and other factors. Enlisting the assistance of an individual with knowledge of social cognitive theory (Bandura, 1977) and its relation to exercise is recommended to augment the training of fitness professionals.

- Following from the previous point, **have the exercisers develop their own reasonably difficult, specific, measurable goals that represent accurate expectations of future performance**. For example, measureable strength gains can be expected after 4–18 weeks of progressive resistance training using 1–3 sets of 6–15 repetitions per set, on average (several studies, as cited by Fleck & Kraemer, 2014, p. 35). Designing a goal involving significant strength improvements in half this time would be unrealistic and lead to reduced self-efficacy; far less challenging goals would also be limited in their helpfulness.
- **Design the resistance-training program involving partners or groups whenever possible.** This has the potential to maximize self-efficacy gains through social persuasion (i.e., encouragement, accountability) as well as the modeling of correct movement forms.
- **Recruit exercise leaders who can serve as identifiable role models for participants**. This will build self-efficacy through vicarious experience (i.e., participants' identification with and modeling of the exercise leader as someone similar to themselves).

Emphasize Additional Physical Activity Modes

In addition to (but not necessarily in place of) weight training, the activities that follow are recommended for their potential to increase muscular strength in older adults when performed with regularity. These include but are certainly not limited to

- Stair-climbing
- Strenuous gardening (i.e., involving carrying, digging, and similar activities)
- Pilates
- Brisk walking or walking on hills
- Yoga
- Tai Chi (see Chapter 10 on Tai Chi to improve balance)

It is important to keep in mind that although the bulk of the empirical literature on building muscular strength and bone density among older adults involves carefully controlled and supervised weight-training programs, similar benefits may be attained through other activities, such as those listed in the preceding text, that provide enjoyment as well as resistance to gravity or other forces on the body. Finally, it is important that resistance training augment rather than replace aerobic forms of physical activity, which benefit health and wellness in numerous ways.

SUMMARY

The benefits of physical activity are available across the human life span, even into advanced old age. Among older adults, regular physical activity—particularly activity that builds musculoskeletal strength—is a key element to successful aging, with benefits that include improvements in body composition, balance, bone health, performance of activities of daily living, and psychological well-being. Individuals designing, supervising, or initiating resistance-training programs for older adults are advised to consult reputable resources (see additional resources listed in the following text in addition to scholarly sources cited in this chapter), develop proficiency of movement patterns under the guidance of certified fitness professionals, and structure physical activities in ways that capitalize on the research that supports self-efficacy as a modifiable determinant of exercise adherence and performance.

Recommended Resources Suitable for Practitioners and General Audiences

Centers for Disease Control and Prevention. (2011). *Growing stronger: Strength training for older adults*. Retrieved from: http://www.cdc.gov/physicalactivity/growingstronger/

Department of Health and Human Services. (2008). *2008 Physical activity guidelines for americans*. Rockville, MD: U.S. Department of Health and Human Services.

Fleck, S. J., & Kraemer, W. J. (2014). *Designing resistance training programs* (4th ed.). Champaign, IL: Human Kinetics.

Signorile, J. F. (2011). *Bending the aging curve: The complete exercise guide for older adults*. Champaign, IL: Human Kinetics.

REFERENCES

Alexander, J. L. (2002). The role of resistance training in weight loss. *Strength and Conditioning Journal*, *24*, 65–69.

American Geriatrics Society Panel on Exercise and Osteoarthritis. (2001). Exercise prescription for older adults with osteoarthritis pain: Consensus practice recommendations. A supplement to the AGS Clinical Practice Guidelines on the management of chronic pain in older adults. *Journal of the American Geriatrics Society*, *49*(6), 808–823.

Bandura. A. (1977). Self-efficacy: Toward a unifying theory of behavioral change. *Psychological Review*, *84*, 191–215.

Berger, C., Goltzman, D., Langsetmo, L., Joseph, L., Jackson, S., Kreiger, N., et al. (2010). Peak bone mass from longitudinal data: Implications for the prevalence, pathophysiology, and diagnosis of osteoporosis. *Journal of Bone and Mineral Research*, *25*(9), 1948–1957. doi:10.1002/jbmr.95

Broskey, N. T., Greggio, C., Boss, A., Boutant, M., Dwyer, A., Schlueter, L., et al. (2014). Skeletal muscle mitochondria in the elderly: Effects of physical fitness and exercise training. *Journal of Clinical Endocrinology & Metabolism*, *99*(5), 1852–1861. doi:10.1210/jc.2013-3983

Chodzko-Zajko, W. J., Proctor, D. N., Fiatarone Singh, M. A., Minson, C. T., Nigg, C. R., Salem, G. J., & Skinner, J. S. (2009). American College of Sports Medicine Position Stand: Exercise and physical activity for older adults. *Medicine & Science in Sports & Exercise*, *41*(7), 1510–1530. doi:10.1249/MSS.0b013e3181a0c95c

Demontiero, O., Vidal, C., & Duque, G. (2012). Aging and bone loss: New insights for the clinician. *Therapeutic Advances in Musculoskeltal Disease*, *4*(2), 61–76. doi:10.1177/1759720X11430858

Donnelly, J. E., Sharp, T., Houmard, J., Carlson, M. G., Hill, J. O., Whately, J. E., & Israel, R. G. (1993). Muscle hypertrophy with large-scale weight loss and resistance training. *American Journal of Clinical Nutrition*, *58*, 561–565.

Fiatarone, M. A., O'Neill, E. F., Ryan, N. D., Clements, K. M., Solares, G. R., Nelson, M. E., et al. (1994). Exercise training and nutritional supplementation for physical frailty in very elderly people. *New England Journal of Medicine*, *330*(25), 1769–1775.

Fleck, S. J., & Kraemer, W. J. (2014). *Designing resistance training programs* (4th ed.). Champaign, IL: Human Kinetics.

Gray, S. E., & Finch, C. F. (2014). Epidemiology of hospital-treated injuries sustained by fitness participants. *Research Quarterly for Exercise and Sport*, *86*(1), 81–87. doi:10.1080/02701367.2014.975177

Green, H. J. (2007). Skeletal muscle adaptation to regular physical activity. In C. Bouchard, S. N. Blair, & W. L. Haskell (Eds.), *Physical activity and health* (pp. 99–125). Champaign, IL: Human Kinetics.

Jo, E. (2013). The clinical application of periodized resistance training during a 12-week hypocaloric treatment for obesity: A joint retrospective and prospective single-center study. *Electronic theses, treatises and dissertations. Paper 8576*. Retrieved from: http://diginole.lib.fsu.edu/etd/8576

Katzmarzyk, P. T., & Janssen, I. (2004). The economic costs associated with physical inactivity an obesity in Canada: An update. *Canadian Journal of Applied Physiology*, *29*(1), 90–115.

Kirkland, J. K., Tchkonia, T., Pirtskhalava, T., Han, J., & Karagiannides, I. (2002). A dipogenesis and aging: Does aging make fat go MAD? *Experimental Gerontology*, *37*(6), 757–767.

Klitgaard, H., Mantoni, M., Schiaffino, S., Ausoni, S., Gorza, L., Laurent-Winter, C., et al. (1990). Function, morphology and protein expression of ageing skeletal muscle: A cross-sectional study of elderly men with different training backgrounds. *Acta Physiologica Scandinavica*, *140*, 41–54.

Konopack, J. F., Marquez, D. X., Hu, L., Elavsky, S., McAuley, E., & Kramer, A. F. (2008). Correlates of functional fitness in older adults. *International Journal of Behavioral Medicine*, *15*, 311–318. doi:10.1080/10705500802365557

Lox, C. L., Martin Ginis, K. A., & Petruzzello, S. J. (2014). *The psychology of exercise: Integrating theory and practice* (4th ed.). Scottsdale, AZ: Holcomb Hathaway.

McAuley, E., & Blissmer, B. (2000). Social cognitive determinants and consequences of physical activity. *Exercise and Sports Science Reviews*, *21*, 85–88.

McAuley, E., Talbot, H. M., & Martinez, S. (1999). Manipulating self-efficacy in the exercise environment in women: Influences on affective responses. *Health Psychology*, *18*(3), 288–294.

McCall, P. (2015). Resistance training. In J. Porcari, C. Bryant, & F. Comana (Eds.), *Exercise physiology* (pp. 412–438). Philadelphia, PA: F. A. Davis.

Motl, R. W., Konopack, J. F., Hu, L., & McAuley, E. (2006). Does self-efficacy influence leg muscle pain during cycling exercise among females? *The Journal of Pain*, *7*, 301–307. doi:10.1016/j.jpain.2005.11.009

Nair, K, S. (2005). Aging muscle. *American Journal of Clinical Nutrition*, *81*, 953–963.

Nelson, M. E., Rejeski, W. J., Blair, S. N., Duncan, P. W., Judge, J. O., King, A., C., et al. (2007). Physical activity and public health in older adults: Recommendation from the American College of Sports Medicine and the American Heart Association. *Circulation*, *116*(9), 1094–1105. doi:10.1161/CIRCULATIONAHA.107.185650

Ormsbee, M. J., Prado, C. M., Ilich, J. Z., Purcell, S., Siervo, M., Folsom, A., & Panton, L. (2014). Osteosarcopenic obesity: The role of bone, muscle, and fat on health. *Journal of Cachexia, Sarcopenia, and Muscle*, *5*(3), 183–192. doi:10.1007/s13539-014-0146-x

Rosenberg, I. H. (1989). Epidemiologic and methodologic problems in determining nutritional status of older persons (Summary comments). *American Journal of Clinical Nutrition*, *50*(5), 1231–1233.

Thompson, P. D. (Ed.). (2014). Preparticipation health screening. In *ACSM's guidelines for exercise testing and prescription* (9th ed., pp. 19–38). Baltimore, MD: American College of Sports Medicine.

Winters-Stone, K. M., Leo, M. C., & Schwartz, A. (2012). Exercise effects on hip bone mineral density in older, post-menopausal breast cancer survivors are age dependent. *Archives of Osteoporosis*, 7, 301–306. doi: 10.1007/s11657-012-0071-6

Zamboni, M., Mazzali, G., Fantin, F., Rossi, F., & De Francesco, V. (2008). Sarcopenic obesity: A new category of obesity in the elderly. *Nutrition, Metabolism, and Cardiovascular Diseases*, *18*(5), 388–395.

CHAPTER 9

Resistance Exercise to Prevent and Manage Sarcopenia and Dynapenia

Timothy D. Law, Leatha A. Clark, and Brian C. Clark

ABSTRACT

For well over 20 centuries, the muscle wasting (sarcopenia) and weakness (dynapenia) that occurs with old age has been a predominant concern for mankind. Exercise has long been suggested as a treatment to combat sarcopenia and dynapenia, as it exerts effects on both the nervous and muscular systems that are critical to positive physiological and functional adaptations (e.g., enhanced muscle strength). For more than two decades, scientists have recognized the profound role that progressive resistance exercise training (RET) can have on increasing muscle strength, muscle size, and functional capacity in older adults. In this review article, we discuss how RET can be used in the management and prevention of sarcopenia and dynapenia. We first provide an overview of the evidence for this notion and highlight certain critical factors—namely, exercise intensity, volume, and progression—that are key to optimizing the resistance exercise prescription. We then highlight how many, if not most, of the commonly prescribed exercise programs for seniors are not the "best practices" and subsequently present easy-to-read guidelines for a well-rounded RET program designed for the management and prevention of sarcopenia and dynapenia, including example training programs for the beginner through programs for the advanced senior resistance exerciser. These guidelines have been written for the academician as well as the student and health-care provider across a variety of disciplines, including those in the long-term care industry, such as wellness instructors or activity directors.

http://dx.doi.org/10.1891/0198-8794.36.205

INTRODUCTION

For well over 20 centuries, the muscle wasting and weakness that occurs with old age has been a predominant concern of mankind. As eloquently reviewed by Narici and Maffulli (Narici & Maffulli, 2010), the Classical Greeks (4th and 5th centuries BC) detested the degrading effects of aging on their bodies and considered it a chronic, incurable, and progressive disease. However, by the 1st century BC and the 1st century AD, the perspective on physical frailty and aging started to change as Cicero and others began to view aging not as an irreversible illness but rather a modifiable condition. In fact, in his "Essay on Old Age" in 44 BC, Cicero argues that "it is our duty . . . to resist old age, to compensate for its defects, to fight against it as we would fight a disease; to adopt a regimen of health; to practice moderate exercise; and to take just enough food and drink to restore our strength." While Cicero's suggestion to use exercise to combat muscle wasting and weakness was logical, it did not truly gain steam in the scientific and medical communities until the latter part of the 20th century. In particular, a series of landmark studies published in the early 1990s by Fiatarone and colleagues in the *Journal of the American Medical Association* (Fiatarone et al., 1990) and the *New England Journal of Medicine* (Fiatarone et al., 1994) highlighted the profound role that progressive resistance exercise training[1] (RET) can have on increasing muscle strength, muscle size, and functional capacity in older adults. For instance, the first of these studies demonstrated that institutionalized nonagenarians (i.e., individuals 90–99 years old) were able to increase their muscle strength, on average, an astounding 174%, their mid-thigh muscle area 9.0%, and their gait speed 48% with 8 weeks of high-intensity progressive RET (Fiatarone et al., 1990). By the start of the 21st century, we knew that muscle fiber types of older adults were able to hypertrophy (~30% increase in size with 16 weeks of high-intensity RET), could transition the fiber type (from type IIX fibers to IIA), and had the capacity to incorporate new nuclei into the fibers (Hikida et al., 2000). These adaptations are comparable to what is observed in younger individuals, suggesting that the muscle of older adults is not limited in its ability to adapt. Some two decades later, there is now evidence indicating that high-intensity RET, when coupled with other targeted multidisciplinary interventions, results in lower mortality, nursing home admissions, and disability compared with usual care after hip fracture (Singh et al., 2012).

With the demographic profile of the United States, and the world for that matter, changing (e.g., more than 14% of the entire U.S population is now greater than 65 years [United States Census Bureau, 2015]), there is a continued and growing interest in developing effective interventional strategies to combat muscle wasting and weakness associated with aging. To date, scientific evidence suggests that high-intensity, progressive RET (also commonly referred to as "strength training") is one of, if not the most, effective interventional strategies to enhance muscle size and strength in the elderly (Bird, Hill, Ball, & Williams, 2009; Chale et al., 2013; Charette et al., 1991; Fiatarone et al., 1990, 1994; Hikida et al., 2000; Kalapotharakos, Diamantopoulos, & Tokmakidis, 2010; Liu & Latham, 2009; Manini et al., 2007; Sylliaas, Brovold, Wyller, & Bergland, 2011; Van Roie, Delecluse, Coudyzer, Boonen, & Bautmans, 2013). Accordingly, in this chapter, we briefly review the current literature regarding the use of RET to prevent and manage sarcopenia and dynapenia, and provide pragmatic advice for patients and practitioners on the resistance exercise prescription for older adults. First, however, we discuss sarcopenia and dynapenia with special attention to their operational definitions.

Sarcopenia is a term, originally proposed by Rosenberg in 1989 (Rosenberg, 1989), specifically referring to the loss of muscle mass associated with aging. However, the meaning of this term has often been extended to the age-related loss of muscle strength and/or physical function. Although sarcopenia is certainly a contributor to muscle weakness, it has been argued that these two terms should not be used interchangeably since this would imply a direct proportionality between the two (Clark & Manini, 2008; Manini & Clark, 2011; Manini, Russ, & Clark, 2012; Narici & Maffulli, 2010; Visser & Schaap, 2011), which is not the case as a variety of other neural and muscular factors contribute to force output that are independent of muscle mass (for review, see Clark & Manini, 2008; Duchateau & Enoka, 2002; Manini & Clark, 2011; Manini et al., 2012; Narici & Maffulli, 2010). Accordingly, the term *dynapenia* was proposed by Clark and Manini in 2008 to specifically refer to the loss of muscle strength and power associated with aging (Clark & Manini, 2008).

While there are semantic debates in the literature, there is progress toward developing criteria/criterion for the diagnosis of clinically significant sarcopenia and/or dynapenia in recent years. For example, the European Working Group on Sarcopenia in Older People incorporates aspects of (a) physical function (i.e., gait speed), (b) muscle strength, and (c) muscle mass into a singular diagnosis of sarcopenia (Cruz-Jentoft et al., 2010). Other criteria, namely, those by the Foundation for the National Institutes of Health's Sarcopenia Working Group, attempted to define low muscle mass and muscle weakness independently using a data-driven approach in a pooled sample of 26,635 older adults (Studenski et al., 2014). While there are significant efforts being put forth by both researchers and practitioners in the development of diagnostic criteria, it is important to note there are no established agreed-upon definition for these common conditions at this time.

RET AND THE MANAGEMENT AND PREVENTION OF MUSCLE WASTING AND WEAKNESS

While sarcopenia and dynapenia are realized to be major clinical problems for older adults, until recently, there has been little widespread support for ways to combat these debilitating conditions. However, research on the effects of exercise and nutrition on sarcopenia and dynapenia has rapidly expanded in the past one to two decades (Sayer et al., 2013). Today, there is still limited evidence suggesting that pharmacologic interventions effectively ameliorate sarcopenia and/or dynapenia. However, there is strong and growing evidence that progressive RET can combat both sarcopenia *and* dynapenia (Burton & Sumukadas, 2010), as RET has a profound effect on virtually all of the physiological mechanisms in the nervous system and the muscular system known to influence strength (Duchateau & Enoka, 2002; Russ, Gregg-Cornell, Conaway, & Clark, 2012). For instance, maximal motor unit discharge rates, a key "neural factor" involved in muscle strength, increased 49% in older adults following only 6 weeks of high-intensity progressive RET (Kamen & Knight, 2004). Non-mass-dependent muscular factors, such as muscle fiber fascicle length and tendon stiffness, have also been observed to increase (10% and 64%, respectively) following RET in older adults (Reeves, Maganaris, & Narici, 2003). Additionally, RET is also a powerful stimulus for inducing muscle hypertrophy as illustrated by 24 weeks of RET, when coupled with modest protein supplementation, increasing thigh muscle cross-sectional area 4.6% in mobility-limited older adults (Chale et al., 2013). Given that there exists widespread evidence that inactivity, which is prevalent in the elderly (Troiano et al., 2008), leads to loss of muscle mass and strength (Clark, 2009), findings of this nature would (or should) lead all scientists and clinicians to support the use of RET for treating, slowing, and/or preventing sarcopenia and dynapenia.

Indeed, the extant literature supports this notion. For instance, a 2009 Cochrane review of 121 trials including over 6,700 participants concluded that "progressive resistance training is an effective intervention for improving physical functioning in older people, including improving strength and the performance of some simple and complex activities" (Liu & Latham, 2009). Most of the trials reviewed involved high-intensity training two to three times per week. Benefits included large positive effects on both muscle mass (hypertrophy) and strength (Liu & Latham, 2009). A functional assessment of gait speed showed a modest improvement, and a strong effect was observed on the ability to rise from a chair (Liu & Latham, 2009).

It is well recognized that the effectiveness of RET for strength and muscle mass improvement is variable across studies, and recent meta-analyses by Peterson and colleagues attempted to identify critical aspects of RET programs, which promote strength adaptation (e.g., the frequency of exercise training, the duration of exercise training, the intensity of exercise training, and the volume of exercise training; Peterson, Rhea, Sen, & Gordon, 2010; Peterson, Sen, & Gordon, 2011). These studies revealed two critical aspects for positive adaptations associated with progressive RET. First, higher intensity RET is associated with greater improvements in muscle strength. Specifically, with each incremental increase in exercise intensity from low intensity (<60% of 1 repetition maximum or 1RM), low/moderate intensity (60%–69% of 1RM), and moderate/high intensity (70%–79% of 1RM) to high intensity (≥80% of 1RM), the average percent change in strength was 5.3%, as shown in Figure 9.1A (Peterson et al., 2010). Second, higher RET volume, defined as the total number of exercise sets performed per session, is associated with greater improvements in lean body mass (LBM) after controlling for a variety of confounders (e.g., age, study duration, gender, training intensity and frequency, etc.), as shown in Figure 9.1B (Peterson et al., 2011). This finding suggests that for every additional 10 sets of exercise performed per session, one can expect, on average, a 0.5 kg increase in LBM (Peterson et al., 2011). It should be noted that this study reported that older individuals experienced a lesser increase in LBM with RET (Peterson et al., 2011). Some scientists have suggested that there are "nonresponders" to progressive RET (Bamman, Petrella, Kim, Mayhew, & Cross, 2007); however, a recent retrospective analysis revealed that while there is a large heterogeneity in the adaptive response to prolonged RET as it relates to changes in strength and mass, the level of responsiveness was strongly affected by the duration of the exercise intervention, with more positive responses following more prolonged exercise training (Churchward-Venne et al., 2015). Accordingly, these findings suggest that there are no true "nonresponders" to the benefits of RET among the elderly and that it should be promoted without restriction to prevent and manage sarcopenia and dynapenia. In Figure 9.2, we present conceptual interactions between physical activity, sarcopenia, dynapenia, fatigability, exercise tolerance, and physical function (Figure 9.2A) and demonstrate how progressive RET can modulate these various phenotypic factors (Figure 9.2B).

THE COMMON PRACTICES ARE NOT THE BEST PRACTICES

Unfortunately, many older people are unable or unwilling to embark on strenuous exercise training programs, and, despite a call from the American Academy of Family Physicians (Physicians, 2015), many seniors are often prescribed "low-dose" resistance exercise programs that are physiologically inadequate to increase gains in muscle mass and strength. In 2004, the National Council on Aging (NCOA) Center for Healthy Aging released a guide entitled *Best Practices*

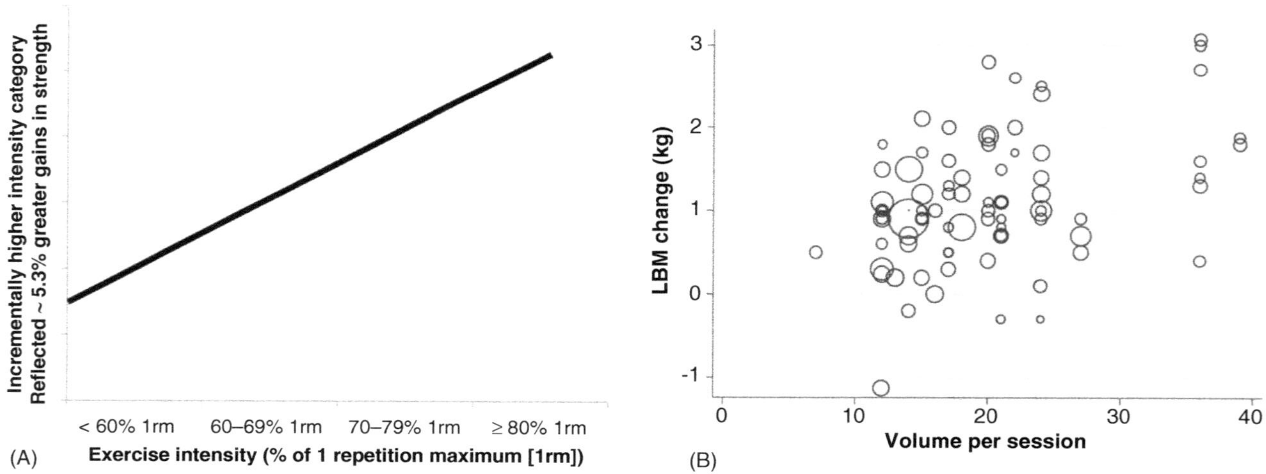

FIGURE 9.1 Higher intensity resistance exercise training is associated with greater improvements in muscle strength (A), and higher volume resistance exercise training is associated with greater improvements in lean body mass (LBM) (B). (A) Peterson et al. (2010) reported in a meta-analysis that with each incremental increase in exercise intensity from low-intensity (<60% of 1RM), low-/moderate-intensity (60%–69% of 1RM), and moderate-/high-intensity (70%–79% of 1RM) to high-intensity (≥80% of 1RM) training, the average percent change in strength was 5.3%. Created from data presented in Peterson et al. (2010). (B) LBM change by training volume (defined as sets per session) when weighted by the number of subjects in a given study using a meta-analytical approach. Reprinted with permission from Peterson et al. (2011).

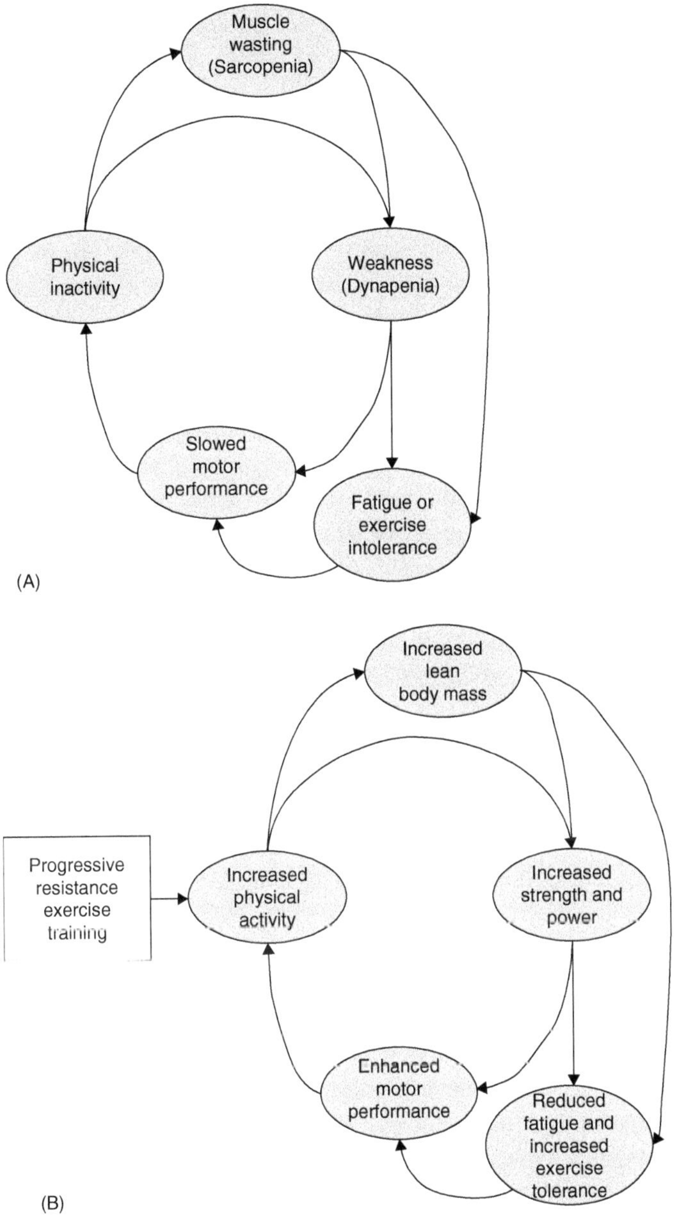

FIGURE 9.2 Conceptual interactions between physical activity, sarcopenia, dynapenia, fatigability, exercise tolerance, and physical function (A) and how progressive resistance exercise training can modulate these various phenotypic factors (B). *Note:* Other influences, such as nutritional, cognitive, and psychological factors, are not shown for clarity. Adapted with permission from Liu and Fielding (2011).

in Physical Activity in order to disseminate information to the public regarding the best practice and evidence-based models that were being employed at a community level (local public or nonprofit organizations) to facilitate older adults in achieving and maintaining functional independence and vitality (NCOA, 2004). A team of experts developed best practice criteria based on expert opinion and findings from the literature and identified 10 community-based programs as national best practice programs. In 2009, Hughes et al. assessed the impact of these 10 best practice physical activity programs for older adults in terms of health-related outcomes (Hughes, Seymour, Campbell, Whitelaw, & Bazzarre, 2009). Not surprisingly, these community-based physical activity programs, which utilized multiple-component physical activity interventions, measurably improved aspects of physical function that are risk factors for disability among older adults. Unfortunately, our anecdotal observation is that there is a large degree of variability in the implementation of physical activity programs in the community-based setting. Common barriers to implementation and participation in community-based exercise programs are program costs, lack of transportation/accessibility, lack of necessary time commitment, unsupportive physical environments, psychological barriers with regard to negative connotations of exercising in the older adults, as well as lack of expertise (Boyette et al., 2002; Mathews et al., 2010; Schutzer et al., 2004). In 2009, Cress et al. identified the key components of best practice physical activity programs for older adult populations as being (a) muscular strength and endurance, (b) balance, (c) cardiovascular endurance, and (d) flexibility (Cress et al., 2005). While many of the existing best practice community programs incorporate these components into their physical activity interventions, very few have adopted the American College of Sports Medicine (ACSM) guidelines for progressive high-intensity RET to promote muscle hypertrophy, strength, and power (ACSM, 2009). An example of one such program is the Go4Life program by the National Institute on Aging (2015). While this program encourages older adults to create personal physical activity programs incorporating all four of these key components, the examples provided for muscular strength training/resistance exercises on the Go4Life website are exercises of very low to moderate intensity for most seniors and are difficult to progress as they utilize wrist weights, TheraBand™, small hand weights, and gravity-reduced body weight resistance exercises. Similarly, our observations indicate that many rehabilitation facilities (including hospitals and short- and long-term stay facilities) have not adopted high-intensity progressive RET into their standard protocol for the prefrail and frail elderly client/patient populations. While many of these facilities offer 60 minutes of therapy twice per day, they commonly use low-intensity exercise (e.g., seated in a wheelchair performing knee extension exercises with ankle weights) in conjunction with some functional training (i.e., wheelchair transfers) and aerobic activity. While the types of exercises mentioned earlier present adequate entry-level exercises for seniors, they are not likely a sufficient stimulus to promote positive muscle growth and adaptation. Accordingly, in the following section, we attempt to provide pragmatic resistance exercise advice for patients and practitioners.

PRAGMATIC RESISTANCE EXERCISE ADVICE FOR PATIENTS AND THE PRACTITIONER

When developing RET programs for older adults, it is important to consider all of the various training-related variables such as frequency, duration, exercises, sets, intensity, repetitions, and progression. Also, many older adults often have existing health issues (e.g., orthopedic limitations and cardiovascular disease) that require special consideration. Therefore, it is highly recommended that older adults who are at risk for RET-induced adverse events receive prior approval from their physician before participating in RET (note: the Physical Activity Readiness Questionnaire [PAR-Q] is a common questionnaire utilized to determine whether an individual should consult a physician before starting a physical activity program). Further, it is suggested that older adults who are beginning a RET program receive proper instruction and supervision by an appropriately trained exercise professional such as a physical therapist or an exercise physiologist.

RET Frequency

Exercise frequency refers to the number of exercise sessions per week. With regard to older adults performing RET, 2–4 days per week are commonly recommended, with training typically being performed on alternating days (e.g., Monday, Wednesday and Friday; Willoughby, 2015). The most common approach for someone beginning a RET program is to perform a "total body" exercise routine whereby all of the major muscle groups are exercised at each exercise session with the "total body" routine being performed 2–3 times per week. An alternative approach, which is more commonly used in more advanced RET programs involves exercising selected muscle groups on 1 or 2 days per week while the remaining are exercised on a separate 1 or 2 days per week (e.g., chest, back, and upper legs on Monday; arms, shoulders, and lower legs on Tuesday; chest, back, and upper legs on Thursday; and arms, shoulders, and lower legs on Friday).

RET Duration

Duration describes the length of each training session. The total duration of RET programs is highly variable and not commonly studied per se as there are many extraneous factors that contribute to duration (e.g., rest time between sets). In general, however, most RET sessions should be able to be completed in 30 minutes to an hour (at an advanced level, more time may be required). The amount of rest taken between sets is a highly influential variable that affects the total duration (alongside the number of sets, exercises, etc.). With respect to between-set rest interval, the ACSM currently recommends rest intervals of 1–2 minutes for training programs designed to stimulate muscular hypertrophy in novice and intermediate healthy resistance exercisers (ACSM, 2009). With this said, many authors have proposed that rest intervals of 30–60 seconds are optimal because they result in the greatest exercise-induced elevations in selected anabolic hormones, notably growth hormones (de Salles et al., 2009; Willardson, 2006). The current literature does not support this notion per se (Henselmans & Schoenfeld, 2014); however, many experienced practitioners anecdotally report more hypertrophic gains with shorter rest intervals.

RET Exercises

Exercises are commonly categorized as either multijoint or unijoint. Multijoint exercises are those in which more than one joint is involved in the exercise, such as the chest press and leg press. Unijoint exercises are those where only one joint is involved, such as bicep curls and leg extensions. For older adults, multijoint exercises should be encouraged (due to their functional relevance) (Willoughby, 2015), although unijoint exercises should not necessarily be discouraged. Additionally, resistance exercise machines (e.g., leg press machines) are recommended for the beginner over free weights (i.e., barbells and dumbbells) as less skill is required when using machines, and the movement restrictions of the machines provide greater safety for the user. As an individual progresses, however, free-weight exercises appropriate for level of skill, training status, and functional capacity are reasonable.

The specific exercises to perform can be highly variable depending on the availability of equipment, but a well-rounded RET program should include exercises that involve all of the "major muscle groups." These muscle groups are commonly defined as the chest, back, arms, shoulders, upper legs (quadriceps, hamstrings, and gluteals), and lower legs (calves). Examples of different exercises for each of these major muscle groups are provided in Table 9.1. One to two exercises per muscle group is adequate for the beginner and intermediate exerciser (Willoughby, 2015), and it should be noted that performing multijoint exercises

TABLE 9.1
Example Exercises for the Major Muscle Groups

Muscle Group	Exercises
Chest	Flat chest press (machine*, barbell**, or dumbbell**)
	Chest flyes (machine*, flat dumbbell flyes**, incline or decline flyes***)
	Incline or decline chest press (machine**, barbell***, or dumbbell***)
	Push-ups (modified with knees on ground** or unmodified with feet on ground***)
Back	Pull-downs or seated cable rows (machine*)
	Chest-supported rows (machine**, barbell***, dumbbell***)
	Pull-ups (with machine body weight assist** or no body weight assist***)
	Shrugs (machine**, barbell***, dumbbell***)
Arms	Seated curls (machine*, barbell**, or dumbbell**)
	Hammer or preacher curls (dumbbell**)
	Triceps extension (machine*, cable press-down*, or prone barbell or dumbbell***)
	Bent-over triceps extension "kickbacks" (dumbbell**)
Shoulders	Overhead press (machine*, barbell***, or dumbbell***)
	Upright rows (machine**, barbell***, or dumbbell***)
	Lateral raises (machine*, barbell***, or cable***)
	Rear deltoid rows/flyes (machine**, barbell***, or dumbbell***)
Upper legs	Leg press (machine*)
	Leg extensions (quadriceps) and curls (hamstrings) (machine*)
	Lunges (no weight**, barbell*** , or dumbbell***)
	Machine squat***
Lower legs	Standing calf raises (no weights*, with additional weight via machine or dumbbells***)
	Seated calf raises (machine*)

Note: Exercises recommended for *the beginner, **an intermediate level, and ***an advanced level. Resistance exercise machines are recommended for the beginner over free weights. As an individual progresses, however, free-weight exercises appropriate for the level of skill, training status, and functional capacity are reasonable. Additionally, multijoint exercises are recommended, as these frequently have higher functional relevance and also result in more than one muscle group being exercised.

results in multiple muscle groups being exercised (e.g., chest press exercises not only the chest [pectoralis] muscles, but also the triceps and the anterior compartment of the shoulder). In general, it is recommended that multijoint exercises be performed before unijoint exercises for a particular muscle group and that within each session, the larger muscle groups be exercised before the smaller muscle groups (Willoughby, 2015).

RET Sets

Significant improvements in muscle strength and size have been observed with the number of sets ranging between one and three (Starkey et al., 1996). We recommend that an individual start with a familiarization period that lasts 1–2 weeks where one set of each exercise is performed with heavy emphasis placed on safety and form. Next, depending on individual need, progression up to three sets in the beginner phase is reasonable when deemed appropriate. With progression to an intermediate and advanced stage, additional sets or additional exercises can be added to increase the overall volume of training (total number of sets per session), which, as illustrated in Figure 9.2B, is critical for hypertrophic gains. Also, as mentioned previously, the interset rest interval is important to consider, and sufficient rest should be taken to avoid excessive fatigue (i.e., enough rest so that the remaining sets can be performed with the appropriate form), but an excessively long rest period should be avoided.

RET Intensity

Intensity refers to the relative amount of weight being lifted (i.e., the percentage of maximum). As illustrated in Figure 9.1A, the RET intensity is a critical factor in determining the amount of neuromuscular adaptation induced via training. Numerous studies have now illustrated that high-intensity RET (e.g., 80+% of 1RM) is tolerated in older adults (Chale et al., 2013; Fiatarone et al., 1994; Reeves et al., 2003; Singh et al., 2012). Accordingly, we suggest that RET intensity should be progressed to "high intensity" as permitted. However, it should be noted that studies have shown intensities ranging from 65% to 75% of maximum will increase strength, and some authors suggest these intensities should be utilized as an attempt to decrease the risk of musculoskeletal injury (Willoughby, 2015).

RET Repetitions

Repetitions refer to the number of times an individual performs a complete movement of a given exercise. The number of repetitions that one can perform is inversely related to the exercise intensity (i.e., the higher the intensity, the fewer repetitions that can be performed). As illustrated in Figure 9.3, if an individual is exercising at 60% of his/her maximum strength, he/she will likely be able to perform between 18 and 32 repetitions to "task failure" using free weights. At 80% of the individual's maximum strength, the number of repetitions to failure is generally between 8 and 15, and at 90%, it is 4–12 repetitions with free weights. The number of repetitions to failure for machines is, generally speaking, slightly higher than with free weights (Figure 9.3) presumably due to free weights requiring more muscles for stabilization and balance compared to a fixed-path machine-lifting task. Understanding these relationships is important, as it provides a mechanism for a trial-and-error approach to be utilized to prescribe the appropriate training load without having to actually test muscle strength (e.g., performing the exercise to task failure within 10–15 repetitions would likely indicate that an individual is exercising at an intensity in the 70%–85% of maximum strength range).

RET Progression

The concept of "progression" refers to gradually overloading, or increasing the stress, placed on the body during exercise. The human body will only respond if it is continually required to exert a greater magnitude of force (or higher volume) to meet higher physiological demands. Thus, in order to continually enjoy improvements in mass, strength, and functional capacity, it is important to consistently incorporate progression and variation into the RET program. There are an ample number of ways to progress a RET program. For instance, one can make adjustments by increasing the frequency, duration, exercises performed, number of exercises for each muscle group, sets, and repetitions. Progression should be a gradual process with adjustments made on a monthly basis commonly recommended (Willoughby, 2015). During progression, it is important for the exercise professional to be aware of the patient's medical limitations and for progression to occur via adjustments in the most appropriate training variables on a case-by-case basis.

In Tables 9.2 to 9.5, we present an example progressive RET program. This program is designed for an older adult without any contraindications for RET training. Modifications would need to be made if certain musculoskeletal, neurological, or mobility limitations precluded an individual from safely performing the program. This program is designed on the assumption that access to typical machine and free-weight resistance exercise equipment is available, but it could be modified as needed based on equipment availability. Additionally, progression could be varied (sped up or slowed down) depending on individual adaptation.

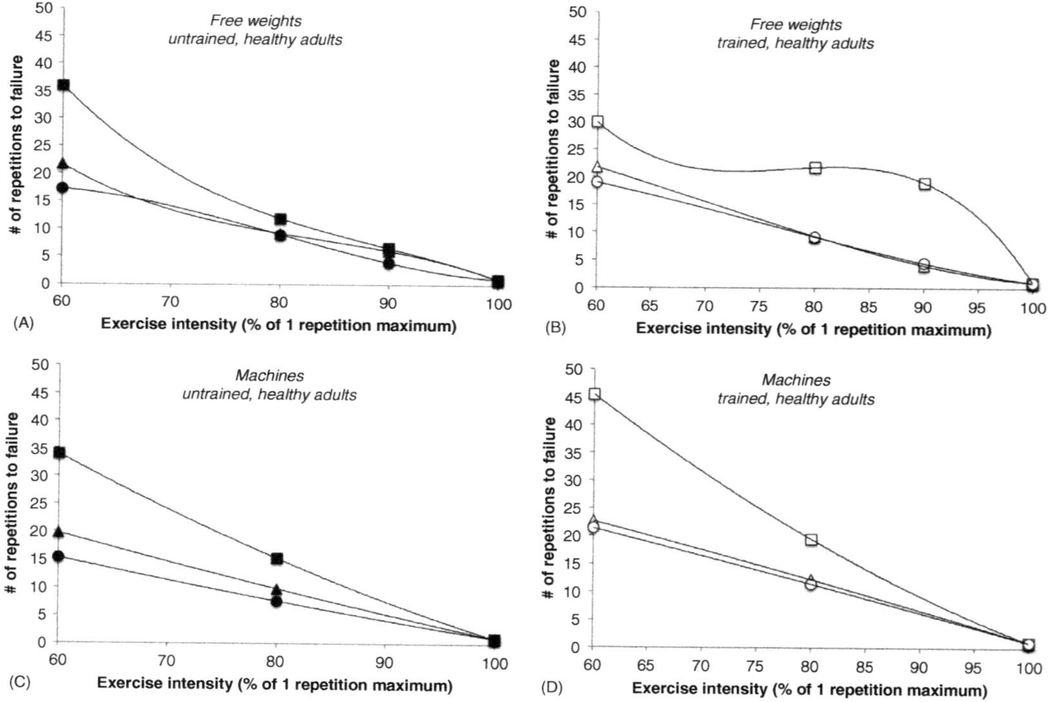

FIGURE 9.3 Relationship between the number of repetitions untrained (A) and trained (B) healthy adults were able to perform *using free weights* at four different resistance exercise intensities (60%, 80%, and 90% of 1RM) for the squat (square), bench press (triangle), and arm curl (circle). Created from data presented in Shimano et al. (2006). Relationship between the number of repetitions untrained (C) and trained (D) healthy adults were able to perform using resistance exercise machines at three different resistance exercise intensities (60%, 80%, and 1RM) for the leg press (square), chest press (triangle), and arm curl (circle). Data represent the mean response for each exercise and intensity, respectively. Created from data presented on Hoeger et al. (1990).

TABLE 9.2
Example Beginner Progressive Resistance Exercise Training Program (Weeks 1–8)

Body Part	Exercise	Sets × Reps
Beginner, Phase I: 50%–60% of 1RM; 2×/Week; 1–2 Weeks; Familiarization Phase		
Chest	Chest press (machine: seated or lying)	1 × 15–20
Back	Seated cable row	1 × 15–20
	Seated cable pull-down	1 × 15–20
Arms	Biceps curl (seated machine)	1 × 15–20
	Triceps extension (seated machine)	1 × 15–20
Shoulders	Overhead press (seated machine)	1 × 15–20
Upper legs	Leg extensions (seated machine)	1 × 15–20
	Leg curl (seated machine)	1 × 15–20
Lower legs	Calf raise (seated machine)	1 × 15–20
	Calf raise (standing)	1 × 15–20
	Rest between sets: 2 minutes (as needed)	**Total sets: 10**
Beginner, Phase II: 60%–69% of 1RM; 2×/Week; 3–8 Weeks		
Chest	Chest press (machine: seated or lying)	1 × 12–18
	Wall push-ups	1 × 12–18
Back	Seated cable row	1 × 12–18
	Seated cable pull-down	1 × 12–18
Arms	Biceps curl (seated machine)	1 × 12–18
	Triceps extension (seated machine)	1 × 12–18
Shoulders	Overhead press (seated machine)	1 × 12–18
Upper legs	Leg extensions (seated machine)	1 × 12–18
	Leg curl (seated machine)	1 × 12–18
Lower legs	Calf raise (seated machine)	1 × 12–18
	Calf raise (standing)	1 × 12–18
	Rest between sets: 90 seconds	**Total sets: 11**

Note: It is suggested that the exercise is performed to, or near, task failure in the range of repetitions provided.

1RM = 1 repetition maximum.

TABLE 9.3
Example Intermediate Progressive Resistance Exercise Training Program (Weeks 9–24)

Body Part	Exercise	Sets × Reps
Intermediate, Phase I: 60%–69% of 1RM; 2×/Week; 9–16 Weeks		
Chest	Chest press (machine: seated or lying)	2 × 12–18
	Wall push-ups	2 × 12–18
	Chest flyes (machine)	2 × 12–18
Back	Seated cable row	2 × 12–18
	Seated cable pull-down	2 × 12–18
Arms	Biceps curl (seated machine)	2 × 12–18
	Triceps extension (seated machine)	2 × 12–18
Shoulders	Overhead press (seated machine)	2 × 12–18
	Lateral raises (seated machine)	2 × 12–18
Upper legs	Leg press (machine)	2 × 12–18
	Leg extensions (seated machine)	2 × 12–18
	Leg curl (seated machine)	2 x 12–18
Lower legs	Calf raise (seated machine)	2 x 12–18
	Calf raise (standing)	2 x 12–18
	Rest between sets: 90 seconds	**Total sets: 28**

Body Part	Exercise	Sets × Reps
Intermediate, Phase II: 70%–79% of 1RM; 3×/Week; 17–24 Weeks		
Chest	Chest press (barbell)	2 × 10–15
	Chest flyes (lying with dumbbells)	2 × 10–15
	Push-ups (knees down)	2 × 10–15
Back	Chest-supported rows (machine)	2 × 10–15
	Pull-ups (machine with body weight assist)	2 × 10–15
Arms	Biceps curl (seated dumbbell)	2 × 10–15
	Triceps extension (cable press-down)	2 × 10–15
	Triceps kickbacks (dumbbells)	2 × 10–15
Shoulders	Overhead press (seated machine)	2 × 10–15
	Lateral raises (seated machine)	2 × 10–15
	Upright rows (barbell or dumbbells)	2 × 10–15

(Continued)

TABLE 9.3
Example Intermediate Progressive Resistance Exercise Training Program (Weeks 9–24) (Continued)

Body Part	Exercise	Sets × Reps
Intermediate, Phase II: 70%–79% of 1RM; 3×/Week; 17–24 Weeks		
Upper legs	Leg press (machine)	2 × 10–15
	Leg Extensions (seated machine)	2 × 10–15
	Lunges (no weight)	2 × 10–15
	Leg curl (seated machine)	2 × 10–15
Lower legs	Calf raise (seated machine)	2 × 10–15
	Calf raise (standing)	2 × 10–15
	Rest between sets: 90 seconds	**Total sets: 34**

Note: It is suggested that the exercise is performed to, or near, task failure in the range of repetitions provided.

1RM = 1 repetition maximum.

TABLE 9.4
Example Advanced Phase I Progressive Resistance Exercise Training Program (Weeks 25–32)

Body Part	Exercise	Sets × Reps
Advanced, Phase I: >80% of 1RM; 3×/Week; 25–32 Weeks		
Chest	Chest press (barbell)	2 × 8–12
	Chest flyes (lying with dumbbells)	2 × 8–12
	Incline chest press (machine)	2 × 8–12
	Push-ups (knees down)	2 × 8–12
Back	Chest-supported rows (machine)	2 × 8–12
	Pull-ups (machine with body weight assist)	2 × 8–12
	Shoulder shrugs (machine)	2 × 8–12
Arms	Biceps curl (seated dumbbell)	2 × 8–12
	Hammer curls (seated dumbbell)	2 × 8–12
	Triceps extension (cable press-down)	2 × 8–12
	Triceps kickbacks (dumbbells)	2 × 8–12
Shoulders	Overhead press (seated machine)	2 × 8–12
	Lateral raises (seated machine)	2 × 8–12

(Continued)

TABLE 9.4
Example Advanced Phase I Progressive Resistance Exercise Training Program (Weeks 25–32) (Continued)

Body Part	Exercise	Sets × Reps
	Rear deltoid flyes (machine or dumbbells)	2 × 8–12
	Upright rows (barbell or dumbbells)	2 × 8–12
Upper legs	Leg press (machine)	2 × 8–12
	Leg extensions (seated machine)	2 × 8–12
	Lunges (no weight)	2 × 8–12
	Leg curl (seated machine)	2 × 8–12
Lower legs	Calf raise (seated machine)	2 × 8–12
	Calf raise (standing)	2 × 8–12
	Rest between sets: 60–90 seconds	**Total sets: 42**

Note: It is suggested that the exercise is performed to, or near, task failure in the range of repetitions provided.

1RM = 1 repetition maximum.

TABLE 9.5
Example Advanced Phase II Progressive Resistance Exercise Training Program (32+ Weeks)

Body Part	Exercise	Sets × Reps
Advanced, Phase II: >80% of 1RM; 4x/Week Split; 32+ Weeks; Monday and Thursday		
Chest	Chest press (barbell or dumbbell)	3 × 6–10
	Incline or decline chest press (barbell or dumbbell)	3 × 6–10
	Chest flyes (lying with dumbbells)	3 × 6–10
	Push-ups	3 × 6–10
Back	Chest-supported rows (barbell or dumbbell)	3 × 6–10
	Pull-ups (with or without assist)	3 × 6–10
	Shoulder shrugs (barbell or dumbbell)	3 × 6–10
Upper legs	Squat (machine)	3 × 6–10
	Leg extensions (seated machine)	3 × 6–10
	Leg curl (seated machine)	3 × 6–10
	Lunges (dumbbell)	3 × 6–10

(Continued)

TABLE 9.5
Example Advanced Phase II Progressive Resistance Exercise Training Program (32+ Weeks) (Continued)

Body Part	Exercise	Sets × Reps
Tuesday and Friday		
Arms	Biceps curl (standing barbell)	3 × 6–10
	Biceps curl (seated dumbbell)	3 × 6–10
	Hammer or preacher curls (seated dumbbell)	3 × 6–10
	Triceps extension (lying with barbell or dumbbell)	3 × 6–10
	Triceps kickbacks (dumbbells)	3 × 6–10
Shoulders	Overhead press (barbell or dumbbell)	3 × 6–10
	Lateral raises (dumbbell or cable)	3 × 6–10
	Rear deltoid flyes (machine or dumbbells)	3 × 6–10
	Upright rows (barbell or dumbbells)	3 × 6–10
Lower legs	Calf raise (seated machine)	3 × 6–10
	Calf raise (standing)	3 × 6–10
	Rest between sets: 60 seconds	**Total sets: 33 sets/day**

Note: This phase goes to four times per week with a "split routine." It is suggested that the exercise is performed to, or near, task failure in the range of repetitions provided.

1RM = 1 repetition maximum.

CONCLUSIONS

A well-designed, progressive RET program is well known to exert positive effects on both the nervous and muscular systems and, ultimately, results in profound enhancements in muscle mass and muscle strength. Accordingly, RET should be considered a first-line treatment strategy for managing and preventing both sarcopenia and dynapenia. While there are many components to an optimal resistance exercise prescription, exercise intensity, exercise volume, and progression are critical factors that deserve strong consideration as this relates to following best practice guidelines. We hope the example RET program presented herein is useful for academicians, students, and healthcare providers across a variety of disciplines, including those in the long-term care industry.

NOTE

1. Progressive RET involves increasing the number of repetitions at a constant load until exceeding an established repetition range (e.g., 12 repetitions). Subsequently, the load is increased and the exercise is performed at the new load until again exceeding the repetition range.

ACKNOWLEDGMENTS

We would like to thank Robert S. Staron, PhD (Ohio University), for his thoughtful critique and input on a draft of this manuscript. This work was supported in part by the following grants from the National Institutes of Health to Brian C. Clark: R01AG044424 from the National Institute on Aging, R01AT006978 from the National Center for Complementary and Integrative Health, and R21AR063909 from the National Institute of Arthritis and Musculoskeletal and Skin Diseases.

REFERENCES

American College of Sports Medicine. (2009). American College of Sports Medicine position stand. Progression models in resistance training for healthy adults. *Medicine and Science in Sports and Exercise, 41*(3), 687–708. doi:10.1249/MSS.0b013e3181915670

Bamman, M. M., Petrella, J. K., Kim, J. S., Mayhew, D. L., & Cross, J. M. (2007). Cluster analysis tests the importance of myogenic gene expression during myofiber hypertrophy in humans. *Journal of Applied Physiology, 102*(6), 2232–2239. doi:10.1152/japplphysiol.00024.2007

Bird, M. L., Hill, K., Ball, M., & Williams, A. D. (2009). Effects of resistance and flexibility-exercise interventions on balance and related measures in older adults. *Journal of Aging and Physical Activity, 17*(4), 444–454.

Boyette, L. W., Lloyd, A., Boyette, J. E., Watkins, E., Furbush, L., Dunbar, S. B., et al. (2002). Personal characteristics that influence exercise behavior of older adults. *Journal of Rehabilitation Research and Development, 39*(1), 95–103.

Burton, L. A., & Sumukadas, D. (2010). Optimal management of sarcopenia. *Clinical Interventions in Aging, 5*, 217–228.

Chale, A., Cloutier, G. J., Hau, C., Phillips, E. M., Dallal, G. E., & Fielding, R. A. (2013). Efficacy of whey protein supplementation on resistance exercise-induced changes in lean mass, muscle strength, and physical function in mobility-limited older adults. *The Journals of Gerontology Series A: Biological Sciences and Medical Sciences, 68*(6), 682–690.doi:10.1093/gerona/gls221

Charette, S. L., McEvoy, L., Pyka, G., Snow-Harter, C., Guido, D., Wiswell, R. A., & Marcus, R. (1991). Muscle hypertrophy response to resistance training in older women. *Journal of Applied Physiology, 70*(5), 1912–1916.

Churchward-Venne, T. A., Tieland, M., Verdijk, L. B., Leenders, M., Dirks, M. L., de Groot, L. C., & van Loon, L. J. (2015). There are no nonresponders to resistance-type exercise training in older men and women. *Journal of the American Medical Directors Association*, *16*, 400–411. doi:10.1016/j.jamda.2015.01.071

Clark, B. C. (2009). In vivo alterations in skeletal muscle form and function after disuse atrophy. *Medicine and Science in Sports and Exercise*, *41*, 1869–1875. doi:10.1249/MSS.0b013e3181a645a6

Clark, B. C., & Manini, T. M. (2008). Sarcopenia ≠ Dynapenia. *The Journals of Gerontology Series A: Biological Sciences and Medical Sciences*, *63*(8), 829–834. doi:10.1093/gerona/63.8.829

Cress, M. E., Buchner, D. M., Prohaska, T., Rimmer, J., Brown, M., Macera, C., et al. (2005). Best practices for physical activity programs and behavior counseling in older adult populations. *Journal of Aging and Physical Activity*, *13*(1), 61–74.

Cruz-Jentoft, A. J., Baeyens, J. P., Bauer, J. M., Boirie, Y., Cederholm, T., Landi, F., et al. (2010). Sarcopenia: European consensus on definition and diagnosis: Report of the European Working Group on Sarcopenia in older people. *Age and Ageing*, *39*(4), 412–423. doi:10.1093/ageing/afq034

de Salles, B. F., Simao, R., Miranda, F., Novaes Jda, S., Lemos, A., & Willardson, J. M. (2009). Rest interval between sets in strength training. *Sports Medicine*, *39*(9), 765–777. doi:10.2165/11315230-000000000-00000

Duchateau, J., & Enoka, R. M. (2002). Neural adaptations with chronic activity patterns in able-bodied humans. *American journal of Physical Medicine & Rehabilitation*, *81*(11, Suppl.), S17–S27. doi:10.1097/00002060-200211001-00004

Fiatarone, M. A., Marks, E. C., Ryan, N. D., Meredith, C. N., Lipsitz, L. A., & Evans, W. J. (1990). High-intensity strength training in nonagenarians. Effects on skeletal muscle. *Journal of the American Medical Association*, *263*(22), 3029–3034.

Fiatarone, M. A., O'Neill, E. F., Ryan, N. D., Clements, K. M., Solares, G. R., Nelson, M. E., et al. (1994). Exercise training and nutritional supplementation for physical frailty in very elderly people. *New England Journal of Medicine*, *330*(25), 1769–1775. doi:10.1056/NEJM199406233302501

Henselmans, M., & Schoenfeld, B. J. (2014). The effect of inter-set rest intervals on resistance exercise-induced muscle hypertrophy. *Sports Medicine*, *44*(12), 1635–1643. doi:10.1007/s40279-014-0228-0

Hikida, R. S., Staron, R. S., Hagerman, F. C., Walsh, S., Kaiser, E., Shell, S., & Hervey, S. (2000). Effects of high-intensity resistance training on untrained older men. II. Muscle fiber characteristics and nucleo-cytoplasmic relationships. *The Journals of Gerontology Series A: Biological Sciences and Medical Sciences*, *55*(7), B347–B354.

Hoeger, W. W. K., Hopkins, D. R., Barette, S. L., & Hale, D. F. (1990). Relationship between repetitions and selected percentages of one repetition maximum. *Journal of Strength and Conditioning Research*, *4*(2), 47–54.

Hughes, S. L., Seymour, R. B., Campbell, R. T., Whitelaw, N., & Bazzarre, T. (2009). Best-practice physical activity programs for older adults: Findings from the national impact study. *American Journal of Public Health*, *99*(2), 362–368. doi:10.2105/AJPH.2007.131466

Kalapotharakos, V. I., Diamantopoulos, K., & Tokmakidis, S. P. (2010). Effects of resistance training and detraining on muscle strength and functional performance of older adults aged 80 to 88 years. *Aging Clinical and Experimental Research*, *22*(2), 134–140.

Kamen, G., & Knight, C. A. (2004). Training-related adaptations in motor unit discharge rate in young and older adults. *The Journals of Gerontology Series A: Biological Sciences and Medical Sciences*, *59*(12), 1334–1338.

Liu, C. K., & Fielding, R. A. (2011). Exercise as an intervention for frailty. *Clinics in Geriatric Medicine*, *27*(1), 101–110.

Liu, C. J., & Latham, N. K. (2009). Progressive resistance strength training for improving physical function in older adults. *Cochrane Database Syst Rev*, (3), CD002759. doi:10.1002/14651858.CD002759.pub2

Manini, T. M., & Clark, B. C. (2011). Dynapenia and aging: An update. *The Journals of Gerontology Series A: Biological Sciences and Medical Sciences*, *67A*, 28–40. doi:10.1093/gerona/glr010

Manini, T., Marko, M., VanArnam, T., Cook, S., Fernhall, B., Burke, J., & Ploutz-Snyder, L. (2007). Efficacy of resistance and task-specific exercise in older adults who modify tasks of everyday life. *The Journals of Gerontology Series A: Biological Sciences and Medical Sciences*, *62*(6), 616–623.

Manini, T. M., Russ, D. W., & Clark, B. C. (2012). The complex relationship between muscle mass and muscle strength. In A. J. Cruz-Jentoft & J. E. Morley (Eds.), *Sarcopenia* (pp. 74–103). Chichester, UK: John Wiley & Sons, Ltd.

Mathews, A. E., Laditka, S. B., Laditka, J. N., Wilcox, S., Corwin, S. J., Liu, R., et al. (2010). Older adults' perceived physical activity enablers and barriers: a multicultural perspective. *Journal of Aging and Physical Activity, 18*(2), 119–140.

Narici, M. V., & Maffulli, N. (2010). Sarcopenia: Characteristics, mechanisms and functional significance. *British Medical Bulletin*, *95*, 139–159. doi:10.1093/bmb/ldq008

National Council on Aging. (2004). *Best practices in physical activity*. Washington, DC: The National Council on Aging. Retrieved from https://www.ncoa.org/wp-content/uploads/BP_PhysicalActivity.pdf

National Institute on Aging. (2015). *Go4Life*. Retrieved April 6, 2015, from https://go4life.nia.nih.gov

Peterson, M. D., Rhea, M. R., Sen, A., & Gordon, P. M. (2010). Resistance exercise for muscular strength in older adults: A meta-analysis. *Ageing Research Reviews*, *9*(3), 226–237. doi:10.1016/j.arr.2010.03.004

Peterson, M. D., Sen, A., & Gordon, P. M. (2011). Influence of resistance exercise on lean body mass in aging adults: Ameta-analysis. *Medicine & Science in Sports & Exercise*, *43*(2), 249–258. doi:10.1249/MSS.0b013e3181eb6265

Physicians, American Academy of Family. (2015). *Choosing wisely: Don't prescribe under-dosed strength training programs for older adults. Instead, match the frequency, intensity, and duration of exercise to the individual's abilities and goals.* Retrieved March 23, 2015, from http://www.aafp.org/afp/recommendations/viewRecommendation.htm?recommendationId=210

Reeves, N. D., Maganaris, C. N., & Narici, M. V. (2003). Effect of strength training on human patella tendon mechanical properties of older individuals. *The Journal of Physiology*, *548*(3), 971–981. doi:10.1113/jphysiol.2002.035576

Rosenberg, I. H. (1989). Summary comments. *The American Journal of Clinical Nutrition*, *50*, 1231–1233.

Russ, D. W., Gregg-Cornell, K., Conaway, M. J., & Clark, B. C. (2012). Evolving concepts on the age-related changes in "muscle quality". *Journal of Cachexia, Sarcopenia and Muscle*, *3*, 95–109. doi:10.1007/s13539-011-0054-2

Sayer, A. A., Robinson, S. M., Patel, H. P., Shavlakadze, T., Cooper, C., & Grounds, M. D. (2013). New horizons in the pathogenesis, diagnosis and management of sarcopenia. *Age and Ageing*, *42*(2), 145–150. doi:10.1093/ageing/afs191

Schutzer, K. A., Graves, B. S. (2004). Barriers and motivations to exercise in older adults. *Preventive Medicine*, *39*(5), 1056–1061.

Shimano, T., Kraemer, W. J., Spiering, B. A., Volek, J. S., Hatfield, D. L., Silvestre, R., et al. (2006). Relationship between the number of repetitions and selected percentages of one repetition maximum in free weight exercises in trained and untrained men. *Journal of Strength and Conditioning Research*, *20*(4), 819–823.

Singh, N. A., Quine, S., Clemson, L. M., Williams, E. J., Williamson, D. A., Stavrinos, T. M., et al. (2012). Effects of high-intensity progressive resistance training and targeted multidisciplinary treatment of frailty on mortality and nursing home admissions after hip fracture: A randomized controlled trial. *Journal of the American Medical Directors Association*, *13*(1), 24–30. doi:10.1016/j.jamda.2011.08.005

Starkey, D. B., Pollock, M. L., Ishida, Y., Welsch, M. A., Brechue, W. F., Graves, J. E., & Feigenbaum, M. S. (1996). Effect of resistance training volume on strength and muscle thickness. *Medicine & Science in Sports & Exercise*, *28*(10), 1311–1320.

Studenski, S. A., Peters, K. W., Alley, D. E., Cawthon, P. M., McLean, R. R., Harris, T. B., et al. (2014). The FNIH sarcopenia project: Rationale, study description, conference recommendations, and final estimates. *The Journals of Gerontology Series A: Biological Sciences and Medical Sciences*, *69*(5), 547–558. doi:10.1093/gerona/glu010

Sylliaas, H., Brovold, T., Wyller, T. B., & Bergland, A. (2011). Progressive strength training in older patients after hip fracture: A randomised controlled trial. *Age and Ageing*, *40*(2), 221–227. doi:10.1093/ageing/afq167

Troiano, R. P., Berrigan, D., Dodd, K. W., Masse, L. C., Tilert, T., & McDowell, M. (2008). Physical activity in the United States measured by accelerometer. *Medicine & Science in Sports & Exercise*, *40*(1), 181–188. doi:10.1249/mss.0b013e31815a51b3

United States Census Bureau. (2015). *USA quick facts from the US Census Bureau*. Retrieved March 23, 2015, from http://quickfacts.census.gov/qfd/states/00000.html

Van Roie, E., Delecluse, C., Coudyzer, W., Boonen, S., & Bautmans, I. (2013). Strength training at high versus low external resistance in older adults: Effects on muscle volume, muscle strength, and force-velocity characteristics. *Experimental Gerontology*, *48*(11), 1351–1361. doi:10.1016/j.exger.2013.08.010

Visser, M., & Schaap, L. A. (2011). Consequences of sarcopenia. *Clinics in Geriatric Medicine*, *27*(3), 387–399. doi:10.1016/j.cger.2011.03.006

Willardson, J. M. (2006). A brief review: Factors affecting the length of the rest interval between resistance exercise sets. *The Journal of Strength and Conditioning Research*, *20*(4), 978–984. doi:10.1519/R-17995.1

Willoughby, D. S. (2015). *Resistance training and the older adult ACSM current comment. current comments are official statements by the American College of Sports Medicine concerning topics of interest to the public at large.* Indianapolis, IN: American College of Sports Medicine.

CHAPTER 10

Tai Chi to Promote Balance Training

Carol E. Rogers

ABSTRACT

In this chapter, the use of Tai Chi (TC) to promote balance training is described. Participating in balance training is recommended for older adults at risk for falls. The *2008 Physical Activity Guidelines for Americans* recommend TC as a muscle-strengthening exercise and state that TC may prevent falls. The majority of TC research in the past 20 years has explored its effect on various balance outcomes. This review of the effect of TC on balance outcomes found significant improvements in static and dynamic balance, fall rates, and fear of falling in mostly healthy adults. There is some evidence that TC improves postural control strategies and intrinsic factors known to affect balance in healthy adults. Studies have included populations with specific diseases, such as vision impairment, cancer, arthritis, poor bone density, Parkinson's disease, polyneuropathy, cognitive impairment, and diabetes, and older adults living in long-term care facilities. Areas of future research include exploration of mechanisms underpinning changes in dynamic and static balance such as postural control strategies and intrinsic factors.

INTRODUCTION

One goal of our aging population is to maintain functional independence and the ability needed to age in place (National Association of Area Agencies on Aging, 2006; World Health Organization, 2002). Poor balance is one of the multiple

http://dx.doi.org/10.1891/0198-8794.36.229

risk factors for falls and decreased function. The types of exercises to reduce falls should include components of balance, flexibility, strength, and some aerobic conditioning (Rubenstein & Josephson, 2006). Therefore, interventions designed to improve balance and reduce falls should consist of all of these components (Spirduso, Francis, & MacRae, 2005). Range of motion exercise is required to promote joint flexibility by extending the length of muscle and coordinating the contraction of muscle groups around a joint (Powers & Howley, 2007). Joint flexibility and coordinated contractions of muscle groups are required to control the center of mass required for static and dynamic balance (Shumway-Cook & Woollacott, 2007). Muscle strength is required to maintain an upright posture. Because older adults may have been sedentary for some time, it is suggested that they begin with balance and muscle-strengthening exercises and gradually advance to aerobic activities (U. S. Department of Health and Human Services, 2008). Participating in regular exercise builds endurance by training the body to respond to increased energy demands (Nieman, 2007).

Tai Chi (TC) is one form of exercise that has demonstrated multiple health outcomes including balance (Howe, 2012). TC is recommended as a training program to promote muscle strengthening (U. S. Department of Health and Human Services, 2008). Previous reviews have reported that TC has improved perceptions and measures of balance (Hackney & Wolf, 2014; Howe, 2012; Logghe et al., 2010; Rogers, Keller, & Larkey, 2010). The purpose of this chapter is to review how TC and similar forms of exercise have improved balance.

WHAT IS TAI CHI?

Mind–body exercise such as TC has increased in popularity in the United States since the 1990s and makes up 30% of the exercise programs in fitness centers (La Forge, 2005). Mind–body practices that blend physical movement or postures and focus on the breath and mind to achieve deep states of relaxation have been defined as *meditative movement* (MM; Larkey, Jahnke, Etnier, & Gonzalez, 2009). Yoga, TC, and Qigong (QG) are examples of MM that are more familiar. One less familiar form, Sign Chi Do, has been studied (Borik, 2004). Two of these forms, TC and QG, are grounded in the principles of traditional Chinese medicine and have been described as equivalent in terms of basic forms and principles and have consistently produced a number of similar health outcomes (Larkey et al., 2009). In Sign Chi Do, sign gestures are used to create the upper body movement (Rogers, Keller, Larkey, & Ainsworth, 2012). Because of the similarity between TC, QG, and Sign Chi Do, they are included in this review.

TC is a multicomponent exercise that employs complex physical movements with cognitive thought processes. In TC, QG, and Sign Chi Do,

TABLE 10.1
Tai Chi Components

Components	Experience in Practice
Breath	Diaphragmatic breath connected with flow of the movement
Meditation effect	Repetitive practice of movement with breath
	Intentional practice of the movement with attention to focus on the movement and a nonjudgmental attitude
Physical form	Engagement of multiple muscle groups
	Slow and controlled transitional leg movements, shifting weight from right to left and front to back with leg stances and flowing motion of arms
	Most forms are from standing position, with adaptations for seated or lying position to progress to standing position

participants practice flowing movements while shifting weight from one foot to the other in front-to-back and side-to-side stepping patterns (Table 10.1). These movements promote ankle joint flexibility. Advanced forms require maintaining a posture while standing on one foot. One of the major components of TC is body posture adjustment (Chodzko-Zajko et al., 2006). Thus, it is not surprising that most of the TC research has been designed to evaluate outcomes on falls and balance.

These forms of exercise have been described as particularly suitable for older adults (Rogers et al., 2010; Rogers, Larkey, & Keller, 2009; Wong, Lin, Chou, Tang, & Wong, 2001), as they are implemented without the strain that is sometimes associated with higher intensity exercise. Older adults self-reported that TC improved balance and that the reasons for initiating a TC class were to improve function and strength as well as maintain fitness (Rogers et al., 2010). They also reported they enjoyed the classes (Jahnke, Larkey, & Rogers, 2010). A growing body of research indicates a wide range of balance outcomes and mechanisms associated with TC. These MM forms of exercise, TC, QG, and Sign Chi Do, as practiced by older adults, are systematically assessed for benefits to improved balance.

The length of intervention classes ranges from 1 week to 12 months, with the preponderance of interventions at 3 to 6 months. Most classes last 60 minutes each, meeting two to three times weekly (ranging from 1 to 7 days/week). TC and QG forms were previously defined as a gentle movement, which indicates they were performed at a low-to-moderate intensity.

TYPES OF TC

A variety of TC and QG styles are practiced. Most of the forms are named after the family of the founder, and for many of the styles, the practice was adapted from larger to smaller number of movements. For example, a Yang form with 108 original movements was adapted to comprise a range of 5–42 movements. Some of the movements were designed for specific populations such as groups with cardiovascular disease or Parkinson's disease (PD). The TC forms used in research, a brief description of the form, the population studied, and author are described in Table 10.2. One study compared the effect of TC to a Vinyasa yoga form developed for balance (Ni et al., 2014).

BALANCE BENEFITS

Balance is multicomponent in nature and therefore exploring the effect of TC on balance is complex. Research in TC has included measuring outcomes of postural stability (static and dynamic); postural control strategies (ankle, hip, step); intrinsic systems (sensory, motor, cognitive); and falls (actual and perceived fear of falling).

Postural Stability

Postural stability is a person's ability to maintain the position of the body, referred to as center of mass, within specific boundaries of space (Spirduso et al., 2005). Multiple studies have explored the effect of TC on measures of static (stationary) and dynamic (moving) balance outcomes expected to improve a person's ability to maintain postural stability during standing and walking activities. Those studies are discussed.

One leg stance (OLS) is a common measure of static balance and measures how long one can stand (up to 60 seconds) on the dominant foot without touching the other foot on the floor (Bohannon, 2006). Other static balance measures include tandem (one foot directly in front of the other with the toe of one foot touching the heel of the other) and semitandem (one foot in front of the other with the big toe of one foot touching the side of the heel of the other).

Cross-sectional studies have reported that experienced TC practitioners show better postural stability than nonpractitioners among healthy older adults (Gyllensten, Hui-Chan, & Tsang, 2010). Time spent in OLS was longer and the medial–lateral displacement of the center of pressure, indicating better balance, was greater for older adults with 8 years of TC experience while practicing a 42-form TC compared to normal walking (Mao, Li, & Hong, 2006). A recent single-group study showed that 48 weeks of TC (Tai Ji Quan: Moving for Better Balance) improved healthy older adults' ability to maintain center of gravity

TABLE 10.2
Forms of Tai Chi Studied

Description	Form Used	Population[a]/Author
Yang[b] Traditional long form has 103 postures Continual slow pace with soft and circular movements	5 form from Cheng Man-Ch'ing's short form	Assisted living
		Vestibulopathy (McGibbon et al., 2005)
	37–short form of Cheng Man-Ch'ing	Healthy
	6 of 24 simplified TC	History of falls (Sattin, Easley, Wolf, Chen, & Kutner, 2005)
		History of falls (Wolf, Sattin, et al., 2003)
	8 form	Visually impaired in long-term care (Chen, Fu, Chan, & Tsang, 2012)
		Healthy (Zhuang, Huang, Wu, & Zhang, 2014)
	8 form (easy TC)	Prefrail (Hass et al., 2004)
		Sedentary (Li, Fisher, Harmer, & McAuley, 2005)
	10 form	Fall risk (Audette et al., 2006)
		Healthy (Wolf, Barnhart, et al., 2003)
		No exercise (Frye, Scheinthal, Kemarskaya, & Pruchno, 2007)
		Healthy (Huang, Yang, & Liu, 2011)
	12 form	Fall risk (Kim, 2009)
		Idiopathic Parkinson's disease (Kim, Kim, Jae, & Son, 2011)
	12 form with fewer leg movements, knee bends, and hand gestures	Long-term care (Chen et al., 2007)

(*Continued*)

TABLE 10.2
Forms of Tai Chi Studied (*Continued*)

Description	Form Used	Population[a]/Author
	24 form	Healthy Chinese (Gyllensten, Hui-Chan, & Tsang, 2010)
		Healthy (Li, Devault, & Van Oteghen, 2007)
		Sedentary (Li et al., 2005)
		Healthy (Li, Xu, & Hong, 2008)
		Fall risk men with osteopenia or osteoporosis (Maciaszek, Osinski, Szeklicki, & Stemplewski, 2007)
		Healthy (Taylor-Piliae et al., 2010)
		Stroke (Taylor-Piliae et al., 2014)
		Healthy (Woo, Hong, Lau, & Lynn, 2007)
		Poor balance (Zhang, IshikawaTakata, Yamazaki, Morita, & Ohta, 2006)
		Healthy men (Yu & Yang, 2012)
		Knee OA (Shen et al., 2008)
	42 form	Experienced TC practitioners (Mao et al., 2006)
	Classical TC (repeated on both sides for 10–15 cycles)	Fall risk with surgical interventions (Gatts & Woollacott, 2006)
	Modified classic	Women with history of cancer (Reid-Arndt, Matsuda, & Cox, 2012)

	Yang combined with Tai Ji Quan principles (Tai Ji Quan: Moving for Better Balance)	Healthy (Li, 2014)
	6 forms of TC from Yang style with single-form repetition and bilateral stepping with body weight transfer.	Parkinson's disease (Hackney & Earhart, 2008)
		Parkinson's disease (Li et al., 2007)
	6-form Yang adapted with positive emotional motivators and hand touch	Dementia (Yao, Giordani, Algase, You, & Alexander, 2013)
	TC ball: more intense Yang style with whole body rotational and multisegmental circular movements	Healthy (Xiao, 2014)
Sun[b] High upright posture, compact movements, and lively footwork	38 Sun-style TC programs with a few Yang forms	Older adults (Voukelatos, Cumming, Lord, & Rissel, 2007)
	Sun style modified for arthritics	Fall risk in residential care (Choi, Moon, & Song, 2005)
	1 form	Women with history of osteoarthritis and no exercise for 1 year (Song, Lee, Lam, & Bae, 2003)
		Women with OA (Song, Roberts, Lee, Lam, & Bae, 2010)
	10 form	Fall risk (Taylor et al., 2012)
	12-movement hybrid of Yang and Sun	Type 2 diabetes and sedentary (Tsang, Orr, Lam, Comino, & Singh, 2007)

(*Continued*)

TABLE 10.2
Forms of Tai Chi Studied (*Continued*)

Description	Form Used	Population[a]/Author
Chen[b]	Full form	Healthy TC practitioners (Ramachandran et al., 2007)
Slow and fast pace with explosive power, circles, and twists	7 form combined with sitting and standing Qigong meditations	Older adults living in community and retirement center (Yang et al., 2007)
	10 form	Sedentary (Wolf, Barnhart, Ellison, & Coogler, 1997)
	Eight Section Brocade Qigong	Frail (Tousignant et al., 2013)
	12- or 18-form TC	History of falling (Ni et al., 2014)
	13 form	Healthy (Lin et al., 2006)
Qigong[c] Generally simpler than TC	Medicinsk sitting and standing positions adapted for study	Coronary artery disease (Stenlund, Lindstrom, Granlund, & Burell, 2005)
Not defined	TC 22 common forms	Polyneuropathy (Quigley et al., 2014)

Note: TC = Tai Chi.

[a]Unless otherwise stated, participants were community living.

[b]Tai Chi and Qigong (2015).

[c]Stenlund, Lindstrom, Granlund, and Burell (2005).

without losing balance (Li, 2014). Another single-group study showed TC practiced with caregivers improved OLS and dynamic balance (Yao, Giordani, Algase, You, & Aexander, 2013).

Many studies have showed that OLS significantly improved following TC compared to control groups (Audette et al., 2006; Choi et al., 2005; Gatts & Woollacott, 2006; Li et al., 2004; Li, Fisher, Harmer, & McAuley, 2005; Li, Fisher, Harmer, & Shirai, 2003; Li, Devault, & Van Oteghen, 2007; Li, Xu, & Hong, 2008; Ni et al., 2014; Quigley et al., 2014; Song, Lee, Lam, & Bae, 2003; Stenlund et al., 2005; Taylor-Piliae et al., 2010; Zhang, IshikawaTakata, Yamazaki, Morita, & Ohta, 2006). In some small studies with strong control groups (i.e., interventions that included some form of exercise that could be expected to also generate improvements), TC still showed improvements in OLS, though not significant (Tsang, Orr, Lam, Comino, & Singh, 2007; Wolf, Barnhart, Ellison, & Coogler, 1997).

In addition to the OLS, TC studies have reported that static balance measures of tandem and semitandem stance significantly improved. For example, tandem stance improved for prefrail older adults living in institutional care settings and persons with PD (Gatts & Woollacott, 2006; Hackney & Earhart, 2008). Two small studies showed nonsignificant improvements in outcomes such as single-leg and tandem stance in healthy older adults and those with diabetes (Li et al., 2008; Tsang et al., 2007).

The effect of TC on dynamic balance required for persons to move about within their environment has also been studied. Timed Up & Go (TUG) is common measure of dynamic balance. The 3-meter TUG test measures combined attributes (muscular strength, flexibility, and balance). It measures the time it takes one to stand from a seated position, walk 10 feet, turn around, and return to the chair and sit down (Podsiadlo & Richardson, 1991).

Many studies reported significant reductions in time for completion of TUG for TC compared to control groups (Audette et al., 2006; Choi et al., 2005; Frye, Scheinthal, Kemarskaya, & Pruchno, 2007; Gatts & Woollacott, 2006; Hackney & Earhart, 2008; Li, 2014; Li et al., 2005; Li et al., 2007; Li, Harmer, Liu, & Chou, 2014; Ni et al., 2014; Quigley et al., 2014; Reid-Arndt, Matsuda, & Cox, 2012; Song et al., 2003; Stenlund et al., 2005; Taylor et al., 2012; Taylor-Piliae et al., 2010; Xiao, 2014; Zhuang, Huang, Wu, & Zhang, 2014; Zhang et al., 2006). Most of the participants in these studies were healthy, community-dwelling older adults at risk for falls. One studied older adults living in a care facility (Choi et al., 2005). Other specific fall risk populations included older adults with polyneuropathy (Quigley et al., 2014) and PD (Hackney & Earhart, 2008; Li et al., 2007).

Measures of functional reach improved following 6 months of TC in healthy adults, 5 days of 90 minutes per day of TC designed for older adults with PD and history of falls, 10 weeks of TC for women with a history of cancer, and 48 weeks of TC with prefrail older adults (Gatts & Woollacott, 2006; Li, Harmer, et al., 2005; Li, Harmer, et al., 2007; Ni et al., 2014; Reid-Arndt et al., 2012; Wolf et al., 2006). One study reported that older adults were able to climb more boxes (simulating stairs) without using the handrail and bend and touch knees without losing balance (Stenlund et al., 2005). Another small study reported significant improvements in a heel-to-toe walking task as a measure of dynamic balance following 6 months of TC compared to a sedentary control group (Li et al., 2007). Composite balance scores such as Berg Balance Scale and Dynamic Gait Index significantly improved (Hackney & Earhart, 2008; Li, Harmer, et al., 2005).

Postural Control Strategies

Research studies have explored ways in which TC affects postural control strategies (ankle, hip, and stepping) used to control body sway (Spirduso et al., 2005). Ankle and hip strategies to maintain balance include activation of muscles around the joints in response to a disturbance in the base of support. Stepping strategies include stepping in different directions in an effort to maintain a person's center of gravity when he or she exceeds the base of support. The ankle and hip strategies are discussed together due to their interaction.

Ankle and Hip

There is some evidence that TC improves joint flexibility required for postural control strategies. One study showed that participating in 16 weeks of TC significantly improved the participant's ability to sense the direction of ankle and knee joints during motion (Li et al., 2008). Five studies reported significant improvements in ankle, knee, and hip flexibility required to move in forward or backward directions (Audette et al., 2006; Chen et al., 2007; Li et al., 2007; Stenlund et al., 2005; Zhuang et al., 2014). A small study comparing TC to brisk walking (N = 19) reported nonsignificant improvements in hip flexibility and knee strength in the TC group (Audette et al., 2006). Two studies reported that trunk flexion improved significantly following an 8-week TC in older adults with a history of poor balance (Song et al., 2003; Zhang et al., 2006).

Some comparison studies have reported significant improvements in knee and ankle strength (Audette et al., 2006; Zhuang et al., 2014). Studies have reported significant improvements in lower body strength measured by chair stands (Frye et al., 2007; Li et al., 2004; Li et al., 2003; Reid-Arndt et al., 2012; Taylor et al., 2012; Zhuang et al., 2014). In another study of prefrail older adults, chair stand time significantly decreased (12.3%) among TC practitioners while it increased (13.7%) in the wellness education control group (Wolf et al., 2006).

Step

Studies have described the typical foot patterns of TC that may contribute to improving balance in older adults. One descriptive study reported that 16 experienced TC practitioners (23 years) support their body by standing on both feet more than one foot while performing a 42-form TC compared to normal walking (Mao, Hong, & Li, 2006). The length of time spent in each form of support (both feet; and right and left foot) was longer; the transition time from one stance to the next was slower; and the stepping direction frequently changed during TC practice. A cross-sectional study showed that experienced TC practitioners (6 years) use better stepping strategies such as slower gait speed and shorter and slower steps, than those not practicing TC, while navigating an obstacle course (Ramachandran, Rosengren, Yang, Hsiao-Wecksler, 2007). They also showed longer time maintaining a position on one leg than the controls.

Gait profiles improved significantly for persons with PD; prefrail and sedentary adults; and persons with vestibulopathy and osteoarthritis (Gatts & Woollacott, 2006, 2007; Hackney & Earhart, 2008; Hass et al., 2004; Kim, Kim, Jae, & Son, 2011; Li, Harmer, et al., 2005; McGibbon et al., 2005; Shen et al., 2008; Zhuang et al., 2014). McGibbon et al. compared TC to vestibular rehabilitation. Zhuang et al. reported longer step length, shorter support phase, and greater sagittal plane range of motion of the hip and ankle joints and stepping distance in all directions except the medial direction of the right leg. Kim et al. attributed improvements in gait initiation to changes in anteroposterior and mediolateral displacement of the center of pressure. Gatts and Woollacott reported that older adults with balance impairment and previous joint surgical procedures demonstrated coordination of muscles surrounding the ankle joint and improved stepping strategies such as increased swing of leg leading to heel strike and step distance following 5 days a week for 3 weeks of TC. Hackney and Earhart reported that backward walking improved significantly.

Gait speed, indicating improved stepping strategies and cardiovascular endurance, significantly improved following TC in eight studies (Li, 2014; Li et al., 2004; Li et al., 2003; Li, Harmer, et al., 2005; Li et al., 2007; Reid-Arndt et al., 2012; Wolf et al., 2006; Zhuang et al., 2014). Some of the participants in those studies had a history of PD or were prefrail older adults (Li et al., 2007; Wolf et al., 2006). Studies have also reported that cardiovascular endurance, measured by 6-minute walk time, which is associated with gait speed, significantly improved following TC and Sign Chi Do (Hackney & Earhart, 2008; Rogers et al., 2012; Taylor-Piliae et al., 2014).

Intrinsic Systems

The mechanics of TC have been studied to determine how it affects intrinsic systems required to maintain static and dynamic balance and mobility. The following subsections discuss how TC affects these systems. Three intrinsic systems (sensory, motor, and cognitive) contribute to the maintenance of balance (Spirduso et al., 2005). The sensory system relies upon input from the vision, somatosensation, and vestibular systems to identify where the body is in space. The motor system offers input to tell the body what it is going to do within that space. Whether the body is standing or moving, speed and accuracy are also important for intrinsic balance. Impairments in the cognitive system affect a person's ability to correctly perceive an appropriate response to the input from the sensory and motor systems.

Sensory Integration

Research studies have explored the effect of TC on the sensory integration system that establishes where a person is in space. Studies have shown improved sensory organization and specifically the visual and vestibular input systems in older adults who completed 12 months of ball TC (Xiao, 2014; Yang et al., 2007; Yu & Yang, 2012). The Yang et al. study showed 2 months of Taiji/QG training increased the base of support, but not the feet-opening angle, suggesting that the improvement was attributed to wider stances. Another study showed improved visual and vestibular scores as well as knee proprioception in visually impaired older adults who completed 16 weeks of TC (Chen, Fu, Chan, & Tsang, 2012).

Motor Integration

The effect of TC on postural stability and postural control were discussed earlier. This section explores more specific motor integration strategies. Postural sway, lateral stability, coordinated stability, and choice stepping reaction time improved more for TC than control (Voukelatos, Cumming, Lord, & Rissel, 2007). Another study showed that TC, yoga, and balance training interventions all improved postural sway in older adults with a history of falling (Ni et al., 2014). Men at fall risk and diagnosed with osteopenia or osteoporosis demonstrated that speed and accuracy of task performance on a stationary force plate platform significantly improved for TC compared to control (Maciaszek, Osinski, Szeklicki, & Stemplewski, 2007).

Healthy older adults diagnosed with balance impairment demonstrated improved control of ankle muscles during walking, reduced cocontraction of agonist and antagonist muscles, and better muscle response organization following TC (Gatts & Woollacott, 2006, 2007). Improved gait was attributed to increased anteroposterior and mediolateral displacement of center of pressure following a 12-week TC intervention in older adults at risk of falling and persons with PD (Kim, 2009; Kim et al., 2011).

Cognitive System

Recent studies have explored the effect of TC on cognition. Outcomes have included global cognition, reaction time, attention, and processing speed. Reaction time and ability to switch attention between different tasks were better for TC and exercise groups compared to sedentary older adults (Fong, Chi, Li, & Chang, 2014). Two single-group studies (*N* = 11 and 38, respectively) reported that TC significantly improved processing speed in older adults with cognitive impairment and healthy males (Chang et al., 2011; Yu & Yang, 2012). Another small study (*n* = 11) reported maintenance of reaction time at 12 months in healthy adults (Li et al., 2007). One large study showed that choice stepping reaction time improved more for the TC group than control (Voukelatos et al., 2007).

Two studies reported improved attention following 10 weeks and 6 months of Yang TC (Reid-Arndt et al., 2012; Taylor-Piliae et al., 2010). In those studies, participants were female cancer survivors and healthy, sedentary adults. Older adults with mild cognitive impairment showed a significant improvement in global cognition scores after 14 weeks of TC compared to a control group (Li, Harmer, Liu, & Chou, 2014). Furthermore, improvement in cognition was associated with improved dynamic balance and confidence in the ability to perform activities.

Falls

Falling and fear of falling are indicators of poor balance. Fear of falling is known to reduce levels of physical activity in an attempt to avoid falling. Of course, this increases the risk of future falling. Studies often report no changes in falls; however, perceptions about fear of falling and the ability to maintain balance in situations representing the ability to move about in one's environment have demonstrated changes. Some studies reported the effect of TC on falls and others reported on fear of falling or level of concern about maintaining balance and falling while completing physical and social activities (Yardley et al., 2005).

Studies have reported up to a 55% lower risk of falls in older adults who completed 6-month TC compared to control groups (Li, Harmer, et al., 2005; Voukelatos et al., 2007; Wolf, Sattin, et al., 2003). Other studies have reported a 30%–66% reduction in falls following TC classes that ranged from 12 to 20 weeks (Lin, Hwang, Wang, Chang, & Wolf, 2006; Taylor et al., 2012; Taylor-Piliae et al., 2014; Tousignant et al., 2013). Some studies showed no significant difference between the groups (Choi et al., 2005; Wolf, Barnhart, et al., 2003; Woo, Hong, Lau, & Lynn, 2007). However, Woo et al. reported lower fall rates for TC compared to resistance training and sedentary controls (25%, 40%, and 51%, respectively) after 12 months of the interventions.

Studies often report no changes in falls. However, perceptions about fear of falling and the ability to maintain balance in situations representing the ability to move about in one's environment are equally important, as older adults who are afraid of falling are reportedly sedentary. Previous reviews have shown confidence in the ability to avoid falls, and fear of falling improved following TC interventions (Logghe et al., 2010; Rogers et al., 2010). Studies demonstrated self-reported fear of falling, and confidence in the ability to maintain balance improved following TC interventions compared to control groups for older adults at risk for falls (Choi et al., 2005; Huang, Yang, & Liu, 2011; Li et al., 2005; Li, Harmer, Liu, & Chou, 2014; Sattin, Easley, Wolf, Chen, & Kutner, 2005; Song, Roberts, Lee, Lam, & Bae, 2010; Wolf, Barnhart, et al., 2003; Xiao, 2014; Zhang et al., 2006).

CONCLUSIONS

State of Science

Following this review of the current literature on TC in the older adult population, it appears that participants are impacted from multiple perspectives. Maintaining balance and subsequent fall reduction risk are important for the maintenance of independence and aging in place for older adults, wherever they live. The evidence presented in this chapter demonstrates that TC reduces fall rates and improves static and dynamic balance as well as fear of falling in mostly healthy older adults.

Many of the studies included healthy older adults living in the community who were prefrail, at risk for falling, and able to stand and walk independently. A few studies included populations with specific diseases such as vision impairment, women with cancer, arthritis, poor bone density, PD, polyneuropathy, cognitive impairment, diabetes, and older adults living in long-term care facilities. Of note, none of the studies reported attrition due to injuries incurred from TC.

All of the studies were conducted in a group format. A group format for older adults provides social contact and is consistent with the ways older adults learn, practice, and maintain new behaviors. It was beyond the scope of this paper to explore all populations studied. However, previous reviews reported that studies have been conducted in multiple countries, thus contributing to the generalizability of TC across geographic populations. These factors, the community group format, and the wide range of populations studied support generalizability of findings across populations in naturalistic settings.

Implications for Practice

Based on the findings of this review, TC is an effective form of exercise for healthy older adults to maintain and improve balance required to maintain independence. Previous reviews have reported that TC is safe for older adults.

Future Research

Recommendations for future research include studies further testing the effect of TC on the specific mechanisms underlying changes in balance such as the postural control strategies and intrinsic systems. Specific populations to include are older adults who may not be able to stand independently such as persons with PD, stroke, arthritis, and diabetic neuropathy; persons with cognitive impairment; and those living in long-term care facilities. Many of the studies were pilot studies and reported small sample sizes and thus were not statistically powered to show significant changes. It is recommended that meta-analyses of outcomes such as postural stability be conducted.

REFERENCES

Audette, J. F., Jin, Y. S., Newcomer, R., Stein, L., Duncan, G., & Frontera, W. R. (2006). Tai Chi versus brisk walking in elderly women. *Age and Ageing, 35*(4), 388–393. doi:10.1093/ageing/afl006

Bohannon, R. W. (2006). Single limb stance times: A descriptive meta-analysis of data from individuals at least 60 years of age. *Topics in Geriatric Rehabilitation, 22*(1), 70–77.

Borik, A. (2004). *Sign Chi Do: The power of mind and body fitness*. Chandler, AZ: SignChiDo Press.

Chang, J. Y., Tsai, P. F., Beck, C., Hagen, J., Huff, D. C., Anand, K., . . . Beuscher, L. (2011). The effect of Tai Chi on cognition in elders with cognitive impairment. *Medsurg Nursing, 20*(2), 63–69.

Chen, E. W., Fu, A. S., Chan, K. M., & Tsang, W. W. (2012). The effects of Tai Chi on the balance control of elderly persons with visual impairment: A randomised clinical trial *Age and Ageing, 41*, 254–259. doi:10.1093/ageing/afr146

Chen, K. M., Li, C. H., Lin, J. N., Chen, W. T., Lin, H. S., & Wu, H. C. (2007). A feasible method to enhance and maintain the health of elderly living in long-term care facilities through long-term, simplified tai chi exercises. *Journal of Nursing Research, 15*(2), 156–164.

Chodzko-Zajko, W., Beattie, L., Chow, R., Firman, J., Jahnke, R., Park, C.-H., et al. (2006). Qi Gong and Tai Chi: Promoting practice that promote healing. *The Journal of Active Aging, 5*(5), 50–56.

Choi, J. H., Moon, J. S., & Song, R. (2005). Effects of Sun-style Tai Chi exercise on physical fitness and fall prevention in fall-prone older adults. *Journal of Advanced Nursing, 51*(2), 150–157. doi:10.1111/j.1365-2648.2005.03480.x

Fong, D. Y., Chi, L. K., Li, F., & Chang, Y. K. (2014). The benefits of endurance exercise and Tai Chi Chuan for the task-switching aspect of executive function in older adults: An ERP study. *Frontiers in Aging Neuroscience, 6*, 295. doi:10.3389/fnagi.2014.00295

Frye, B., Scheinthal, S., Kemarskaya, T., & Pruchno, R. (2007). Tai Chi and low impact exercise: Effects on the physical functioning and psychological well-being of older people. *Journal of Applied Gerontology, 26*(5), 433–453. doi:10.1177/0733464807306915

Gatts, S. K., & Woollacott, M. H. (2006). Neural mechanisms underlying balance improvement with short term Tai Chi training. *Aging-Clinical & Experimental Research, 18*(1), 7–19.

Gatts, S. K., & Woollacott, M. H. (2007). How Tai Chi improves balance: Biomechanics of recovery to a walking slip in impaired seniors. *Gait & Posture, 25*(2), 205–214.

Gyllensten, A. L., Hui-Chan, C. W. Y., & Tsang, W. W. N. (2010). Stability limits, single-leg jump, and body awareness in older Tai Chi practitioners. *Archives of Physical Medicine and Rehabilitation, 91*(2), 215–220.

Hackney, M. E., & Earhart, G. M. (2008). Tai Chi improves balance and mobility in people with Parkinson disease. *Gait & Posture, 28*(3), 456–460. doi:10.1016/j.gaitpost.2008.02.005

Hackney, M. E., & Wolf, S. L. (2014). Impact of Tai Chi chu'an practice on balance and mobility in older adults: An integrative review of 20 years of research. *Journal of Geriatric Physical Therapy, 37*(3), 127–135. doi:10.1519/JPT.0b013e3182abe784

Hass, C. J., Gregor, R. J., Waddell, D. E., Oliver, A., Smith, D. W., Fleming, R. P., & Wolf, S. L. (2004). The influence of Tai Chi training on the center of pressure trajectory during gait initiation in older adults. *Archives of Physical Medicine and Rehabilitation, 85*(10), 1593–1598.

Howe, T. E. (2012). Exercise for improving balance in older people. *Cochrane Database of Systematic Reviews,* (11), CD004963. doi:10.1002/14651858.CD004963.pub3

Huang, T. T., Yang, L. H., & Liu, C. Y. (2011). Reducing the fear of falling among community-dwelling elderly adults through cognitive-behavioural strategies and intense Tai Chi exercises: A randomized controlled trial. *Journal of Advanced Nursing, 67*(5), 961–971. doi:10.1111/j.1365-2648.2010.05553.x

Jahnke, R., Larkey, L., & Rogers, C. E. (2010). Dissemination and benefits of a replicable Tai Chi and Qigong program for older adults. *Geriatric Nursing, 31*(4), 272–280. doi:10.1016/j.gerinurse.2010.04.012

Kim, H. -D. (2009). Effects of Tai Chi exercise on the center of pressure trace during obstacle crossing in older adults who are at a risk of falling. *Journal of Physical Therapy Science, 21*(1), 49–54. doi:10.1589/jpts.21.49

Kim, H.-D., Kim, T.-Y., Jae, H. D., & Son, S.-T. (2011). The effects of Tai Chi based exercise on dynamic postural control of Parkinson's disease patients while initiating gait. *Journal of Physical Therapy Science, 23*(2), 265–269. doi:10.1589/jpts.23.265

La Forge, R. (2005). Aligning mind and body: Exploring the disciplines of mindful exercise. *ACSMs Health & Fitness Journal, 9*(5), 7–14. doi:10.1097/00135124-200509000-00006

Larkey, L., Jahnke, R., Etnier, J., & Gonzalez, J. (2009). Meditative movement as a category of exercise: Implications for research. *Journal of Physical Activity & Health, 6*(2), 230–238.

Li, F. (2014). The effects of Tai Ji Quan training on limits of stability in older adults. *Clinical Interventions in Aging, 9*, 1261–1268. doi:10.2147/cia.s65823

Li, F., Fisher, K. J., Harmer, P., Irbe, D., Tearse, R. G., & Weimer, C. (2004). Tai chi and self-rated quality of sleep and daytime sleepiness in older adults: A randomized controlled trial. *Journal of American Geriatrics Society, 52*(6), 892–900. doi:10.1111/j.1532-5415.2004.52255.x

Li, F., Fisher, K. J., Harmer, P., & McAuley, E. (2005). Falls self-efficacy as a mediator of fear of falling in an exercise intervention for older adults. *Journals of Gerontology. Series B: Psychological Sciences and Social Sciences, 60B*(1), P34–P40.

Li, F., Fisher, K. J., Harmer, P., & Shirai, M. (2003). A simpler eight-form easy Tai Chi for elderly adults. *Journal of Aging and Physical Activity, 11*(2), 206–218.

Li, F., Harmer, P., Fisher, K. J., McAuley, E., Chaumeton, N., Eckstrom, E., & Wilson, N. L. (2005). Tai chi and fall reductions in older adults: A randomized controlled trial. *Journals of Gerontology.Series A: Biological Sciences and Medical Sciences, 60A*(2), 187–194.

Li, F., Harmer, P., Fisher, K. J., Xu, J., Fitzgerald, K., & Vongjaturapat, N. (2007). Tai Chi-based exercise for older adults with Parkinson's disease: A pilot-program evaluation. *Journal of Aging & Physical Activity, 15*(2), 139–151.

Li, F., Harmer, P., Liu, Y., & Chou, L. S. (2014). Tai Ji Quan and global cognitive function in older adults with cognitive impairment: A pilot study. *Archives of Gerontology and Geriatrics, 58*(3), 434–439. doi:10.1016/j.archger.2013.12.003

Li, J. X., Xu, D. Q., & Hong, Y. (2008). Effects of 16-week Tai Chi intervention on postural stability and proprioception of knee and ankle in older people. *Age and Ageing, 37*(5), 575–578. doi:10.1093/ageing/afn109

Li, Y., Devault, C. N., & Van Oteghen, S. (2007). Effects of extended Tai Chi intervention on balance and selected motor functions of the elderly. *American Journal of Chinese Medicine, 35*(3), 383–391.

Lin, M. R., Hwang, H. F., Wang, Y. W., Chang, S. H., & Wolf, S. L. (2006). Community-based tai chi and its effect on injurious falls, balance, gait, and fear of falling in older people. *Physical Therapy, 86*(9), 1189–1201.

Logghe, I. H. J., Verhagen, A. P., Rademaker, A. C. H. J., Bierma-Zeinstra, S. M. A., van Rossum, E., Faber, M. J., & Koes, B. W. (2010). The effects of Tai Chi on fall prevention, fear of falling and balance in older people: A meta-analysis. *Preventive Medicine, 51*(3–4), 222–227. doi:http://dx.doi.org/10.1016/j.ypmed.2010.06.003

Maciaszek, J., Osinski, W., Szeklicki, R., & Stemplewski, R. (2007). Effect of Tai Chi on body balance: Randomized controlled trial in men with osteopenia or osteoporosis. *American Journal of Chinese Medicine, 35*(1), 1–9. doi:10.1142/s0192415x07004564

Mao, D. W., Hong, Y., & Li, J. X. (2006). Characteristics of foot movement in Tai Chi exercise. *Physical Therapy, 86*(2), 215–222.

Mao, D. W., Li, J. X., & Hong, Y. (2006). The duration and plantar pressure distribution during one-leg stance in Tai Chi exercise. *Clinical Biomechanics, 21*(6), 640–645. doi:10.1016/j.clinbiomech.2006.10.008

McGibbon, C. A., Krebs, D. E., Parker, S. W., Scarborough, D. M., Wayne, P. M., & Wolf, S. L. (2005). Tai Chi and vestibular rehabilitation improve vestibulopathic gait via different neuromuscular mechanisms: Preliminary report. *BioMed Central Neurology, 5*(1), 3. doi:10.1186/1471-2377-5-3

National Association of Area Agencies on Aging. (2006). *The maturing of America: Getting communities on track for an aging population*. Washington, DC: Author. Retrieved from http://www.livable.org/storage/documents/reports/AIP/maturing_of_america.pdf

Ni, M., Mooney, K., Richards, L., Balachandran, A., Sun, M., Harriell, K., . . . Signorile, J. F. (2014). Comparative impacts of Tai Chi, balance training, and a specially-designed yoga program on balance in older fallers. *American Congress of Rehabilitation Medicine, 95*, 1620–1628. doi:10.1016/j.apmr.2014.04.022

Nieman, D. C. (2007). *Exercise testing and prescription: A health-related approach* (6th ed.). Boston, MA: McGraw-Hill.

Podsiadlo, D., & Richardson, S. (1991). The timed "up & go": A test of basic functional mobility for frail elderly persons. *Journal of American Geriatrics Society, 39*(2), 142–148.

Powers, S. K., & Howley, E. T. (2007). *Exercise phisiology: Theory and application to fitness and performance* (6th ed.). New York, NY: McGraw Hill.

Quigley, P. A., Bulat, T., Schulz, B., Friedman, Y., Hart-Hughes, S., Richardson, J. K., & Barnett, S. (2014). Exercise interventions, gait, and balance in older subjects with distal symmetric polyneuropathy. *American Journal of Physical Medicine and Rehabilitation, 93*(1), 1–16. doi:10.1097/PHM.0000000000000052

Ramachandran, A. K., Rosengren, K. S., Yang, Y., & Hsiao-Wecksler, E. T. (2007). Effect of Tai Chi on gait and obstacle crossing behaviors in middle-aged adults. *Gait & Posture, 26*(2), 248–255. doi:10.1016/j.gaitpost.2006.09.005

Reid-Arndt, S. A., Matsuda, S., & Cox, C. R. (2012). Tai Chi effects on neuropsychological, emotional, and physical functioning following cancer treatment: A pilot study. *Complementary Therapies in Clinical Practice, 18*(1), 26–30. doi:http://dx.doi.org/10.1016/j.ctcp.2011.02.005

Rogers, C., Keller, C., & Larkey, L. K. (2010). Perceived benefits of meditative movement in older adults. *Geriatric Nursing, 31*(1), 37–51. doi:10.1016/j.gerinurse.2009.10.002

Rogers, C. E., Keller, C., Larkey, L. K., & Ainsworth, B. E. (2012). A randomized controlled trial to determine efficacy of Sign Chi do exercise on adaptation to aging. *Research in Gerontological Nursing, 5*(2), 101–113. doi:10.3928/19404921-20110706-01

Rogers, C. E., Larkey, L. K., & Keller, C. (2009). A review of clinical trials of tai chi and qigong in older adults. *Western Journal of Nursing Research, 31*(2), 245–279. doi:10.1177/0193945908327529

Rubenstein, L. Z., & Josephson, K. R. (2006). Falls and their prevention in elderly people: What does the evidence show? *The Medical Clinics of North America, 90*, 807–824.

Sattin, R. W., Easley, K. A., Wolf, S. L., Chen, Y., & Kutner, M. H. (2005). Reduction in fear of falling through intense Tai Chi exercise training in older, transitionally frail adults. *Journal of American Geriatrics Society, 53*(7), 1168–1178. doi:10.1111/j.1532-5415.2005.53375.x

Shen, C.-L., James, C. R., Chyu, M.-C., Bixby, W. R., Brismee, J.-M., Zumwalt, M. A., & Poklikuha, G. (2008). Effects of Tai Chi on gait kinematics, physical function, and pain in elderly with knee osteoarthritis--A pilot study. *American Journal of Chinese Medicine, 36*(2), 219–232. doi:10.1142/s0192415x08005734

Shumway-Cook, A., & Woollacott, M. H. (2007). *Motor control: Translating research into clinical practice* (3rd ed.). Philadelphia, PA: Lippincott Williams & Wilkins.

Song, R., Lee, E.-O., Lam, P., & Bae, S.-C. (2003). Effects of tai chi exercise on pain, balance, muscle strength, and perceived difficulties in physical functioning in older women with osteoarthritis: A randomized clinical trial. *Journal of Rheumatology, 30*(9), 2039–2044.

Song, R., Roberts, B. L., Lee, E. O., Lam, P., & Bae, S. C. (2010). A randomized study of the effects of t'ai chi on muscle strength, bone mineral density, and fear of falling in women with osteoarthritis. *The Journal of Alternative and Complementary Medicine, 16*(3), 227–233. doi:10.1089/acm.209.0165

Spirduso, W. W., Francis, K. L., & MacRae, P. G. (2005). *Physical dimensions of aging* (2nd ed.). Champaign, IL: Human Kinetics.

Stenlund, T., Lindstrom, B., Granlund, M., & Burell, G. (2005). Cardiac rehabilitation for the elderly: Qi Gong and group discussions. *European Journal of Cardiovascular Prevention and Rehabilitation, 12*(1), 5–11. doi:10.1097/00149831-200502000-00002

Tai Chi and Qigong. (2015, June 7). Tai Chi Chuan Forms. Retrieved from http://www.taichiandqigong.com/taichiforms.php

Taylor, D., Hale, L., Schluter, P., Waters, D. L., Binns, E. E., McCracken, H., . . . Wolf, S. L. (2012). Effectiveness of Tai Chi as a community-based falls prevention intervention: A randomized controlled trial. *Journal of the American Geriatrics Society, 60*, 841–848. doi:10.1111/j.1532-5415.2012.03928.x

Taylor-Piliae, R. E., Hoke, T. M., Hepworth, J. T., Latt, L. D., Najafi, B., & Coull, B. M. (2014). Effect of Tai Chi on physical function, fall rates and quality of life among older stroke survivors. *American Congress of Rehabilitation Medicine, 95*, 816–824. doi:10.1016/j.apmr.2014.01.001

Taylor-Piliae, R. E., Newell, K. A., Cherin, R., Lee, M. J., King, A. C., & Haskell, W. L. (2010). Effects of Tai Chi and western exercise on physical and cognitive functioning in healthy community-dwelling older adults. *Journal of Aging and Physical Activity, 18*(3), 261–279.

Tousignant, M., Corriveau, H., Roy, P.-M., Desrosiers, J., Dubuc, N., & Hebert, R. (2013). Efficacy of supervised Tai Chi exercises versus conventional physical therapy exercises in fall prevention for frail older adults: A randomized controlled trial. *Disability and Rehabilitation, 35*(17), 1429–1435. doi:10.3109/09638288.2012.737084

Tsang, T., Orr, R., Lam, P., Comino, E. J., & Singh, M. F. (2007). Health benefits of Tai Chi for older patients with type 2 diabetes: The "Move It for Diabetes Study"- A randomized controlled trial. *Clinical Interventions in Aging, 2*(3), 429–439.

U. S. Department of Health and Human Services. (2008). *Physical activity guidelines advisory committee report. Part G. Section 6: Functional health.* Retrieved from http://www.health.gov/PAGuidelines/Report/G6

Voukelatos, A., Cumming, R. G., Lord, S. R., & Rissel, C. (2007). A randomized, controlled trial of tai chi for the prevention of falls: The central Sydney Tai Chi trial. *Journal of the American Geriatrics Society, 55*(8), 1185–1191. doi:10.1111/j.1532-5415.2007.01244.x

Wolf, S. L., Barnhart, H. X., Ellison, G. L., & Coogler, C. E. (1997). The effect of Tai Chi Quan and computerized balance training on postural stability in older subjects. Atlanta FICSIT group. Frailty and injuries: Cooperative Studies on intervention techniques. *Physical Therapy, 77*(4), 371–381.

Wolf, S. L., Barnhart, H. X., Kutner, N. G., McNeely, E., Coogler, C., Xu, T., & Atlanta Ficsit Group. (2003). Selected as the best paper in the 1990s: Reducing frailty and falls in older persons: An investigation of tai chi and computerized balance training. *Journal of American Geriatrics Society, 51*(12), 1794–1803. doi:10.1046/j.1532-5415.2003.51566.x

Wolf, S. L., O'Grady, M., Easley, K. A., Guo, Y., Kressig, R. W., & Kutner, M. (2006). The influence of intense Tai Chi training on physical performance and hemodynamic outcomes in transitionally frail, older adults. *Journals of Gerontology. Series A-Biological Sciences and Medical Sciences, 61*(2), 184–189.

Wolf, S. L., Sattin, R. W., Kutner, M., O'Grady, M., Greenspan, A. I., & Gregor, R. J. (2003). Intense Tai Chi exercise training and fall occurrences in older, transitionally frail adults: A randomized, controlled trial. *Journal of American Geriatrics Society, 51*(12), 1693–1701. doi:10.1046/j.1532-5415.2003.51552.x

Wong, A. M., Lin, Y., Chou, S., Tang, F., & Wong, P. (2001). Coordination exercise and postural stability in elderly people: Effect of Tai Chi Chuan. *Archives of Physical Medicine and Rehabilitation, 82*(85), 608–612. doi:10.1053/apmr.2001.22615

Woo, J., Hong, A., Lau, E., & Lynn, H. (2007). A randomised controlled trial of Tai Chi and resistance exercise on bone health, muscle strength and balance in community-living elderly people. *Age and Ageing, 36*(3), 262–268. doi:10.1093/ageing/afm005

World Health Organization. (2002). *Active Ageing: A policy framework.* Paper presented at the Second World Assembly on Ageing, Madrid, Spain.

Xiao, C. M. (2014). Effects of long-term Tai Chi ball practice on balance performance in older adults. *Journal of American Geriatrics Society, 62*(5), 984–985. doi:10.1111/jgs.12805

Yang, Y., Verkuilen, J. V., Rosengren, K. S., Grubisich, S. A., Reed, M. R., & Hsiao-Wecksler, E. T. (2007). Effect of combined Taiji and Qigong training on balance mechanisms: A randomized controlled trial of older adults. *Medical Science Monitor, 13*(8), CR339–CR348.

Yao, L., Giordani, B. J., Algase, D. L., You, M., & Alexander, N. B. (2013). Fall risk-relevant functional mobility outcomes in dementia following dyadic Tai Chi exercise. *Western Journal of Nursing Research, 35*(3), 281–296. doi:10.1177/0193945912443319

Yardley, L., Beyer, N., Hauer, K., Kempen, G., Piot-Ziegler, C., & Todd, C. (2005). Development and initial validation of the Falls Efficacy Scale-International (FES-I). *Age and Ageing, 34*(6), 614–619. doi:10.1093/ageing/afi196

Yu, D.-H., & Yang, H.-X. (2012). The effect of Tai Chi intervention on balance in older males. *Journal of Sport and Health Science, 1*(1), 57–60. doi:10.1016/j.jshs.2012.03.001

Zhang, J., IshikawaTakata, K., Yamazaki, H., Morita, T., & Ohta, T. (2006). The effects of Tai Chi Chuan on physiological function and fear of falling in the less robust elderly: An intervention study for preventing falls. *Archives of Gerontology and Geriatrics, 42*(2), 107–116. doi:10.1016/j.archger.2005.06.007

Zhuang, J., Huang, L., Wu, Y., & Zhang, Y. (2014). The effectiveness of a combined exercise intervention on physical fitness factors related to falls in community-dwelling older adults. *Clinical Interventions in Aging, 9*, 131–140. doi:10.2147/CIA.S56682

CHAPTER 11

The Theoretical Basis for Engagement in Physical Activity Among Older Adults

Claudio R. Nigg and Zoe Durand

ABSTRACT

Theories have been used increasingly over the past few decades to help understand, explain, and promote physical activity of older adults. We organize and present examples of theories in overlapping categories of belief–attitude (e.g., Theory of Planned Behavior); competence (e.g., Self-Efficacy Theory); control (e.g., Self-Determination Theory); stage based (e.g., Transtheoretical Model); and ecological (e.g., Social Ecological Model) and summarize the literature applying the theories to older adult physical activity. These theories provide guidance on intervention development, underlying mechanisms of change, and explain when an intervention is or is not effective. When making decisions about which theory to choose, we recommend defining the behavior as specifically as possible (e.g., walking, endurance activities, balance exercise, and preventing falls), establishing the population in question (e.g., gender, ethnicity/race, rural/urban, age, socioeconomic status, and acculturation status), the setting (e.g., free-living, senior center, nursing home, and senior living complex), and the intervention channels available (e.g., telephone, print, technology–web based, face-to-face, and group based). Choosing a theory carefully and appropriately will inevitably lead to an increased chance of understanding and success.

http://dx.doi.org/10.1891/0198-8794.36.251

WHAT IS THEORY?

Over half a century ago, Lewin (1951) noted that "there is nothing as practical as a good theory." This implies that an important starting point for the understanding and promotion of health-related behavior is the study of its theory.

A theory is a set of interrelated concepts (or constructs or variables), their definitions, and propositions that are a systematic representation of phenomena by specifying variable relationships in order to explain and predict phenomena (Nigg, 2012). Researchers using theory to understand, explain, and promote physical activity of older adults have adopted theories and models based largely from individual psychological approaches to understanding health behaviors (US Department of Health and Human Services, 2005). These theories and models typically stem from general, social, educational, and health domains.

We present some of the leading theoretical frameworks that have been applied to older adults' physical activity and place them into a classification system to facilitate understanding (Biddle & Mutrie, 2008; Biddle & Nigg, 2000; Nigg, 2012). Presented is a heuristic with overlap between categories, which may reflect different theory types, such as continuous approaches (e.g., Theory of Planned Behavior [TPB]) and stage models (e.g., Transtheoretical Model [TTM]) that assume discontinuity, at least for some variables. Armitage and Conner (2000) separate "motivational" and "behavioral enaction" frameworks. The former include a set of variables to predict behavior. Usually intention or motivation is central and typically mediates the influences of the behavioral predictors, whereas behavioral enaction models address the translation of intentions into behavior by postintentional variables, such as implementation intentions (discussed later). The categorizations are belief–attitude; competence; control; stage based; and ecological. Examples of theories and models are presented in these categories along with literature applying these to older adult physical activity.

BELIEF–ATTITUDE APPROACHES

Attitude has been incorporated into numerous models adopted to understand health behavior, as attitudes predict behavior. However, there often is an attitude–behavior gap. Over the past 30 years, social cognitive approaches have attempted to resolve this disparity. Current theories incorporate attitude in parallel to other important belief-based constructs to understand behavioral mechanisms.

Health Belief Model and Protection Motivation Theory

The Health Belief Model (HBM) and Protection Motivation Theory (PMT) are both belief-based approaches. The HBM is a commonly used integrative approach to understanding health behaviors. It was developed to explain why people fail to adopt behaviors that will prevent disease. Today it provides an overarching model for why people do or do not undertake various health behaviors such as getting screenings done for early cancer diagnosis or engaging in heart-healthy diets. The HBM proposes that certain factors combine to motivate a person to change his or her behavior for a health reason: possessing a certain level of motivation and knowledge, viewing the condition as threatening to self, being convinced of the efficacy of a preventive action or "treatment," and seeing few difficulties in undertaking the action (see Figure 11.1). These factors are affected by socioeconomic and demographic factors and can be modified through "cues to action" such as media messages or the illness of a close friend (Janz & Becker, 1984).

The HBM may be best used in conjunction with other theories and tools of behavior change. One reason for this is that while the overall HBM can predict behavior change, effect sizes vary greatly for different aspects of the model and in different environments. For example, prospective studies tend to have significantly smaller effect sizes than retrospective studies. The HBM is oriented to reducing the risk of disease, and the majority of HBM research has involved preventing new illnesses or preventing complications of existing conditions. Application of the HBM alone to physical activity is problematic because many people initiate physical activity for motives other than avoiding illness. Motivation to avoid illness and associated symptoms (e.g., pain from arthritis) often increases with age, however, making the HBM well suited for older adults.

PMT has some similarities with the HBM but was originally developed to explain the influence of fear or "fear appeals" on health behavior change. PMT explains that the intentions to adopt health behaviors ("protection motivation") arise from how an individual views a threat ("threat appraisal") and his or her

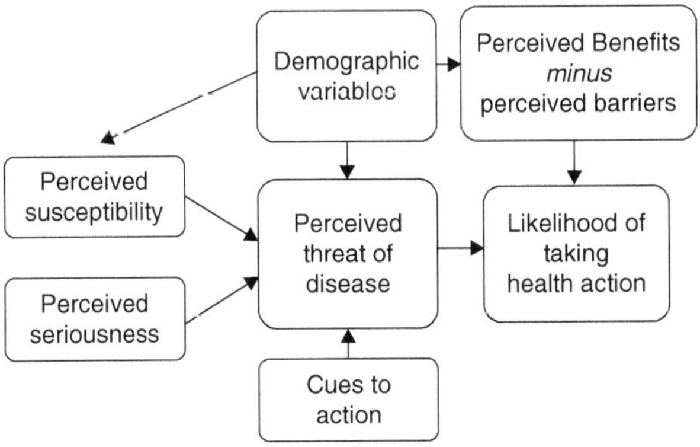

FIGURE 11.1 The Health Belief Model.

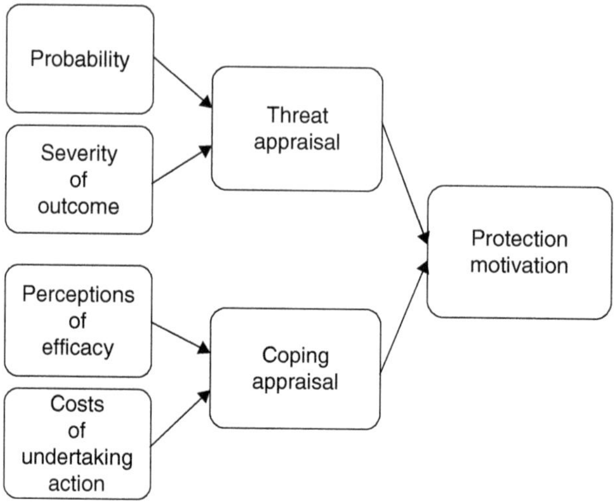

FIGURE 11.2 Protection Motivation Theory.

ability to respond to that threat ("coping appraisal"). "Threat appraisal" encompasses perceptions of the probability and possible severity of illness. "Coping appraisal" encompasses perceptions of the efficacy of an action to counteract illness and the ease or difficulty of undertaking that action, as illustrated in Figure 11.2 (Rogers, 1983).

While PMT was originally developed to evaluate the role of fear, research shows that the self-efficacy component of PMT is a stronger predictor of health behavior change than the fear/threat component. Nonetheless, PMT as a whole can help elucidate constructs in motivation.

Review of HBM and PMT Applied to Older Adults' Physical Activity

Health Belief Model

Some constructs of the HBM predict physical activity in older adults. Studies on physical activity in older adults showed that high exercise adherence is predicted by the desire to improve physical health (Pentecost & Taket, 2011), perceived efficacy of exercise in preventing illness, and perceived threat of illness if exercise is not undertaken (Hill et al., 2011). A cue to action in the form of a reminder from a health-care worker can predict initiation or increase of short-term physical activity (Al-Ali & Haddad, 2004; Hill et al., 2011).

In older adults, the desire to improve their health through physical activity is weighed against the fear that physical activity may cause a fall or other injury. In this case, perceived barriers are more associated with physical activity than perceived threats are (Koch, 2002). Perceived lack of safety is a common barrier in this population, but older adults' confidence in the safety of physical activity can be increased through HBM-based personal coaching and group activities (Fitzpatrick et al., 2008). Additional common barriers to exercise are the belief that exercise is not needed and the expectation or experience of pain during exercise (Hill et al., 2011). HBM may be used to explore peoples' attitudes and beliefs and craft messages that focus on emphasizing the benefits, efficacy, and strategies for the safety of physical activity to aid in providing tailored health education for older adults.

Protection Motivation Theory

Research in PMT in older adults has shown that threat appraisal and coping appraisal may be targeted in different ways to motivate physical activity. Threat appraisal can stimulate intention to exercise in general, but for some conditions people may become fatigued from an overload of threat appraisal messages that cause this approach to lose its efficacy. Even if perceptions of threat are already high, however, people can still be persuaded to take action through coping appraisal messages that the action is viable and effective (Ritland & Rodriguez, 2014). Coping appraisal approaches show differences in effectiveness by gender. Older men may respond more to physical activity messages targeting self-efficacy and response efficacy while older women may respond more to physical activity messages targeting self-efficacy and response costs (Ruthig, 2014). Coping appraisal and other PMT constructs have predicted physical activity in the short term (6 months) but not the long term (1 year; Tulloch et al., 2009).

Theories of Reasoned Action and Planned Behavior

The Theory of Reasoned Action (TRA) is based on the assumption that attitudes and subjective/social normative factors predict intentions, which are the immediate determinants of behavior. Attitude is a function of the behavioral beliefs and the evaluation of the likely outcomes of the behavior. A subjective norm is a function of the beliefs of significant others and how much one is motivated to comply with such beliefs of people. The TPB modified the TRA by accounting for peoples' perceptions of their ability to perform a behavior or "perceived behavioral control." The TPB is better equipped than the TRA to explain behaviors where volitional control is relatively low (Ajzen, 1991). The two models are shown in Figure 11.3. Measurement of TRA/TPB variables should be specific and congruent with the behavior being addressed.

Review of TPB/TRA Applied to Older Adults' Physical Activity

The attitude component of the TRA/TPB predicts physical activity better than other components for middle-aged adults, but subjective norms and perceived behavioral control are the best predictors for older adults (Kosma, 2014; Rhodes,

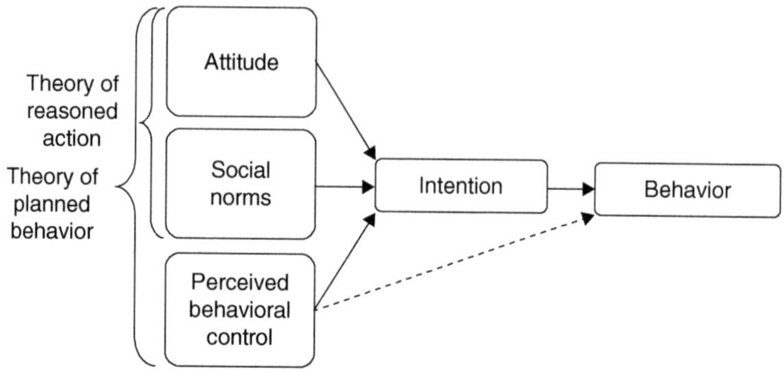

FIGURE 11.3 Theory of Reasoned Action/Theory of Planned Behavior.

Blanchard, & Blacklock, 2008). Subjective norms and behavioral control are predictors of physical activity participation in both male and female older adults (Dean, Farrell, Kelley, Taylor, & Rhodes, 2007; Rhodes, Blanchard, & Blacklock, 2008). A recent randomized controlled trial (RCT) applied the TPB to adjust perceptions of subjective norms and behavioral control and was effective in short-term increase of physical activity among older adults (White et al., 2012). These studies suggest the need for socially supportive settings promoting physical activity for older adults (Kosma, 2014). Another approach is to increase older adults' perceptions of the subjective norms of physical activity, for example, a paid media campaign significantly increased the number of older adult walkers in a community (Reger et al., 2002).

Meta-analyses have shown that attitude affects intention and intention affects exercise behavior. In young and middle-aged populations, the effect of attitude is twice that of subjective norms. In older adults, however, subjective norms and behavioral control have strong effects on motivation while attitude has a small or no effect. In the TPB, perceived behavioral control is "the perceived ease or difficulty of performing the behavior." In older adults, this may imply that regardless of how much individuals want to undertake a health behavior or what social influences they perceive to be encouraging them to do so, they must believe that they are capable of the behavior before they will initiate it. Perceived behavioral control must closely approximate actual control for perceived control to accurately predict behavior. Perceived behavioral control may predict behavior through the intermediary of increasing intention.

While the TRA and TPB models have been successful in predicting intentions and behavior, predicting behavior is usually weaker. As unidirectional models, however, the TRA and TPB are only used for predicting future behavior and do not explain past actions. Additionally, their focus solely on social psychological perceptions may weaken their applicability to all populations.

Implementation Intentions

One reason why the TRA and TPB do not fully explain if and how intentions are translated into action is that people often do not carry out their intentions. It may also be that other competing goal-directed behaviors increase in priority over the original intended behavior. Social cognitive theories (like TRA/TPB) do not address the challenges associated with enactment of intentions, and as a result may not fully explain the intention–behavior relationship.

Motivational techniques such as the TRA and TBP focus on increasing intention levels but do not facilitate the enactment of intentions. Volitional techniques, in contrast, increase the probability that these strong intentions will be converted into action without changing intentions. Combining motivational techniques with volitional techniques is theoretically based and increases uptake and retention of health behaviors.

For example, a combination of a rational decision-making strategy, or decisional balance sheet (weighing up the pros and cons), combined with implementation intentions was more effective in promoting physical activity behavior than either of the strategies alone. This provides evidence for two distinct phases of behavior change: a predecisional, motivational phase during which people decide whether or not to perform a behavior, and a postdecisional, volitional, or implemental phase during which people plan when and where they will convert their intentions into behavior. Interventions may be most effective at promoting health behaviors when they combine motivational and volitional techniques.

Review of Implementation Intentions Applied to Older Adults' Physical Activity

An RCT of an implementation intention intervention on prostate cancer survivors showed that participants in the implementation intention group significantly doubled the amount of physical activity compared to the standard physical activity recommendation group. The intervention group applied implementation intention to create specific plans for how, where, and when they would become more physically active. Results about the best way to apply implementation intention were mixed: Participants in a telephone-administered intervention participated more fully in the implementation intention but showed no change in physical activity, while participants in a self-administered intervention participated less in the implementation intention but demonstrated a significant increase in physical activity (McGowan, North, & Courneya, 2013).

COMPETENCE-BASED APPROACHES

Recent research on social cognitive perspectives in individual motivation has drawn extensively on Self-Efficacy Theory (SET). SET has had great impact on behavior change research and theory, but achievement motivation and self-presentation are sometimes employed as other confidence and competence-related perspectives.

Self-Efficacy Theory

SET was originally a general theory of behavior explaining how a person's beliefs in his or her own abilities interact with his or her goals and achievements. SET explains behavior through (a) a person's self-efficacy, the belief that he or she has the ability to perform a behavior that will result in an expected outcome, and (b) a person's outcome expectations, the expected consequences of successful behavior enactment (Bandura, 1997). Four main factors influence self-efficacy and outcome expectancy. In order of influence, they are mastery experiences (behavioral), modeling (cognitive), verbal persuasion (social), and interpretation of emotional/physiological arousal (physiological), as illustrated in Figure 11.4.

The theory recognizes that self-efficacy beliefs and outcome expectancies need to be specific to the behavior. Furthermore, the more specific identification of behaviors leads to less ambiguity and stronger relationships of behavior with

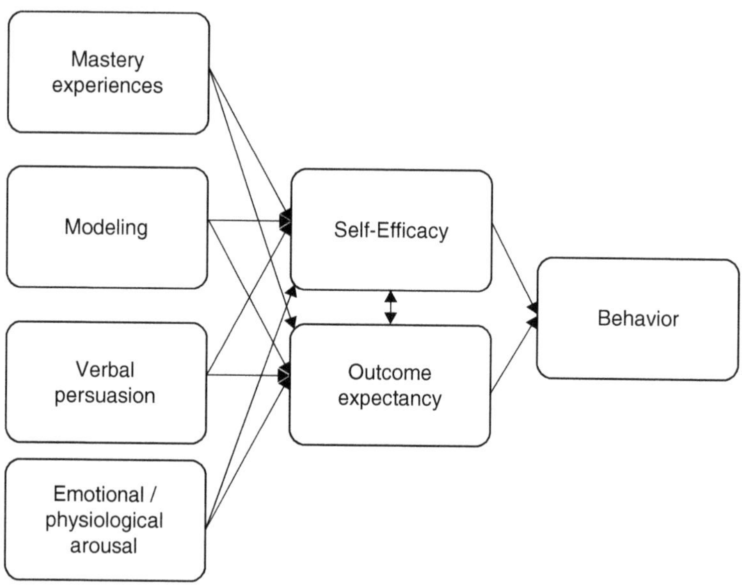

FIGURE 11.4 Self-Efficacy Theory.

self-efficacy and outcome expectancies. Therefore, efficacy is specific to each behavioral situation rather than being assessed as a trait. The theory has some generalizability to health behaviors other than the behavior under study and is more generalizable to more closely related behaviors. For example, if one has high efficacy for vegetable intake, one is more likely to have higher efficacy for fruit intake than for portion control.

SET has been one of the more popular and successful theories. In fact, the self-efficacy construct has been added to the HBM, PMT, and TTM (see later) after their original conceptualizations, where it is one of the more important constructs. A weakness of SET is the assessment variation for different investigations. However, the support found using different assessments also points to the universality of the theory.

Effort, potential barriers, and behavioral self-regulation must be associated with the behavior under study in order for self-efficacy to be assessed in any meaningful way. For example, "easy" habitual behaviors, such as handwashing, are likely to be unrelated to feelings of efficacy, whereas "difficult" health behaviors requiring planning, effort, and the overcoming of considerable barriers tend to be more highly associated with efficacy beliefs.

Review of SET Applied to Older Adults' Physical Activity

Self-efficacy has been shown to have a cross-cultural reciprocal effect on physical activity in older adults where self-efficacy increases physical activity, which, in turn, increases self-efficacy (Allison & Keller, 2004; Perkins, Multhaup, Perkins, & Barton, 2008). Increased self-efficacy is also related to better balance, which may improve the benefits of physical activity and prevent falls that would decrease physical activity (Chao, Scherer, Wu, Lucke, & Montgomery, 2013). Self-efficacy in older adults may be increased through self-administered workbooks (Jones, Mandy, & Partridge, 2009), cooperative discussions with a counselor (Chao et al., 2013), or physical activity (McAuley et al., 2006). However, some self-efficacy techniques that are effective in younger people, such as setting behavioral goals and self-monitoring behavior, are not as effective in older adults (French, Olander, Chisholm, & Mc Sharry, 2014).

CONTROL-BASED THEORIES

Changes in health behaviors are thought to be associated with the need for personal control of our lifestyles. This is supported through the common terminology of many contemporary diseases linked with premature mortality as "lifestyle related." The label "lifestyle related" implies the need for personal control and change through the message that we, as individuals, are at least partly responsible for our health and well-being. We are becoming increasingly aware, however, that social determinants play a large role in health. It is clear that perceptions of control, which may be influenced by social determinants, are important psychological correlates of health-related behavior at the individual level.

Self-Determination Theory

Cognitive Evaluation Theory involves the processing of information concerning rewards. This feedback can reinforce the behavior if rewards have a positive motivational effect but can undermine the behavior if rewards are seen to be controlling or repressive. Edward Deci and Richard Ryan (1985) have proposed their "Self-Determination Theory" (SDT) as an approach to intrinsic motivation that expands on Cognitive Evaluation Theory. In contrast to approaches in which intrinsic and extrinsic motivation are mutually exclusive, SDT proposes that all types of motivation form a continuum. Different types of extrinsically regulated behavior are located along this continuum according to their specific motivators. In addition to intrinsic motivation, there are three main types of extrinsic motivation: external, introjected, and identified regulation. *External regulation* is in response to a perceived necessity, often controlled by rewards and threats, and reflects feelings of "need." *Introjected regulation* is in response to internal accountability or the desire for approval from others and reflects feelings of "ought." The individual is acting out of avoidance of negative feelings, such as guilt, or to seek approval from others for his or her behavior. *Identified regulation* is in response to a desired reward, is a type of self-determination, and reflects feelings of "want."

In contrast to these forms of extrinsic motivation, intrinsic motivation is in response to enjoyment and reflects feelings of "like." The individual participates in the action for the sake of the action itself or for the feelings that he or she experiences while participating. Intrinsic and self-determination contribute more to higher levels of intention and sustained involvement than external and introjected regulation because they are likely to involve stronger feelings of personal investment and autonomy. These four behavioral regulations contribute to a "relative autonomy index" (RAI), with higher scores reflecting more intrinsic and self-determined reasons for the health behavior. A-motivations refers to a complete lack of motivation. The RAI reflects a person's perceived locus of causality (rather than locus of *control*) and involves autonomy and choice (see Figure 11.5).

In response to research on different types of motivation, SDT has been expanded to include different types of extrinsic motivation and the role of need satisfaction. The main challenge for practitioners in applying SDT is to create an environment that supports autonomy and self-determined forms of motivation for health behaviors.

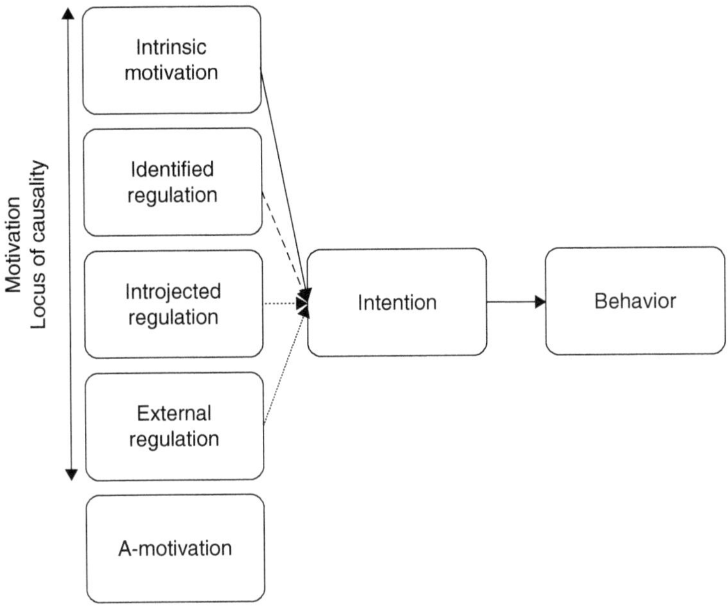

FIGURE 11.5 Self-determination theory.

Review of SDT Applied To Older Adults' Physical Activity

Self-determination research has only recently been applied to older adults' physical activity and has been shown to predict physical activity adherence (Resnick et al., 2010). Physical activity among older adults may be increased through SDT-based coaching (Van Hoecke, Delecluse, Bogaerts, & Boen, 2014), possibly through the mechanism of increased motivation (Lee et al., 2015). SDT based approaches have been shown to be effective with both partially active and sedentary older adults (Van Hoecke et al., 2014).

STAGE-BASED MODELS

Not all theoretical approaches are continuous models like the ones discussed thus far. There are also stage-based models, where constructs are represented as discrete stages rather than as continuous variables. The most widely used "stage" conceptualization is the TTM. The TTM was originally developed to treat addictive behaviors such as smoking and drug use in psychotherapy. Today it is often offered as a coherent framework to help understand behavior adoption.

TTM of Behavior Change

The TTM incorporates cognitive, behavioral, and temporal aspects as a comprehensive model of behavior change. The overall model is an aggregate of four components: (a) stages of change, (b) processes of change, (c) decisional balance, and (d) self-efficacy (Prochaska et al., 2002). The stage of change is the time dimension along which behavior change occurs. The stages are precontemplation (PC)—no intention to engage in the health behavior; contemplation (C)—intending to engage in the health behavior, usually within the next 6 months; preparation (P)—immediate intention (within the next 30 days) and commitment to engage in the health behavior (sometimes along with small behavioral changes); action (A)—engaging in the health behavior but for less than 6 months; and maintenance (M)—engaging in the health behavior for some time (more than 6 months).

Successful behavior change (progression to maintenance) rarely occurs on the first try, and relapse to earlier stages is expected. Clear and concise definition of the target behavior is beneficial to developing a plan based on the TTM and learning from regression to earlier stages of change.

The strategies used to progress along the stages of change are called the processes of change, which may be experiential or behavioral. Experiential processes gather information through experiences and include consciousness raising, social liberation, dramatic relief, self- reevaluation, and environmental reevaluation. Behavioral processes gather information through the environment and actions and include counterconditioning, stimulus control, helping relationships, self-liberation, and reinforcement management. Earlier stages of change tend to be more influenced by experiential processes, while later stages tend to be more influenced by behavioral processes (see Figure 11.6).

Decisional balance and self-efficacy are particularly important to the TTM. Decisional balance is the evaluation of the costs (cons) and benefits (pros) of engaging in a behavior. Results of the TTM over various health behaviors indicate that a person's perceived pros increase as higher stages are reached while his or her cons decrease. People generally perceive pros to outweigh cons if they surpass the contemplation or preparation stage (see Figure 11.6). Self-efficacy is a person's belief in the ability to engage in a behavior, given barriers. Self-efficacy usually increases across the stages (see Figure 11.6).

There has been a great amount of research on the TTM. Early research is dominated by measurement development followed by validation and, more recently, intervention studies. The TTM is appealing to practitioners because it provides concrete strategies (the processes) on which intervention strategies should be used for each stage.

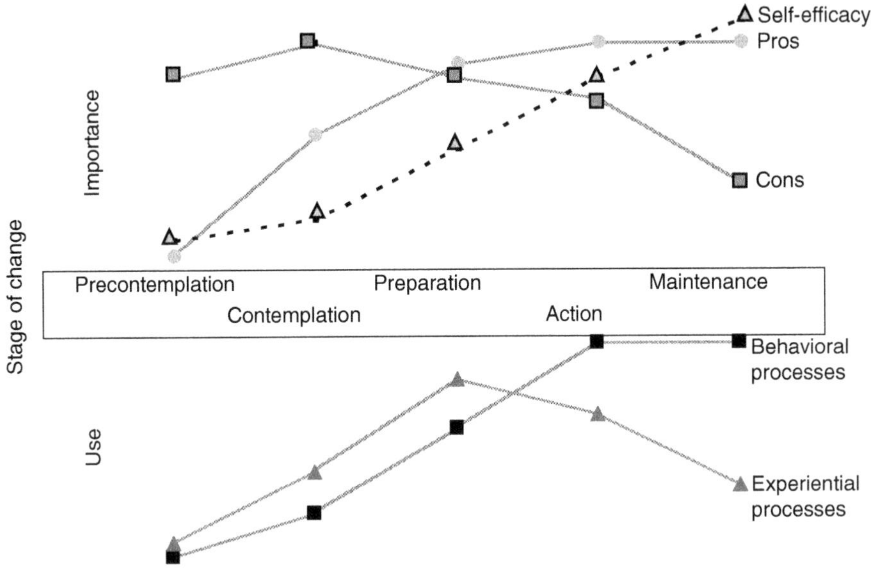

FIGURE 11.6 Transtheoretical Model of Behavior Change.

Review of TTM Applied to Older Adults' Physical Activity

As a whole, the TTM is moderately effective in predicting physical activity change in older adults with the self-efficacy component being a better predictor than decisional balance or stage of change (Cheung et al., 2007). The stage-of-change component of the TTM, however, has been successfully used as an indicator for which a health promotion approach will be most appropriate for that person (Burbank, Reibe, Padula, & Nigg, 2002; Clark et al., 2011). For example, stages of change have been used to increase recruitment (Hildebrand & Neufeld, 2009), adherence (Lach, Everard, Highstein, & Brownson, 2004) and frequency of participation (Märki, Bauer, Nigg, Conca-Zeller, & Gehring, 2006) in physical activity interventions among older adults. This approach with the TTM has been shown to be especially effective in non-face-to-face interventions with older adults, such as interventions conducted through printed materials or over the phone (Müller & Khoo, 2014).

Stage models offer the possibility of individual- or group-tailored programs and treatments that will be more effective and efficient than interventions standardized for the general population. Through identifying and altering particular factors (for example, self-efficacy), empirically supported models are useful for encouraging behavior change by helping people move from one stage to the next.

Therefore, theory provides an essential guide for interventions to develop best practices for successful health behavior change.

THE HEALTH ACTION PROCESS APPROACH

The Health Action Process Approach (HAPA, Schwarzer et al., 2007) is a *hybrid model* of integrated continuous and stage model assumptions. The HAPA additionally integrates motivational and behavior-enabling model elements (see Figure 11.7).

While the HAPA integrates these previously different approaches, it also makes a distinction between a motivation phase and a volition/postdecision phase of health behavior change. These two need to be distinct because individuals experience a shift of mindset when moving from predecision (motivational) to postdecision (volitional) phase. When people commit themselves to an intention to exercise, for example, they enter the volitional phase. The volitional phase is divided into two subphases where people either have made the decision and begun action (actors) or have made the decision but not begun action (intendors). These three total phases or stages are shown in Figure 11.7.

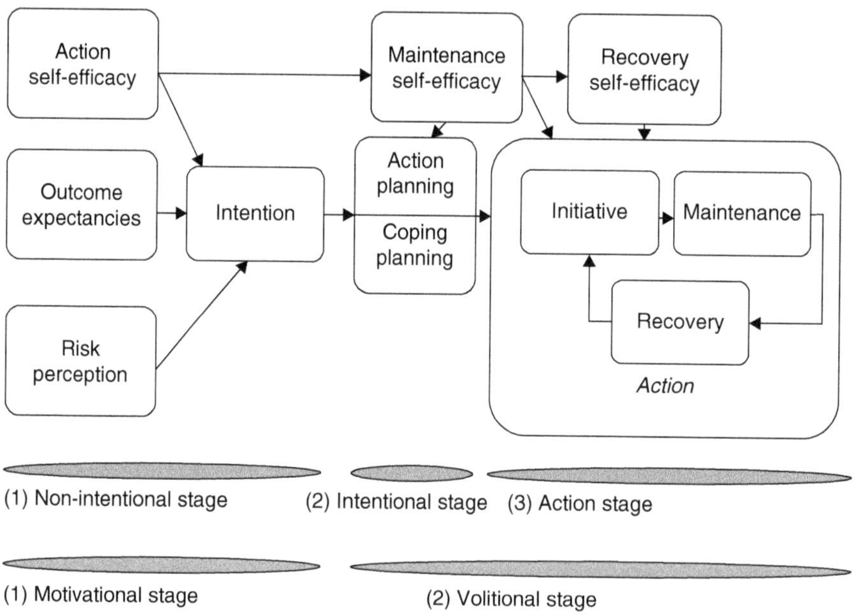

FIGURE 11.7 The Health Action Process Approach.

The (a) *nonintentional* stage is a motivational, intention-developing stage similar to the contemplation stage in the TTM. The (b) *intentional stage* is a primary volitional, planning/preparation stage, where the intention has been formed but action has not been begun (or at least not reached the recommended level). The (c) *action stage* is a secondary volitional stage where activity has reached the recommended goal behavior level. The HAPA is still relatively young and is not yet supported by a diverse array of research.

Review of HAPA Applied to Older Adults' Physical Activity

There is a paucity of research on the HAPA solely in older adults, but several recent studies have been conducted. An observational study found that predictors of physical activity among older adults vary by HAPA stage, with action self-efficacy and risk perception predicting physical activity intention in the motivational phase and physical activity intention and coping self-efficacy predicting physical activity behavior in the volitional phase (Caudroit, Stephan, & Le Scanff, 2011). Another, currently ongoing, RCT is using a HAPA-based intervention to increase physical activity among older adults with limited mobility. This study teaches home-based exercises and provides personal counseling with different approaches for people in motivational and volitional phases (Hinrichs et al., 2011); results are yet to be published. The importance of a wider set of influences, including the broader social, environmental, and cultural context of behaviors, however, is acknowledged.

THE SOCIAL ECOLOGICAL APPROACH

Environmental approaches are important parts of a holistic strategy for addressing preventable chronic disease because health behaviors are influenced by environmental, community, and societal factors beyond an individual's motivation (Glanz et al., 2002). Environmental approaches include policies, programs, or organizational practices that influence behaviors by, for example, increasing the desirability of outdoor spaces for safe physical activity or the affordability of recreation/fitness centers. Environmental approaches seek to "make it easier" for people to engage in healthy behaviors and tend to have wide-reaching effects. One benefit of ecological approaches is that they are easy to integrate with existing developments. For example, new trails and pathways can be easily connected to other parks, schools, libraries, and public lands.

Ecological approaches account for developmental, psychosocial, and behavioral characteristics beyond individual psychology. This broad approach offers the opportunity to improve the environment for health behaviors, including physical activity, to be sustained and reinforced through factors external to the individual. Interventions that target individuals, in contrast, often have limited success in sustaining health behaviors over the long term. Individually targeted interventions provide the momentum to initially alter individual behavior, but after the intervention ends, social and environmental factors drive a return to previous behaviors. Social ecological models (SEMs) of health behaviors focus on improving social and environmental factors alongside influencing individuals to increase the chances of long-term maintenance.

Individuals and environments have synergistic effects on each other, and SEMs capitalize on this interdependency. With a social ecological approach, interventions made at any level (within, between, or outside of individuals) will have implications for all other parts of the system. This offers the opportunity for novel points of intervention. Structural ecological models primarily aim to change behavior beyond an individual's level and influence the social and physical environment in which the interventions are placed. Social ecological interventions are typically conducted within existing structures such as organizations, communities, and schools.

The policy and environmental components of the SEM need more research to establish best practices. However, they do appear to be effective at changing the shared environment and may extend into the homes of many individuals. These interventions bring health professionals into interaction with other sectors of the population that they typically would not collaborate with professionally. For example, school principals, community agencies and organizations, legislators, and the mass media have not typically been actively involved in orchestrating interventions based on other approaches. However, implementing interventions based on ecological models (e.g., environmental and policy changes) is typically time and resource intensive. These interventions often require a great deal of planning and collaboration with professional, governmental, and community partners.

Review of SEM Applied to Older Adults' Physical Activity

Consistent with the SEM, older adults describe environmental, structural, and organizational factors as well as personal barriers to physical activity (Bethancourt, Rosenberg, Beatty, & Arterburn, 2014). Perceived neighborhood problems (Bowling, Barber, Morris, & Ebrahim, 2006; Michael & Carlson, 2009) and limited opportunities for social activities (Yeom, Fleury, & Keller, 2008) were noted to be associated with low levels of physical activity among older adults. This suggests that resources at personal, social, environmental, and policy levels may increase opportunities for older adults to engage in physical activity (Hurley, Lyle, & Hyner, 2013). For example, the SEM was recently used to promote physical activity through community-based senior games (Cardenas, Henderson, & Wilson, 2009).

CONCLUSION

Applying theory to facilitate physical activity among older adults is recommended for several reasons including providing guidance on intervention development, understanding underlying mechanisms of change, and explaining when an intervention is or is not effective (Nigg et al., 2002). The application of theory to older adults' physical activity is growing and has shown positive results across several theories/models. Plus, newer models show promise. When making decisions about which theory to choose, we recommend defining the behavior as specifically as possible (e.g., walking, endurance activities, balance exercise, and preventing falls), establishing the population in question (e.g., gender, ethnicity/race, rural/urban, age, socioeconomic status, and acculturation status), the setting (e.g., free-living, senior center, nursing home, and senior living complex), and the intervention channels available (e.g., telephone, print, technology–web based, face-to-face, and group based). Choosing a theory carefully and appropriately will inevitably lead to an increased chance of understanding and success.

REFERENCES

Ajzen, I. (1991). The theory of planned behavior. *Organizational Behavior and Human Decision Processes, 50,* 179–211.

Al-Ali, N., & Haddad, L. G. (2004). The effect of the health belief model in explaining exercise participation among Jordanian myocardial infarction patients. *Journal of Transcultural Nursing, 15*(2), 114–121.

Allison, M. J., & Keller, C. (2004). Self-efficacy intervention effect on physical activity in older adults. *Western Journal of Nursing Research, 26*(1), 31–46.

Armitage, C. J., & Conner, M. (2000). Social cognition models and health behaviour: A structured review. *Psychology and Health, 15,* 173–189.

Bandura, A. (1997). *Self-efficacy: The exercise of control.* New York, NY: Freeman.

Bethancourt, H. J., Rosenberg, D. E., Beatty, T., & Arterburn, D. E. (2014). Barriers to a facilitators of physical activity program use among older adults. *Clinical Medicine & Research, 12*(1–2). doi:10.3121/cmr.2013.1171

Biddle, S. J. H., & Mutrie, N. (2008). *Psychology of physical activity: Determinants, well-being, and interventions* (2nd ed.). London: Routledge.

Biddle, S. J. H., & Nigg, C. R. (2000). Theories of exercise behavior. *International Journal of Sport Psychology, 31,* 290–304.

Bowling, A., Barber, J., Morris, R., & Ebrahim, S. (2006). Do perceptions of neighbourhood environment influence health? Baseline findings from a British survey of aging. *Journal of Epidemiology & Community Health, 60,* 476–483.

Burbank, P. M., Reibe, D., Padula, C. A., & Nigg, C. (2002). Exercise and older adults: Changing behavior with the transtheoretical model. *Orthopaedic Nursing, 21*(4), 51–61.

Cardenas, D., Henderson, K. A., & Wilson, B. E. (2009). *Journal of Aging and Physical Activity*, *17*(2), 135–153.

Caudroit, J., Stephan, Y., & Le Scanff, C. (2011). Social cognitive determinants of physical activity among retired older individuals: An application of the health action process approach. *British Journal of Health Psychology*, *16*(2), 404–417.

Chao, Y. Y., Scherer, Y. K., Wu, Y. W., Lucke, K. T., & Montgomery, C. A., (2013). The feasibility of an intervention combining self-efficacy theory and Wii Fit exergames in assisted living residents: A pilot study. *Geriatric Nursing*, *34*(5), 377–382.

Cheung, C., Wyman, J., Gross, C., Peters, J., Findorff, M., & Stock, H. (2007). Exercise behavior in older adults: A test of the transtheoretical model. *Journal of Aging and Physical Activity*, *15*(1), 103–118.

Clark, P. G., Blissmer, B. J., Greene, G. W., Lees, F. D., Riebe, D. A., & Stamm, K. E. (2011). Maintaining exercise and healthful eating in older adults: The SENIOR project II: Study design and methodology. *Contemporary Clinical Trials*, *32*(1), 129–139.

Dean, R. N., Farrell, J. M., Kelley, M. L., Taylor, M. J., & Rhodes, R. E. (2007). Testing the efficacy of the theory of planned behavior to explain strength training in older adults. *Journal of Aging & Physical Activity*, *15*, 1–12.

Deci, E. L., & Ryan, R. M. (1985). *Intrinsic motivation and self-determination in human behavior*. New York, NY: Plenum Press.

Fitzpatrick, S. E., Reddy, S., Lommel, T. S., Fischer, J. G., Speer, E. M., Stephens, H., . . . Johnson, M. A. (2008). Physical activity and physical function improved following a community-based intervention in older adults in Georgia senior centers. *Journal of Nutrition for the Elderly*, *27*(1–2), 135–154.

French, D. P., Olander, E. K., Chisholm, A., & Mc Sharry, J. (2014). Which behaviour change techniques are most effective at increasing older adults' self-efficacy and physical activity behaviours? A systematic review. *Annals of Behavioral Medicine*, *48*(2), 225–234.

Glanz, K., Rimer, B. K., & Lewis, F. M. (Eds.). (2002). *Health behavior and health education: Theory, research and practice*. San Francisco, CA: Jossey-Bass.

Hildebrand, M., & Neufeld, P. (2009). Recruiting older adults into a physical activity promotion program: Active living every day offered in a naturally occurring retirement community. *Gerontologist*, *49*(5), 702–210.

Hill, A. M., Hoffmann, T., McPhail, S., Beer, C., Hill, K. D., Brauer, S. G., & Haines, T. P. (2011). Factors associated with older patients' engagement in exercise after hospital discharge. *Archives of Physical Medicine and Rehabilitation*, *92*, 1395–1403.

Hinrichs, T., Moschny, A., Brach, M., Wilm, S., KlaaBen-Mielke, R., Trampisch, M., & Platen, P. (2011). Effects of an exercise programme for chronically ill and mobility-restricted elderly with structured support by the general practitioner's practice (HOMEfit) —Study protocol of a randomised controlled trial. *Trials*, *12*, 263. doi:10.1186/1745-6215-12-263

Hurley, K. S., Lyle, R. M., & Hyner, G. C. (2013). Physical activity attitudes, beliefs, and practices among adults 50 and older: Baseline community assessment. *International Quarterly of Community Health Education*, *34*(3), 235–254.

Janz, N. K., & Becker, M. H. (1984). The health belief model: A decade later. *Health Education Quarterly, 11*, 1–47.

Jones, F., Mandy, A., & Partridge, C. (2009). Changing self-efficacy in individuals following a first time stroke: Preliminary study of a novel self-management intervention. *Clinical Rehabilitation, 23*(6), 522–533.

Koch, J. (2002). The role of exercise in the African-American woman with Type 2 diabetes mellitus: Application to the health belief model. *Journal of the American Academy of Nurse Practitioners, 14*(3), 126–129.

Kosma, M. (2014). An expanded framework to determine physical activity and falls risk among diverse older adults. *Research on Aging, 36*(1), 95–114.

Lach, H. W., Everard, K. M., Highstein, G., & Brownson, C. A. (2004). Application of the transtheoretical model to health education for older adults. *Health Promotion Practice*, 5(1), 88–93.

Lee, M., Kim, M. J., Suh, D., Kim, J., Jo, E., & Yoon, B. (2015). Feasibility of a self-determination theory-based exercise program in community-dwelling South Korean older adults: Experiences from a 13-month trial. *Journal of Aging and Physical Activity* (Advance online publication).

Lewin, K. (1951). Problems of research in social psychology. In D. Cartwright (Ed.), *Field theory in social science: Selected theoretical papers* (p. 169). New York, NY: Harper Row.

Märki, A., Bauer, G. F., Nigg, C. R., Conca-Zeller, A., & Gehring, T. M. (2006). Transtheoretical model-based exercise counselling for older adults in Switzerland: Quantitative results over a 1-year period. *Sozial und Praventivmedizin, 51*(5), 273–280.

McAuley, E., Konopack, J. F., Motl, R. W., Morris, K. S., Doerksen, S. E., & Rosengren, K. R. (2006). Physical activity and quality of life in older adults: Influence of health status and self-efficacy. *Annals of Behavioral Medicine, 31*(1), 99–103.

McGowan, E. L., North, S., & Courneya, K. S. (2013). Randomized controlled trial of a behaviour change intervention to increase physical activity and quality of life in prostate cancer survivors. *Annals of Behavioral Medicine*, 46(3), 382–393.

Michael, Y. L., & Carlson, N. E. (2009). Analysis of individual social-ecological mediators and moderators and their ability to explain effect of a randomized neighbourhood walking intervention. *International Journal of Behavioral Nutrition and Physical Activity*, 6, 49. doi:10.1186/1479-5868-6-49

Müller, A. M., & Khoo, S. (2014). Non-face-to-face physical activity interventions in older adults: A systematic review. *International Journal of Behavioral Nutrition, and Physical Activity, 11*(1), 35. doi:10.1186/1479-5868-11-35

Nigg, C. R. (2012). Behavior modification: A summary of theories and models of behavior change. In J. M. Rippe (Ed.), *Encyclopedia of lifestyle medicine and health*. Thousand Oaks, CA: SAGE.

Nigg, C. R., Allegrante, J. P., & Ory, M. (2002). Theory-comparison and multiple-behavior research: Common themes advancing health behavior research. *Health Education Research, 17*, 670–679.

Pentecost, C., & Taket, A. (2011). Understanding exercise uptake and adherence for people with chronic conditions: A new model demonstrating the importance of exercise identity, benefits of attending and support. *Health Education Research, 26*(5), 908–922.

Perkins, J. M., Multhaup, K. S., Perkins, H. W., & Barton, C. (2008). Self-efficacy and participation in physical and social activity among older adults in Spain and the United States. *Gerontologist, 48*(1), 51–58.

Prochaska, J. O., Redding, C. A., & Evers, K. E. (2002). The transtheoretical model and stages of change. In K. Glanz, B. K. Rimer, & F. M. Lewis (Eds.), *Health behavior and health education: Theory, research and practice* (pp. 99–120). San Francisco, CA: Jossey-Bass.

Reger, B., Cooper, L., Booth-Butterfield, S., Smith, H., Bauman, A., Wootan, M., . . . Greer, F. (2002). Wheeling walks: A community campaign using paid media to encourage walking among sedentary older adults. *Preventive Medicine, 35*(3), 285–292.

Resnick, B., Michael, K., Shaughnessy, M., Kopunek, S., Nahm, E. S., & Macko, R. F. (2010). Motivators for treadmill exercise after stroke. *Topics Stroke Rehabilitation, 15*(5), 494–502.

Rhodes, R. E., Blanchard, C. M., & Blacklock, R. E. (2008). Do physical activity beliefs differ by age and gender? *Journal of Sport & Exercise Psychology, 30*(3), 412–423.

Ritland, R., & Rodriguez, L. (2014). The influence of antiobesity media content on intention to eat healthily and exercise: A test of ordered protection motivation theory. *Journal of Obesity* (Advance online publication), *2014*, 1–10. doi:10.1155/2014/954784

Rogers, R. W. (1983). Cognitive and physiological processes in fear appeals and attitude change: A revised theory of protection motivation. In J. R. Cacioppo & R. E. Petty (Eds.), *Social psychology: A sourcebook* (pp. 153–176). New York, NY: Guilford Press.

Ruthig, J. C. (2014). Health risk perceptions and exercise in older adulthood: An application of protection motivation theory. *Journal of Applied Gerontology* (Advance online publication). pii: 0733464814544214

Schwarzer, R., Schüz, B., Ziegelmann, J. P., Lippke, S., Luszczynska, A., & Scholz, U. (2007). Adoption and maintenance of four health behaviors: Theory-guided longitudinal studies on dental flossing, seat belt use, dietary behavior, and physical activity. *Annals of Behavioral Medicine, 33*(2), 156–166.

Tulloch, H., Reida, R., D'Angeloa, M. S., Plotnikoff, R. C., Morrina, L., Beatona, L., . . . Pipe, A. (2009). Predicting short and long-term exercise intentions and behaviour in patients with coronary artery disease: A test of protection motivation theory. *Psychology & Health, 24*(3), 255–269.

U.S. Department of Health and Human Services, National Institutes of Health. (2005, September). *Theory at a glance: A guide for health promotion practice* (2nd ed.). National Cancer Institute. Retrieved from http://www.nci.nih.gov/PDF/481f5d53-63df-41bc-bfaf-5aa48ee1da4d/TAAG3.pdf

Van Hoecke, A. S., Delecluse, C., Bogaerts, A., & Boen, F. (2014). The long-term effectiveness of need-supportive physical activity counseling compared with a standard referral in sedentary older adults. *Journal of Aging and Physical Activity*, 22(2), 186–198.

White, K. M., Terry, D. J., Troup, C., Rempel, L. A., Norman, P., Mummery, K., . . . Kenardy, J. (2012). An extended theory of planned behavior intervention for older adults with type 2 diabetes and cardiovascular disease. *Journal of Aging and Physical Activity*, *20*(3), 281–299.

Yeom, H. A., Fleury, J., & Keller, C. (2008). Risk factors for mobility limitation in community-dwelling older adults: A social ecological perspective. *Geriatric Nursing*, *29*(2), 133–140.

CHAPTER 12

Psychosocial Factors Associated With Physical Activity in Older Adults

Mary L. Greaney, Faith D. Lees, Bryan J. Blissmer, Deborah Riebe, and Phillip G. Clark

ABSTRACT

Overwhelming evidence supports the health benefits of physical activity and the negative health consequences associated with physical inactivity. Nonetheless, the vast majority of older adults (65+ years of age) are insufficiently active. There is an array of psychosocial factors associated with physical activity among older adults. This chapter provides an overview of several of these key psychosocial factors that may be unique to older adults and are amenable to change through intervention. They should be considered when developing interventions to increase or maintain physical activity participation, regardless of intervention setting. Expanding our understanding of, and addressing psychosocial factors associated with, physical activity among older adults may strengthen programs designed to increase physical activity in this age group, which can lead to both reduced chronic diseases and disabilities and increased quality of life.

INTRODUCTION

Overwhelming evidence supports the benefits of physical activity in attenuating the physiologic changes associated with aging, promoting cognitive and psychological well-being, improving physical function, preventing and managing

http://dx.doi.org/10.1891/0198-8794.36.273

chronic disease, increasing longevity, and reducing the risk of falls (American College of Sports Medicine, 2014; Chodzko-Zajko, Schwingel, & Park, 2009; Nelson et al., 2007). Conversely, physical inactivity can have significant negative health consequences (American College of Sports Medicine et al., 2009; Chodzko-Zajko et al., 2009; Nelson et al., 2007) including increasing the risk factors associated with chronic disease that result in poorer health, more visits to the doctor, more medication, and increased health-care costs. All of these outcomes place a burden on the health-care system (Wang, Pratt, Macera, Zheng, & Heath, 2004). Two out of every three older adults have multiple chronic conditions (Centers for Disease Control and Prevention, 2013), many of which could be attenuated by participation in regular physical activity.

Despite the known benefits of physical activity and the risks associated with inactivity, the vast majority of older adults (65+ years of age) are insufficiently active. In 2010, only 11% reported participating in 150 minutes of leisure-time aerobic activities and two bouts of muscle-strengthening activities per week as recommended by the 2008 Federal physical activity guidelines (American College of Sports Medicine et al., 2009; Physical Activity Guidelines Advisory Committee, 2008), making older adults the least physically active of all age groups in the United States. Physical activity declines with age: fourteen percent of people aged 65–74 met the guidelines for leisure-time aerobic and muscle-strengthening activities compared to 4% of those 85+ years of age (Federal Interagency Forum on Aging-Related Statistics, 2012). Men are more active than their female counterparts, with 13.6% meeting both activity recommendations compared to 8% of women (Federal Interagency Forum on Aging-Related Statistics, 2012).

On average, nearly 10,000 people in the United States turn 65 each year, and it is projected that the number of older adults will double to 72 million over the next 25 years—accounting for about 20% of the U.S. population by 2030 (Centers for Disease Control and Prevention, 2013). The rapidly aging U.S. population poses an unprecedented public health challenge, and addressing this challenge will require increased financial resources and changes to existing infrastructure to provide needed services. Public health interventions designed to promote healthful behaviors including physical activity among the older adult population are needed (Birkel et al., 2015; Centers for Disease Control and Prevention, 2013). Adopting and maintaining physical activity is essential to postpone or prevent chronic disease. Yet, it can be challenging for health-care experts and clinicians to develop intervention programs to assist older adults in adopting and maintaining regular physical activity due to many factors such as existing health-related problems, functional limitations, and safety concerns (e.g., accessible and safe walking areas; Chodzko-Zajko, 2014). Thoughtful approaches are needed to promote and maintain physical activity in this age group, as older adults may carry a lifetime of habits and attitudes that may inhibit physical activity.

There is a vast array of psychosocial factors associated with physical activity among older adults. The purpose of this chapter is not to discuss all of these potential elements, but rather to provide an overview of several key psychosocial factors that may be unique to older adults and are amenable to change through intervention. Although the focus is on modifiable factors at the individual and interpersonal level, we recognize the importance of nonmodifiable factors (e.g., sex, age, socioeconomic status). Individuals working to promote physical activity need to be cognizant of nonmodifiable factors due to their potential impact on physical activity. Nonmodifiable factors should be taken into account when designing interventions and health promotion strategies, as recommended activities may require modifications. For each factor discussed in the following sections, we provide a brief review of the current literature and highlight interventions that have successfully incorporated the factor and/or suggest possible intervention strategies. We have used an ecological model (McLeroy, Bibeau, Steckler, & Glanz, 1988; Sallis et al., 2006) to frame our discussion, which is focused on the individual and interpersonal levels. Additionally, throughout this chapter, we use *physical activity* as an umbrella term that includes unstructured exercise, leisure-time physical activity, physical activity for transport, physical activity associated with caring for one's house, and so forth, as well as planned/structured exercise activity.

INDIVIDUAL-LEVEL FACTORS

Adults, including older adults, face many common challenges such as lack of time that may make it difficult to become physically active or to maintain a physically active lifestyle. In addition, there are many individual-level psychosocial factors associated with physical activity participation (e.g., intention to be physically active, satisfaction with physical activity) that are common to many adults, including older adults. This section highlights individual-level factors that may be particularly salient to older adults, including fear of falling, perceptions regarding appropriateness of physical activity, physical activity intentions, motivation, and self-efficacy.

Fear of Falling

Approximately 30% of older adults report having fallen at least once (Masud & Morris, 2001; Talbot, Musiol, Witham, & Metter, 2005), placing them at an increased risk of being disabled, hospitalized, admitted to nursing homes

(Gill, Murphy, Gahbauer, & Allore, 2013), or dying. Due to the frequency of falls and the negative physical and psychological outcomes associated with falling, many older adults have a fear of falling (Austin, Devine, Dick, Prince, & Bruce, 2007; Murphy, Williams, & Gill, 2002). Fear of falling includes psychosocial concerns such as fear, anxiety, loss of confidence, and impaired perception of ability to walk without falling, and impacts individuals who have previously fallen and those who have not (Scheffer, Schuurmans, van Dijk, van der Hooft, & de Rooij, 2008; Zijlstra et al., 2007). Both qualitative studies (Lees, Clark, Nigg, & Newman, 2005; Mathews et al., 2010) and quantitative studies (Jefferis et al., 2014; Murtagh et al., 2015) have found that fear of falling is associated with reduced physical activity. For example, the Irish Longitudinal Study on Ageing determined that participants (n = 4,892) who had not fallen and were not afraid of falling were less likely to be physically inactive compared to those who had fallen or were afraid of falling (Murtagh et al., 2015). Fear of falling is associated with restriction of activity (Howland et al., 1998; Tinetti, Mendes de Leon, Doucette, & Baker, 1994) and curtails participation in social activities contributing to social isolation (Zijlstra et al., 2007), which, in turn, is associated with decreased physical activity. This decrease in physical activity can lead to a downward spiral, with older adults becoming less physically active due to fear of falling, which, in turn, makes them even more fearful to be physically active.

Being physically active may reduce fear of falling. A recent meta-analysis conducted by Kendrick et al. (2014) that included 30 intervention studies with community-dwelling older adults found modest evidence that exercise interventions reduced the fear of falling, although there was insufficient evidence to determine if fear of falling was reduced beyond the intervention period. This study is consistent with an earlier review (Gilespie et al., 2012) that suggested that group and home-based programs including strength and balance exercises help prevent falls among older adults living in the community. Home-based programs have traditionally focused on increasing aerobic activity such as brisk walking; thus, there is a need to emphasize strength and balance. Given the negative outcomes associated with the fear of falling and the potential benefits of participating in physical activity in reducing this fear, intervention efforts should be directed toward older adults who are afraid of falling, regardless of fall history. The Centers for Disease Control and Prevention (CDC) is now in the process of creating partnerships with community-based organizations such as YMCAs to implement effective fall prevention programs (Ehrenreich et al., 2015). The CDC has also created STEADI (Stopping Elderly Accidents, Deaths and Injuries), an intervention to be implemented by health-care providers, which is available on their website (www.cdc.gov). Additionally, individuals working with older adults should discuss strategies to minimize fall risk. For example, health-care providers could discuss the potential risks associated with throw rugs and low lighting, especially for older adults with vision impairments. Older adults should be advised to conduct home audits to identify potential fall risks and to devise strategies to overcome these potential risks as home hazard assessment and modification result in decreased falls (Gillespie et al., 2003). The AARP provides tools to assess home and community environments (www.aarp/housing).

Perceptions Regarding Appropriateness of Physical Activity for Older Adults

An individual's implicit attitudes toward aging and assigned gender roles influence participation in physical activity. Existing social norms influence whether older adults exercise and also the type of physical activities in which they engage. Research supports that the more the older adults endorse negative aging stereotypes, the less likely they are to exercise (Sánchez Palacios, Trianes Torres, & Blanca Mena, 2009). The Aging and Stereotypes and Exercise Scale (Chalabaev et al., 2013) may be a useful measure to understand older adults' attitudes regarding exercise. There is also some work suggesting that these biases impact not only older adults but also health professionals. For example, research has found that physicians are less likely to recommend physical activity to older patients than to middle-aged patients (Austin, Qu, & Shewchuk, 2013). It is important that health profession training programs address and attempt to combat aging stereotypes as they may undermine older adults' attitudes regarding exercise. The theory of reasoned action posits that positive attitudes and subjective norms are associated with intention to perform the behavior (Fishbein & Ajzen, 2010). An individual's attitude toward physical activity is a strong predictor of intentions to engage in the behavior (French et. al., 2005). Therefore, older adults who believe that being physically active is appropriate behavior for people their age are more likely to be physically active than those who think it is more suitable for younger adults and children. Without appropriate role models, older adults may not consider the idea that they can and should be physically active throughout their life span. The lack of role models may be particularly salient for women in this current cohort of older adults who were in high school and college prior to Title IX of the Education Amendments Act of 1972 ("Education Amendments Act of 1972," 1972) and more likely perceive physical activity as behavior more appropriate for males than females. Title IX prohibits discrimination "on the basis of sex in any federally funded education program or activity," and requires federally funded education programs or activities to offer equitable athletic opportunities to men and women. When designing interventions, it is important to consider strategies to counter these implicit attitudes that may be undermining activity levels. Use of vignettes, video examples, and exercise leaders with similar characteristics may all help counter negative attitudes.

Intentions

The theory of planned behavior postulates that the intention to engage in a behavior is the immediate and important predictor of behavior, assuming that the individual has the needed abilities, resources, and opportunities to perform the behavior (Ajzen, 1991). Yet, intentions alone do not guarantee initiation or maintenance of behavior, as evidenced by the gap between intentions and behavior (Godin & Conner, 2008). Developing implementation intentions may increase the likelihood of meeting physical activity goals (e.g., exercising regularly). An implementation intention specifies when, where, and how the goal will be achieved (Gollwitzer, 1999). For example, an individual may say to himself/herself, "I will walk for 30 minutes each morning in my neighborhood immediately after finishing breakfast." Implementation intentions may strengthen the relationship of intention to behavior by engaging not just motivation but also decision-making and planning systems, and interventions with older adults focusing on implementation intentions show promise. A study of older women aged 61–89 years (n = 75) determined that those who were randomized to a weekly implementation intentions for physical activity intervention (vs. implementation intentions intervention for an alternate behavior or a control group) reported more physical activity over the 4-week intervention. Women with stronger executive function benefited the most from the intervention, supporting the notion that effects may be operating through the engagement of higher order cognitive processes (Hall, Zehr, Paulitzki, & Rhodes, 2014).

Self-Efficacy

Self-efficacy, an individual's belief in his/her capabilities to complete a course of action or perform a behavior, is a central construct in social cognitive theory. It is one of the strongest predictors of physical activity (Hu, Motl, McAuley, & Konopack, 2007; McAuley, 1993), including physical activity among older adults (Resnick, Orwig, Magaziner, & Wynne, 2002; van Stralen, De Vries, Mudde, Bolman, & Lechner, 2009). Self-efficacy affects choice of activities, effort exerted, and perseverance in overcoming barriers and difficulties when participating in selected activities (Bandura, 1997). Older adults with higher levels of exercise self-efficacy are more active than individuals with lower levels (McAuley, 1993). Within the physical activity and exercise realm, self-efficacy has been conceptualized as the confidence to perform exercise/physical activity (task self-efficacy) and barrier self-efficacy (self-regulatory efficacy), the confidence to be physically active in the face of common barriers such as lack of time, illness/poor health, and inclement weather. Older adults may have low self-efficacy to be physically active due to limited experience in physical activity, lack of familiarity with current gym equipment, and lack of physical activity role models. It is important to recognize that the first step is to instill in older adults the belief that they can complete the desired bout of activity, as without that initial belief, barrier efficacy is meaningless.

Exercise self-efficacy and barrier self-efficacy are malleable; therefore, interventions to promote physical activity/exercise often include components designed to increase these factors. Increasing physical activity will lead to increased exercise self-efficacy. There are a number of approaches outlined using the primary sources of efficacy judgments that can be used to increase exercise self-efficacy, such as the use of small steps, the start low, go slow concept of exercise, and positive feedback. Similarly, an individual's barrier self-efficacy can be increased by developing strategies to overcome potential barriers. For example, an older adult living in a low-rise apartment building who has low self-efficacy to be physically active during inclement weather could be encouraged to walk the hallways in his/her apartment building when the weather is not hospitable to walking outside. Changes in barrier self-efficacy are associated with changes in physical activity (Rejeski et al., 2003). Barrier self-efficacy can be increased by having older adults develop strategies to overcome obstacles to being physically active. Both exercise self-efficacy and barrier self-efficacy predict maintenance of exercise behavior (McAuley & Blissmer, 2000; McAuley, Jerome, Elavsky, Marquez, & Ramsey, 2003; Neupert, Lachman, & Whitbourne, 2009; Sallis et al., 1986); thus, it is essential to develop both.

INTERPERSONAL-LEVEL FACTORS

Several interpersonal-level psychosocial factors associated with physical activity may become increasingly important as a result of changing social networks due to advancing age and morbidity. Changing social networks may alter physical activity participation through changes in informal social support, while formal social support may have a greater influence on physical activity participation. Social support, broadly defined, refers to the supportive actions from members of an individual's social network, and this support can be offered through informal (e.g., family, friends) or formal (e.g., health-care providers) networks. These factors and examples are discussed in detail in the following section.

Changing Social Networks

Aging is associated with a decrease in the size of the aging adult's social networks, due to relocation, morbidity, and mortality. The decreasing network size results in increased loneliness and in isolation, both of which negatively impact opportunities and motivation for exercise. A longitudinal study of adults aged 50–68 found that loneliness was associated with declines in physical activity over 2 years (Hawkley, Thisted, & Cacioppo, 2009). Older adults who participate in physical activity with others have increased opportunities for social interaction and access to resources to expand social interactions (McAuley, Jerome, Marquez, Elavsky, & Blissmer, 2003). Older adults may find social interaction offered through group exercise to be appealing, and socialization offered by exercise programs may promote retention (Belza et al., 2004; Chiang, Seman, Belza, & Tsai, 2008).

Walking groups provide opportunities for conversation and socialization, and a meta-analysis determined that walking groups increase physical activity, with a greatest effect in older adults compared to younger adults (Kassavou, Turner, & French, 2013). Given the positive relationship between opportunities for socialization and physical activity for older adults, communities and organizations should consider strategies to increase attendance at available group activities and increase available programs and facilitate the development of peer-led activities. There is a need to expand the reach of existing programs, and one possible way to do this may be through the use of trained peer leaders who have access to community space (e.g., room at senior center or school gymnasium after hours). Programs may need to consider different walking speed and ability.

Informal Social Support

Due to changing social networks, older adults may have less informal social support for physical activity. There are several types of social support. Instrumental support is tangible support (e.g., providing rides to an exercise program), while emotional support is the expression of caring, love, and empathy (e.g., encouragement). Informational support is the provision of advice and suggestions. A recent study (n = 138) determined that older adults with low levels of social support were more likely to incorrectly believe that they met physical activity recommendations, when they did not (Visser, Brychta, Chen, & Koster, 2014). Although results of interventions are not entirely consistent (Hogan, Linden, & Najarian, 2002), perceived social support for exercise (Litt, Kleppinger, & Judge, 2002; McAuley, Jerome, Elavsky, et al., 2003) as well as general social support (Mathews et al., 2010; Schutzer & Graves, 2004; van Stralen et al., 2009) have been identified as key factors associated with both adoption and maintenance of exercise behaviors.

Increasing social support among older adults may be an important strategy for promoting and maintaining physical activity. Physical activity interventions for older adults that are framed in both social cognitive theory and group dynamics have resulted in increased activity (Brawley, Rejeski, & King, 2003). Social support offered by group programs is associated with increases in socialization as well as exercise adherence (Cress et al., 2005; Williams & Lord, 1995). A study of adults aged 65–85 (n = 309) determined that individuals with low social support were less likely to be physically active even if self-efficacy was high; participants with low self-efficacy were less likely to be active even with social support (Warner, Ziegelmann, Schuz, Wurm, & Schwarzer, 2011). This finding suggests that interventions should work to increase both self-efficacy and social support. Furthermore, qualitative studies with sedentary African American men have identified that having a peer who serves as "buddy" or partner increases the motivation to be physically active (Bopp et al., 2007; Griffith, King, & Ober Allen, 2013). Additionally, studies have determined that middle-aged and older African American men prefer to be physically active in a social setting, and physical activities that involve family and the community may be preferable (Hooker, Wilcox, Rheaume, Burroughs, & Friedman, 2011). Social support for physical activity can be fostered in a variety of ways, including peer-led group exercise classes, community walking groups, and wellness coaching/counseling. Furthermore, support does not have to be offered in person, but can be facilitated by technology—Internet groups, e-mails from staff, online counseling, and telephonic support.

For many older adults, social support from members of their faith communities is second only to that offered by family (Koenig, Moberg, & Kvale, 1988). Social support available within faith communities may promote healthful behaviors (Koenig, 2012). Analyses of data from the National Health and Nutrition Examination Survey determined that European American and Mexican American women aged 60+ who attended church frequently participate in more leisure-time physical activity than those who attended church infrequently (Gillum, 2006). Faith-based interventions have been efficacious in promoting physical activity among older African Americans (Duru, Sarkisian, Leng, & Mangione, 2010; Tussing-Humphreys, Thomson, Mayo, & Edmond, 2013) and may be an important strategy for the promotion of physical activity among Latinos (Bopp, Fallon, & Marquez, 2011; Martinez, Arredondo, Perez, & Baquero, 2009). Future research should continue to explore promoting physical activity through faith-based organizations.

Formal Social Support

Physicians and health-care providers have a valuable opportunity to interact with their older adult patients to promote physical activity (King, 2001). They may be an important source of formal social support (Hinrichs & Brach, 2012) for older adults in the United States. Physicians are viewed as a valued source for health-related information and their counsel may serve as a catalyst for increasing physical activity (Kreuter, Chheda, & Bull, 2000; Petrella, Koval, Cunningham, & Paterson, 2003). One objective of *Healthy People 2020* is to increase the number of physician office visits that include physical activity education or counseling (U.S. Department of Health and Human Services, 2011). The U.S. Preventive Services Task Force found that behavioral counseling in this setting has a limited effect on increasing physical activity among adults free of cardiovascular disease (CVD), hypertension, hyperlipidemia, or diabetes (U.S. Preventive Services Task Force, 2012) and recommended that patients who are overweight and have additional the risk factors for CVD be offered or referred to intensive behavioral counseling to promote healthy eating and physical activity to prevent CVD (LeFevre & U.S. Preventive Services Task Force, 2014). A meta-analysis found that behavioral counseling of medium-to-high intensity could lead to increases in self-reported physical activity behaviors, although long-term follow-up was very limited (Lin,O'Connor, Whitlock, & Beil, 2010). A recent systematic review found that promotion of physical activity in primary care was associated with small-to-moderate increases in self-reported physical activity at 12 months (Orrow, Kinmonth, Sanderson, & Sutton, 2012). The American Heart Association and the American College of Sports Medicine recently implemented the "Exercise is Medicine" initiative to promote physicians prescribing exercise (Exercise is Medicine, n.d.).

Physician counseling may be limited due to a lack of certainty about the efficacy of physical activity counseling on physical activity, feeling uncomfortable about counseling, and lack of time, training, and reimbursement (Hebert, Caughy, & Shuval, 2012). Group medical visits may be a possible solution to reimbursement concerns. These visits, usually conducted by a physician or nurse practitioner and focused on a condition (e.g., diabetes management), include an individual assessment and an educational session for the entire group (Jaber, Braksmajer, & Trilling, 2006). Group visits could provide opportunities for increased formal and informal social support. Additionally, the Treat and Reduce Obesity Act of 2013 ("Treat and Reduce Obesity Act of 2013," 2013) expands obesity prevention efforts first funded by the Affordable Care Act (Koh & Sebelius, 2010) to include reimbursement for obesity counseling for obese adults. Counseling could increase formal support for physical activity and might encourage obese older adults without health conditions that would limit participation to increase their physical activity.

It is important to note that not all social support—whether it is from family, friends, or health-care professionals—is conducive to promoting physical activity. These individuals may encourage sedentary behaviors due to internalizing beliefs that physical activity should decline with advancing age. For example, results of a focus group study suggest that husbands of Latina women may disapprove of their participation in physical activity, although this research was not specific to older adults (Ramirez, Chalela, Gallion, & Velez, 2007). A problem that often arises in older adults is the issue of overprotectiveness, in which family members may not allow older adults to do activities out of concern for their safety or health. These concerns can undermine self-efficacy and future exercise participation (Berkhuysen, Nieuwland, Buunk, Sanderman, & Rispens, 1999). In an interesting study in a cardiac rehabilitation program, where overprotectiveness is often a concern, spouses who exercised with the patient felt less overprotective, which led to greater adherence (Erling & Oldridge, 1985).

CONCLUSION

Although we have focused on malleable factors, the importance of nonmodifiable psychosocial factors that are associated with physical activity should be considered by those working to promote or maintain physical activity among older adults. For example, religiosity may be extremely valuable for addressing physical activity, as the majority of older adults (69%), especially racial/ethnic minorities, state that religion is very important in their life (Pew Forum, 2008). With aging, the neighborhood in which one resides becomes increasingly important. Declining health and physical impairments associated with aging increase the time spent in one's neighborhood. It has been hypothesized that perceived neighborhood safety is associated with physical activity, although the research has yielded inconsistent results (Foster & Giles-Corti, 2008; Foster, Knuiman, Hooper, Christian, & Giles-Corti, 2014; Humpel, Owen, & Leslie, 2002). Nonetheless, a cross-sectional study analyzing data from the 2004 Health and Retirement Study of older adults aged 50+ determined that those perceiving their neighborhood as safe had an 8% higher mean rate of leisure-time physical activity, compared to older adults who perceived their neighborhood as unsafe, after controlling for socioeconomic status (Tucker-Seeley, Subramanian, Li, & Sorensen, 2009).

There are other psychosocial factors that have had minimal examination and warrant further exploration. For example, resilience, the ability to bounce back from an adverse event (Ryff & Singer, 2003), is a modifiable factor that provides a buffer from negative events and consequences (Clark et al., 2011; Clark, Burbank, Greene, Owens, & Riebe, 2010). Resilience may be increasingly important with age due to the increased likelihood of facing multiple adverse events with age, such as the death of a spouse or hospitalization (Campbell-Sills, Cohan, & Stein, 2006). Older adults with higher levels of resilience may be able to return to their previous level of functioning after an adverse event, while those who are less resilient may be unable to do so. It is possible that resilience is associated with physical activity behaviors of older adults. A study examining the maintenance of healthful behaviors (exercise and fruit and vegetable intake) among older adults determined that a person's level of resilience is associated with his/her level of physical activity (Mlinac, Lees, Stamm, Saint, & Mulligan, 2014), although the direction of this association is not clear.

This review presents psychosocial constructs that individuals and groups may want to consider when developing interventions to increase or maintain physical activity participation among older adults, regardless of intervention setting. This discussion is not exhaustive, and there are a number of existing reviews examining correlates and/or determinants of physical activity initiation and/or maintenance (van Stralen et al., 2009) and interventions designed to increase physical activity among older adults that can be consulted (Conn, Minor, Burks, Rantz, & Pomeroy, 2003; King, 2001; King, Rejeski, & Buchner, 1998; Taylor et al., 2004; van der Bij, Laurant, & Wensing, 2002). It is, however, important to note that older adults are a diverse and heterogeneous group, and there may be differences in psychosocial factors based on age (e.g., adults aged 65–74 vs. adults aged 85+), race/ethnicity, income, socioeconomic status, location (urban, suburban, or rural), and presence or type of disability. Expanding our understanding of, and addressing psychosocial factors associated with, physical activity among older adults will be important for promoting and maintaining physical activity within this population, which will likely lead to reduced chronic diseases and disabilities associated with inactivity while increasing the quality of life.

REFERENCES

Ajzen, I. (1991). The theory of planned behavior. *Organizational Behavior and Human Decision Processes, 50*, 179–211.

American College of Sports Medicine. (2014). Benefits of Regular Physical Activity and/or Exercise. In L. S. Pescatello, R. Arena, D. Riebe, & P. Thompson (Eds). *ACSM's guidelines for exercise testing and prescription*. Baltimore, MD: LippincottWilliams & Wilkins.

American College of Sports., Chodzko-Zajko, W. J., Proctor, D. N., Fiatarone Singh, M. A., Minson, C. T., Nigg, C. R., . . . Skinner, J. S. (2009). American College of Sports Medicine position stand. Exercise and physical activity for older adults. *Medicine and Science Sports Exercise, 41*(7), 1510–1530.

Austin, N., Devine, A., Dick, I., Prince, R., & Bruce, D. (2007). Fear of falling in older women: A longitudinal study of incidence, persistence, and predictors. *Journal of American Geriatrics Society, 55*(10), 1598–1603.

Austin, S., Qu, H., & Shewchuk, R. M. (2013). Health care providers' recommendations for physical activity and adherence to physical activity guidelines among adults with arthritis. *Preventing Chronic Disease, 10*, E182.

Bandura, A. (1997). *Self-efficacy: The exercise of control*. New York, NY: Freeman.

Belza, B., Walwick, J., Shiu-Thornton, S., Schwartz, S., Taylor, M., & LoGerfo, J. (2004). Older adult perspectives on physical activity and exercise: Voices from multiple cultures. *Preventing Chronic Disease, 1*(4), A09.

Berkhuysen, M. A., Nieuwland, W., Buunk, B. P., Sanderman, R., & Rispens, P. (1999). Change in self-efficacy during cardiac rehabilitation and the role of perceived overprotectiveness. *Patient Education and Counseling, 38*(1), 21–32.

Birkel, R., Dessem, E., Eldridge, S., Kulinski, K., Lachenmayr, S., Spafford, M., . . .Zenker, W. (2015). Improving lives through evidence-based health promotion programs: A national priority. *Frontiers in Public Health, 2*, 255.

Bopp, M., Fallon, E. A., & Marquez, D. X. (2011). A faith-based physical activity intervention for Latinos: Outcomes and lessons. *American Journal of Health Promotion, 25*(3), 168–171.

Bopp, M., Lattimore, D., Wilcox, S., Laken, M., McClorin, L., Swinton, R., . . . Bryant, D. (2007). Understanding physical activity participation in members of an African American church: A qualitative study. *Health Education Research, 22*(6), 815–826.

Brawley, L. R., Rejeski, W. J., & King, A. C. (2003). Promoting physical activity for older adults: The challenges for changing behavior. *American Journal Preventive Medicine, 25*(3 Suppl. 2), 172–183.

Campbell-Sills, L., Cohan, S. L., & Stein, M. B. (2006). Relationship of resilience to personality, coping, and psychiatric symptoms in young adults. *Behaviour Research and Theraphy, 44*(4), 585–599.

Centers for Disease Control and Prevention. (2013). *The state of aging and health in America 2013*. Atlanta, GA: Centers for Disease Control and Prevention.

Chalabaev, A., Emile, M., Corrion, K., Stephan, Y., Clement-Guillotin, C., Pradier, C., & d'Arripe-Longueville, F. (2013). Development and validation of the aging stereotypes and exercise scale. *Journal of Aging and Physical Activity, 21*(3), 319–334.

Chiang, K. C., Seman, L., Belza, B., & Tsai, J. H. (2008). "It is our exercise family": Experiences of ethnic older adults in a group-based exercise program. *Preventing Chronic Disease, 5*(1), A05.

Chodzko-Zajko, W. (Ed.). (2014). *ACSM's exercise for older adults*. Baltimore, MD: Lippincott Williams & Wilkins.

Chodzko-Zajko, W., Schwingel, A., & Park, H. E. (2009). Succesful aging: The role of physical activity. *American Journal of Lifestyle Medicine, 3*(1), 20–28.

Clark, P. G., Blissmer, B. J., Greene, G. W., Lees, F. D., Riebe, D. A., & Stamm, K. E. (2011). Maintaining exercise and healthful eating in older adults: The SENIOR Project II: Study design and methodology. *Contemporary Clinical Trials, 32*(1), 129–139.

Clark, P. G., Burbank, P., Greene, G., Owens, N., & Riebe, D. (2010). What do we know about resilience in older adults? An exploration of some facts, factors, and facets. In B. Resnick, K. Roberto, & L. Gwyther (Eds.), *Resilience in aging: Concepts, research, and outcomes*. New York, NY: Springer.

Conn, V. S., Minor, M. A., Burks, K. J., Rantz, M. J., & Pomeroy, S. H. (2003). Integrative review of physical activity intervention research with aging adults. *Journal of American Geriatrics Society, 51*(8), 1159–1168.

Cress, M. E., Buchner, D. M., Prohaska, T., Rimmer, J., Brown, M., Macera, C., . . . Chodzko-Zajko, W. (2005). Best practices for physical activity programs and behavior counseling in older adult populations. *Journal of Aging and Physical Actitvity, 13*(1), 61–74.

Duru, O. K., Sarkisian, C. A., Leng, M., & Mangione, C. M. (2010). Sisters in motion: A randomized controlled trial of a faith-based physical activity intervention. *Journal of American Geriatrics Society, 58*(10), 1863–1869.

Ehrenreich, H., Pike, M., Hohman, K., Kaniewski, M., Longjohn, M., Myers, G., & Lee, L. (2015). CDC and YMCA: A promising partnership for delivering fall prevention programing. *Frontiers in Public Health, 2*, 235.

Erling, J., & Oldridge, N. B. (1985). Effect of a spousal-support program on compliance with cardiac rehabilitation. *Medicine and Science in Sports and Exercise, 15*, 120.

Education Amendments Act of 1972. (1972). Retrieved May 25, 2015 from www.justice.gov/crt/about/cor/coord/titleix.php

Exercise is Medicine. (n.d.). *Exercise is medicine*. Retrieved March 18, 2015, from http://www.exerciseismedicine.org

Federal Interagency Forum on Aging-Related Statistics. (2012). Older Americans 2012: Key indicators of well-being. *Federal Interagency Forum on Aging-Related Statistics*. Washington, DC: U.S. Government Printing Office.

Fishbein, M., & Ajzen, I. (2010). *Predicting and changing behavior: The reasoned action approach*. New York: Psychology Press.

Foster, S., & Giles-Corti, B. (2008). The built environment, neighborhood crime and constrained physical activity: An exploration of inconsistent findings. *Preventive Medicine, 47*(3), 241–251.

Foster, S., Knuiman, M., Hooper, P., Christian, H., & Giles-Corti, B. (2014). Do changes in residents' fear of crime impact their walking? Longitudinal results from RESIDE. *Preventive Medicine, 62*, 161–166.

French, D. P., Sutton, S., Hennings, S. J., Mitchell, J., Wareham, N. J., Griffin, S., . . . Kinmonth, A. L. (2005). The importance of affective beliefs and attitudes in the theory of planned behavior: Predicting intention to increase physical activity. *Journal of Applied Social Psychology, 35*(9), 1824–1848.

Gilespie, L. D., Robertson, M. C., Gillespie, W. J., Sherrington, C., Gates, S., Clemson, L. M., & Lamb, S. E. (2012). Interventions for preventing falls in older people living in the community. *Cochrane Database of Systematic Reviews*, (9), CD007146.

Gill, T. M., Murphy, T. E., Gahbauer, E. A., & Allore, H. G. (2013). Association of injurious falls with disability outcomes and nursing home admissions in community-living older persons. *American Journal of Epidemiology, 178*(3), 418–425.

Gillespie, L. D., Gillespie, W. J., Robertson, M. C., Lamb, S. E., Cumming, R. G., & Rowe, B. H. (2003). Interventions for preventing falls in elderly people. *Cochrane Database Systematic Reviews*, (4), CD000340.

Gillum, R. F. (2006). Frequency of attendance at religious services and leisure-time physical activity in American women and men: The third National Health and Nutrition Examination Survey. *Annals of Behavioral Medicine, 31*(1), 30–35.

Godin, G., & Conner, M. (2008). Intention-behavior relationship based on epidemiologic indices: An application to physical activity. *American Journal of Health Promotion, 22*(3), 180–182.

Gollwitzer, P. M. (1999). Implementation intentions: Strong effects of small plans. *American Journal of Psychology, 54*(7), 493–503.

Griffith, D. M., King, A., & Ober Allen, J. (2013). Male peer influence on African American men's motivation for physical activity: Men's and women's perspectives. *American Journal of Mens Health, 7*(2), 169–178.

Hall, P. A., Zehr, C., Paulitzki, J., & Rhodes, R. (2014). Implementation intentions for physical activity behavior in older adult women: An examination of executive function as a moderator of treatment effects. *Annals of Behavior Medicine, 48*(1), 130–136.

Hawkley, L. C., Thisted, R. A., & Cacioppo, J. T. (2009). Loneliness predicts reduced physical activity: Cross-sectional & longitudinal analyses. *Health Psychology, 28*(3), 354–363.

Hebert, E. T., Caughy, M. O., & Shuval, K. (2012). Primary care providers' perceptions of physical activity counselling in a clinical setting: A systematic review. *British Journal of Sports Medicine, 46*(9), 625–631.

Hinrichs, T., & Brach, M. (2012). The general practitioner's role in promoting physical activity to older adults: A review based on program theory. *Current Aging Science, 5*(1), 41–50.

Hogan, B. E., Linden, W., & Najarian, B. (2002). Social support interventions: Do they work? *Clinical Psychology Review, 22*(3), 383–442.

Hooker, S. P., Wilcox, S., Rheaume, C. E., Burroughs, E. L., & Friedman, D. B. (2011). Factors related to physical activity and recommended intervention strategies as told by midlife and older African American men. *Ethnicity & Disease, 21*(3), 261–267.

Howland, J., Lachman, M. E., Peterson, E. W., Cote, J., Kasten, L., & Jette, A. (1998). Covariates of fear of falling and associated activity curtailment. *Gerontologist, 38*(5), 549–555.

Hu, L., Motl, R. W., McAuley, E., & Konopack, J. F. (2007). Effects of self-efficacy on physical activity enjoyment in college-aged women. *International Journal of Behavioral Medicine, 14*(2), 92–96.

Humpel, N., Owen, N., & Leslie, E. (2002). Environmental factors associated with adults' participation in physical activity: A review. *American Journal of Preventive Medicine, 22*(3), 188–199.

Jaber, R., Braksmajer, A., & Trilling, J. S. (2006). Group visits: A qualitative review of current research. *Journal of the American Board of Family Medicine, 19*(3), 276–290.

Jefferis, B. J., Iliffe, S., Kendrick, D., Kerse, N., Trost, S., Lennon, L. T., . . . Whincup, P. H. (2014). How are falls and fear of falling associated with objectively measured physical activity in a cohort of community-dwelling older men? *BMC Geriatrics, 14*, 114.

Kassavou, A., Turner, A., & French, D. P. (2013). Do interventions to promote walking in groups increase physical activity? A meta-analysis. *International Journal of Behavioral Nutrition and Physical Activity, 10*, 18.

Kendrick, D., Kumar, A., Carpenter, H., Zijlstra, G. A., Skelton, D. A., Cook, J. R., et al. (2014) Exercise for reducing fear of falling in older people living in the community. *Cochrane Database of Systematic Reviews.*

King, A. C. (2001). Interventions to promote physical activity by older adults. *The Journals of Gerontology. Series A, Biological Sciences and Medicine Sciences, 56*(Spec No 2), 36–46.

King, A. C., Rejeski, W. J., & Buchner, D. M. (1998). Physical activity interventions targeting older adults. A critical review and recommendations. *American Journal of Preventive Medicine, 15*(4), 316–333.

Koenig, H. G. (2012). Religion, spirituality, and health: The research and clinical implications. *ISRN Psychiatry, 2012*, 278730.

Koenig, H. G., Moberg, D. O., & Kvale, J. N. (1988). Religious activities and attitudes of older adults in a geriatric assessment clinic. *Journal of the American Geriatrics Society, 36*(4), 362–374.

Koh, H. K., & Sebelius, K. G. (2010). Promoting prevention through the Affordable Care Act. *The New England Journal of Medicine, 363*(14), 1296–1299.

Kreuter, M. W., Chheda, S. G., & Bull, F. C. (2000). How does physician advice influence patient behavior? Evidence for a priming effect. *Archives of Family Medicine, 9*(5), 426–433.

Lees, F. D., Clark, P. G., Nigg, C. R., & Newman, P. (2005). Barriers to exercise behavior among older adults: A focus-group study. *Journal of Aging and Physical Activity, 13*(1), 23–33.

LeFevre, M. L., & U.S. Preventive Services Task Force. (2014). Behavioral counseling to promote a healthful diet and physical activity for cardiovascular disease prevention in adults with cardiovascular risk factors: U.S. Preventive Services Task Force Recommendation Statement. *Annals of International Medicine, 161*(8), 587–593.

Lin, J. S., O' Connor, E., Whitlock, E.P., & Beil, T. L. (2010) Behavioral counseling to promote physical activity and a healthful diet to prevent cardiovascular disease in adults: A systematic review for the U.S. Preventive Services Task Force. *Annals of International Medicine, 153*(11), 736–750.

Litt, M. D., Kleppinger, A., & Judge, J. O. (2002). Initiation and maintenance of exercise behavior in older women: Predictors from the social learning model. *Journal of Behavioral Medicine, 25*(1), 83–97.

Martinez, S. M., Arredondo, E. M., Perez, G., & Baquero, B. (2009). Individual, social, and environmental barriers to and facilitators of physical activity among Latinas living in San Diego County: Focus group results. *Family & Community Health, 32*(1), 22–33.

Masud, T., & Morris, R. O. (2001). Epidemiology of falls. *Age and Ageing, 30*(Suppl. 4), 3–7.

Mathews, A. E., Laditka, S. B., Laditka, J. N., Wilcox, S., Corwin, S. J., Liu, R., . . . Logsdon, R. G. (2010). Older adults' perceived physical activity enablers and barriers: A multicultural perspective. *Journal of Aging and Physical Activity, 18*(2), 119–140.

McAuley, E. (1993). Self-efficacy and the maintenance of exercise participation in older adults. *Journal of Behavioral Medicine, 16*(1), 103–113.

McAuley, E., & Blissmer, B. (2000). Self-efficacy determinants and consequences of physical activity. *Exercise and Sport Sciences Reviews, 28*(2), 85–88.

McAuley, E., Jerome, G. J., Elavsky, S., Marquez, D. X., & Ramsey, S. N. (2003). Predicting long-term maintenance of physical activity in older adults. *Preventive Medicine, 37*(2), 110–118.

McAuley, E., Jerome, G. J., Marquez, D. X., Elavsky, S., & Blissmer, B. (2003). Exercise self-efficacy in older adults: Social, affective, and behavioral influences. *Annals of Behavioral Medicine, 25*(1), 1–7.

McLeroy, K. R., Bibeau, D., Steckler, A., & Glanz, K. (1988). An ecological perspective on health promotion programs. *Health Education Quarterly, 15*(4), 351–377.

Mlinac, M., Lees, F., Stamm, K. E., Saint, J., & Mulligan, J. (2014). Maintaining late life health behaviors: Comparing clinician rating and self-reported resilience. *Topics in Geriatric Rehabilitation, 30*(3), 188–194.

Murphy, S. L., Williams, C. S., & Gill, T. M. (2002). Characteristics associated with fear of falling and activity restriction in community-living older persons. *Journal of the American Geriatrics Society, 50*(3), 516–520.

Murtagh, E. M., Murphy, M. H., Murphy, N. M., Woods, C., Nevill, A. M., & Lane, A. (2015). Prevalence and correlates of physical inactivity in community-dwelling older adults in Ireland. *PLOS One, 10*(2), e0118293.

Nelson, M. E., Rejeski, W. J., Blair, S. N., Duncan, P. W., Judge, J. O., King, A. C., . . . American Heart Association. (2007). Physical activity and public health in older adults: Recommendation from the American College of Sports Medicine and the American Heart Association. *Circulation, 116*(9), 1094–1105.

Neupert, S. D., Lachman, M. E., & Whitbourne, S. B. (2009). Exercise self-efficacy and control beliefs: Effects on exercise behavior after an exercise intervention for older adults. *Journal of Aging and Physical Activity, 17*(1), 1–16.

Orrow, G., Kinmonth, A. L., Sanderson, S., & Sutton, S. (2012). Effectiveness of physical activity promotion based in primary care: Systematic review and meta-analysis of randomised controlled trials. *BMJ, 344*, e1389.

Pew Forum. (2008). *Religious beliefs and practices: Diverse and politically relevant.* Washington, DC: Pew Research Center.

Physical Activity Guidelines Advisory Committee. (2008). *Physical activity guidelines advisory committee report, 2008*. Washington, DC: U.S. Department of Health and Human Services.

Petrella, R. J., Koval, J. J., Cunningham, D. A., & Paterson, D. H. (2003). Can primary care doctors prescribe exercise to improve fitness? The Step Test Exercise Prescription (STEP) project. *American Journal of Preventive Medicine, 24*(4), 316–322.

Ramirez, A. G., Chalela, P., Gallion, K., & Velez, L. F. (2007). Energy balance feasibility study for Latinas in Texas: A qualitative assessment. *Preventive Chronic Disease, 4*(4), A98.

Rejeski, W. J., Brawley, L. R., Ambrosius, W. T., Brubaker, P. H., Focht, B. C., Foy, C. G., & Fox, L. D. (2003). Older adults with chronic disease: Benefits of group-mediated counseling in the promotion of physically active lifestyles. *Health Psychology, 22*(4), 414–423.

Resnick, B., Orwig, D., Magaziner, J., & Wynne, C. (2002). The effect of social support on exercise behavior in older adults. *Clinical Nursing Research, 11*(1), 52–70.

Ryff, C. D., & Singer, B. (2003). The role of emotion on pathways to positive health. In R. J. Davidson, K. R. Scherer, & H. H. Goldsmith (Eds.), *Handbook of affective sciences*. New York, NY: Oxford University Press.

Sallis, J. F., Cervero, R. B., Ascher, W., Henderson, K. A., Kraft, M. K., & Kerr, J. (2006). An ecological approach to creating more physically active communities. *Annual Review of Public Health, 27*, 297–322.

Sallis, J. F., Haskell, W. L., Fortmann, S. P., Vranizan, K. M., Taylor, C. B., & Solomon, D. S. (1986). Predictors of adoption and maintenance of physical activity in a community sample. *Preventive Medicine, 15*(4), 331–341.

Sánchez Palacios, C., Trianes Torres, M. V., & Blanca Mena, M. J. (2009). Aging negative stereotypes and their relationship with sociodemographic variables over 65 elderly. *Revista Espanola de Geriatria Gerontologia, 44*(3), 124–129.

Scheffer, A. C., Schuurmans, M. J., van Dijk, N., van der Hooft, T., & de Rooij, S. E. (2008). Fear of falling: Measurement strategy, prevalence, risk factors and consequences among older persons. *Age and Ageing, 37*(1), 19–24.

Schutzer, K. A., & Graves, B. S. (2004). Barriers and motivations to exercise in older adults. *Preventive Medicine, 39*(5), 1056–1061.

Talbot, L. A., Musiol, R. J., Witham, E. K., & Metter, E. J. (2005). Falls in young, middle-aged and older community dwelling adults: Perceived cause, environmental factors and injury. *BMC Public Health, 5*, 86.

Taylor, A. H., Cable, N. T., Faulkner, G., Hillsdon, M., Narici, M., & Van Der Bij, A. K. (2004). Physical activity and older adults: A review of health benefits and the effectiveness of interventions. *Journal of Sports Sciences, 22*(8), 703–725.

Tinetti, M. E., Mendes de Leon, C. F., Doucette, J. T., & Baker, D. I. (1994). Fear of falling and fall-related efficacy in relationship to functioning among community-living elders. *Journal of Gerontology, 49*(3), M140–M147.

Treat and Reduce Obesity Act of 2013, S.1184, 113th Congress. (2013). Retrieved May 11, 2015 from congress.gov/bill/113th-congress/senate-bill/1184

Tucker-Seeley, R. D., Subramanian, S. V., Li, Y., & Sorensen, G. (2009). Neighborhood safety, socioeconomic status, and physical activity in older adults. *American Journal of Preventive Medicine, 37*(3), 207–213.

Tussing-Humphreys, L., Thomson, J. L., Mayo, T., & Edmond, E. (2013). A church-based diet and physical activity intervention for rural, lower Mississippi Delta African American adults: Delta Body and Soul effectiveness study, 2010–2011. *Preventive Chronic Disease, 10*, E92.

U.S. Department of Health and Human Services, Office of Disease Prevention and Health Promotion. (2011). *Healthy People 2020*. Retrieved May 1, 2015 from http://www.healthypeople.gov/2020/topics-objectives/topic/physical-activity/objectives

U.S. Preventive Services Task Force. (2012). *Healthful diet and physical activity for cardiovascular disease prevention in adults: Behavioral counseling: Recommendation summary*. Retrieved May 1, 2015 from uspreventiveservicestaskforce.org/Page/Topic/recommendation-summary/healthful-diet-and-physical-activity-for-cardio vascular-disease-prevention-in-adults-behavioral-counseling

van der Bij, A. K., Laurant, M. G., & Wensing, M. (2002). Effectiveness of physical activity interventions for older adults: A review. *American Journal of the Preventive Medicine, 22*(2), 120–133.

van Stralen, M. M., De Vries, H., Mudde, A. N., Bolman, C., & Lechner, L. (2009). Determinants of initiation and maintenance of physical activity among older adults: A literature review. *Health Psychology Review, 3*(2), 147–207.

Visser, M., Brychta, R. J., Chen, K. Y., & Koster, A. (2014). Self-reported adherence to the physical activity recommendation and determinants of misperception in older adults. *Journal of Aging Physical Activity, 22*(2), 226–234.

Wang, G., Pratt, M., Macera, C. A., Zheng, Z. J., & Heath, G. (2004). Physical activity, cardiovascular disease, and medical expenditures in U.S. adults. *Annals of Behavioral Medicine, 28*(2), 88–94.

Warner, L. M., Ziegelmann, J. P., Schuz, B., Wurm, S., & Schwarzer, R. (2011). Synergistic effect of social support and self-efficacy on physical exercise in older adults. *Journal of Aging and Physical Activity, 19*(3), 249–261.

Williams, P., & Lord, S. R. (1995). Predictors of adherence to a structured exercise program for older women. *Psychology Aging, 10*(4), 617–624.

Zijlstra, G. A., van Haastregt, J. C., van Rossum, E., van Eijk, J. T., Yardley, L., & Kempen, G. I. (2007). Interventions to reduce fear of falling in community-living older people: A systematic review. *Journal of American Geriatrics Society, 55*(4), 603–615.

CHAPTER 13

Incorporating Function and Physical Activity Across All Settings

Barbara Resnick and Marie Boltz

ABSTRACT

The majority of older adults do not engage in regular physical activity. In surveys of community dwelling, among older adults age 75 and above, one in three men and one in two women engage in no physical activity. These rates are even lower among those who are hospitalized or institutionalized in nursing homes or assisted living settings. Moreover, those living in institutional settings demonstrate a decline in function that exceeds what would be expected based on disease states. Limited activity and functional decline place older adults at risk for pain associated with contractures, pressure sores, and decreased sense of well-being and overall quality of life. We propose a Function Focused Care approach that encourages caregivers to engage older adults in function and physical activity during all care interactions. This approach can be implemented using a four-step approach and practical, cost-neutral approaches. This chapter delineates the ways in which to implement Function Focused Care across all settings, describes outcomes associated with this approach, and provides ways in which to overcome the setting-specific challenges.

http://dx.doi.org/10.1891/0198-8794.36.293

Physical activity is any bodily movement produced by skeletal muscles that requires energy expenditure (World Health Organization, 2014). Functional activities for older adults such as bathing, dressing, and walking are important components of overall physical activity. It is well known that physical inactivity has significant negative health outcomes increasing the risk of cardiovascular disease, cancers, diabetes, and depression, among other problems (Blair, 2009). Conversely, meta-analyses have shown that physical activity can improve bone health and function, decrease fall risk, and reduce disease risk and progression, among other positive outcomes (Cress et al., 2005; Desveaux, Beauchamp, Goldstein, & Brooks, 2014; Netz, Wu, Becker, & Tennenbaum, 2005; Silva, Eslick, & Duque, 2013; Windle, Hughes, Linck, Russell, & Woods, 2010). This is true even for chronically ill or frail older adults for whom it is often falsely believed that physical activity will exacerbate versus ameliorate underlying health problems (Clegg, Barber, Young, Forster, & Iliffe, 2012). Although current recommendations for the amount of daily physical activity that older individuals should engage in have been established by the American Heart Association and the American College of Sports Medicine (i.e., 30 minutes daily of moderate-level physical activity; American College of Sports Medicine and the American Heart Association, 2013), substantial benefits can be achieved at even relatively low levels of exercise intensity (Cornelissen & Fagard, 2005; Singh, 2002; Tudor-Locke et al., 2011).

Unfortunately, the majority of older adults do not engage in regular physical activity. In surveys of community-dwelling older adults age 75 and above, one in three men and one in two women engage in no physical activity (Centers for Disease Control, 2014). These rates are even lower among those who are hospitalized or institutionalized in nursing homes or assisted living settings (Boltz, Resnick, Capezuti, & Shabbat, 2011; Brown, Redden, Flood, & Allman, 2009; Galik, Resnick, Hammersla, & Brightwater, 2014; Król-Zielińska, Kusy, Zieliński, & Osiński, 2011).

CHALLENGES TO PARTICIPATION IN FUNCTION AND PHYSICAL ACTIVITY AMONG OLDER ADULTS

There are many challenges and barriers to adherence to regular physical activity among older individuals. These include such things as providers not recommending participation or discouraging participation in physical activity or activity programs (Trinh, Wilson, Williams, & Sum, 2012); lack of belief in the benefits associated with physical activity and the importance it has in maintaining function (Horne & Tierney, 2012); intrapersonal factors such as comorbidities, genetics, age, gender, and mood (Dolansky, Stepanczuk, Charvat, & Moore, 2010; Hawley-Hague et al., 2014; Hyman, Oden, & Wagner, 2010);

interpersonal factors such as social support to engage in physical activity (Horne & Tierney, 2012; Moody, Hale, & Waters, 2012; Siceloff, Coulon, & Wilson, 2014; Tung, Cooke, & Moyle, 2013); lack of environmental resources such as flat open spaces to ambulate, bike paths, and opportunities to swim; access to age-appropriate exercise equipment (Ferrer, Cruz, Burge, Bayles, & Castilla, 2014; Horne & Tierney, 2012; Sangster et al., 2013); or the all too common experience of having chronic pain and lack of belief that the physical activity may actually decrease rather than exacerbate pain (Stubbs et al., 2013). Similar to the unpleasant sensation of pain associated with exercise, many older adults fear falling, whether or not they have previously sustained a fall (Schepens, Sen, Painter, & Murphy, 2012). As with pain, exercise interventions are one of the best ways in which to decrease the risk of falling and the fear of falling among older adults (Kumar et al., 2014).

Motivation is a particularly critical component in adhering to regular physical activity and participation in functional activities (Janssen, Dugan, Karavolos, Lynch, & Powell, 2014). Motivation is the inner urge that moves or prompts a person to action. Motivation refers to the need, drive, or desire to act in a certain way to achieve a certain end. In addition to motivation, older adults need to be physically resilient in order to remain optimally engaged in functional and physical activity. Resilience is defined as one's ability to "bounce back" or respond appropriately to challenging experiences. The challenging experience can be used as a learning opportunity and can facilitate growth for the individual. For example, older adults who utilize the experience of a hip fracture or acute cardiac event as an opportunity to adhere to rehabilitation services offered and change their lifestyle and increase their physical activity would be noted to be physically resilient. While there are likely genetic components to motivation and resilience (Rana et al., 2014), there are interventions that can be implemented to strengthen resilience and motivate individuals to engage in functional and physical activity, as shown in Table 13.1.

Along with motivation and resilience, cognitive challenges are also commonly noted as a barrier to engagement in physical activity. Approximately 50% of all nursing home residents in the United States have dementia, and many of these individuals exhibit challenging behavioral symptoms such as apathy and a lack of willingness to engage in any activity, physical aggression, agitation, and resistance to care. Concerns about exacerbating these symptoms and difficulty following even a single-step command makes engaging these individuals in regular physical activity particularly difficult (Chung, 2012; Galik et al., 2014). Moreover, older adults with cognitive impairment are also likely to experience other challenges noted such as fear of falling, pain, and an underlying lack of motivation or resilience.

TABLE 13.1

Interventions to Strengthen Motivation and Physical Resilience

Psychosocial	Behavioral
Acknowledge the event/the loss	Engage the individual in the behaviors necessary to overcome the physical challenge experienced (e.g., exercising; going to therapy)
Help the individual figure out a plan of care/take control of the challenging event	Break down activities into successful small steps (transfer to standing position prior to walking)
Provide appropriate resources to engage in the plan of care	Provide immediate verbal reinforcement for behaviors completed
Strengthen self-efficacy using verbal encouragement, role modeling, and elimination of unpleasant sensations around the activity to be performed (e.g., going to therapy after a hip fracture)	Integrate the long-term behavior change necessary to utilize the challenge as a learning experience and one of growth (long-term exercise program following a hip fracture)
Help the individual develop problem-solving techniques	Work with the individual to identify physical goals that will lead to physical growth
Review prior successes in overcoming challenging situations	
Help the individual find meaning in the challenging experience	

FUNCTION FOCUSED CARE

Function Focused Care is proposed as a way in which to help assure that older adults engage in function and physical activity across all settings of care. Function Focused Care is a philosophy of care that focuses on evaluating the older adult's underlying capability with regard to function and physical activity and helping him or her optimize maintaining abilities. The goal is to ensure that the individual performs his or her functional tasks such as bathing and dressing at the highest level possible and continually increases time spent in physical activity. Examples of Function Focused Care interactions are shown in Table 13.2 and include such things as using verbal cues during bathing so the older individual performs the tasks rather than the direct care worker (DCW) bathing the individual, having the individual walk or self-propel to the bathroom rather than using a urinal, or going to an exercise class.

TABLE 13.2

Examples of Function Focused Care Activities

Activity	Examples of Function Focused Care Performed	Examples of When Function Focused Care Is Not Performed
Bed mobility	– Asks or encourages the individual to move in bed. – Gives him or her time to move. – Gives step-by-step cues on how to move in bed. – Places individual's hands to facilitate independent movement—e.g., on guardrail.	– Asks the individual to move in bed but does not allow time for him or her to respond. – Moves the individual—pulls the individual up using the bedsheet or rolls the individual over. – Discourages or stops older adult from moving in the bed.
Transfer from one surface to another	– Asks or encourages the individual to transfer and allows sufficient time for movement. – Gives step-by-step cues on how to transfer—e.g., "Slide to the edge of the chair." – Places hands to facilitate independent movement—e.g., places hands on walker.	– Transfers/lifts the individual with no encouragement for him or her to participate in the transfer. – Discourages or stops the individual from performing the transfer.

(*Continued*)

TABLE 13.2
Examples of Function Focused Care Activities (Continued)

Activity	Examples of Function Focused Care Performed	Examples of When Function Focused Care Is Not Performed
Mobility (ambulation/ wheelchair)	– Encourages the individual to walk or independently propel the wheelchair and gives him or her time to perform activity. – Gives step-by-step cues to help the individual walk—e.g., "Move your left foot forward, now move your right foot." – Assist, ask, and/or encourage use of assistive devices.	– Utilizes wheelchair instead of encouraging ambulation. – Discourages or stops the individual from walking or self-propelling the wheelchair.
Physical activity/ exercise	– Encourages the individual to go to an exercise class, park farther from a store, walk daily. – Takes the individual to an exercise class. – Exercises with the individual. – Utilizes outdoor areas to encourage physical activity.	– Discourages participating in physical activity. – Encourages sedentary behavior. – Propagates a fear of falling by encouraging individuals to sit…or they might fall. – Locks access to outdoor areas.

THEORETICAL MODEL TO GUIDE INTEGRATION OF THE FUNCTION FOCUSED CARE ACROSS ALL CARE SETTINGS

To optimize integration of a Function Focused Care approach into all care settings in which older adults live, it is helpful to use a theoretical model. The model combines the Social Ecological Model (Gregson et al., 2003) and Social Cognitive Theory (Bandura, 1997). The Social Ecological Model includes a focus, at the center, on intrapersonal factors such as the individual's age, comorbidities, genetics, education, mood, and underlying capability. The next component of the model to consider includes the interpersonal relationships and interactions that individuals have in all settings. This might include interactions with family, peers, or staff. Social Cognitive Theory and the sources of information proposed by Bandura (Bandura, 1997) that are known to influence behavior are extremely helpful in directing interpersonal interactions that can influence functional and physical activity. Social cognitive theory is based on self-efficacy and outcome expectations with the central theme being that the more strongly one believes in his or her ability to perform a course of action and successfully complete an activity, the more likely he or she will be to perform that activity. In addition, outcome expectations also influence behavior. If the individual believes that performance of the activity will have a positive outcome (e.g., if I diet I will lose weight and my clothes will fit better; or if I exercise I will be able to carry my groceries better), then he or she will be more likely to perform the activity. There are four sources of information or four ways in which we can interact with individuals to strengthen self-efficacy or outcome expectations. These sources of information and examples for how they can be used with older adults are shown in Table 13.3.

The next component of the Social Ecological Model to consider is the environment, particularly the physical environment. Environments can be evaluated for how they positively or negatively influence an individual's willingness to engage in functional or physical activity. Table 13.4 provides an example of one assessment tool for the environment. Particular consideration should be given to chair and bed height, which can facilitate or impair transfers (Kuo, 2013; Shinichi & Takayoshi, 2007), and access to outdoors for walking and other types of physical activity. Chair and bed height should be between 80% and 120% of the individual's lower leg length or there should not be more than a 20% difference between the individual's lower leg length and the height of the chair. Access to outdoors, particularly gardens and places to walk should be evaluated as they may not only help physical activity but may also improve behavioral symptoms associated with dementia (Whear et al., 2014).

TABLE 13.3

Informational Sources Used to Guide Interpersonal Interactions

Informational Source	Examples of Use
Performance of the activity	– Set up situations in which the individual can *successfully* complete the activity such as walking a few steps; going to an exercise class; participating in some aspects of bathing such as washing one's face.
Verbal encouragement and positive reinforcement	– Provide ongoing verbal encouragement to perform an activity and encourage continuation of engagement in the activity. – Provide positive reinforcement for any level of activity done. – Repeatedly ask about exercise activities at follow-up interactions. – Avoid negative encouragement to remain sedentary: Avoid stating, "Don't get up, you might fall." – Engage individuals in walking when they seem ready and willing to do so.
Role or self-modeling	– Tell older individuals about your physical activity/exercise. – Tell individuals about others like them who exercise. – Remind individuals of what they are able to do because they have done so previously.
Physiological feedback/affective states experienced during an activity	– Anticipate and eliminate unpleasant sensations around an activity such as pain, fear of falling, and shortness of breath. – Optimize positive outcomes associated with physical activity (feeling better, energized, less pain). – Make exercise activities pleasant and fun.

TABLE 13.4

Assessment of Environment for Factors That Influence Function and Physical Activity

Item	Present	Not Present
1. Evidence of area for walking that is clear of clutter		
2. Evidence of area for walking that has rest spots available		
3. Evidence of area for walking that is pleasant		
4. Evidence of pleasant destination areas		
5. Evidence of cues in the environment to encourage physical activity		
6. Evidence of supplies (i.e., safe assistive devices) to encourage function and activity		
7. Chair heights in rooms and hallways appropriate (between 80% and 120% of the individual's lower leg length as measured from the floor to the individual's patella or less than a 20% difference between the height of the chair and the lower leg length of an individual [knee to ankle])		
8. Bed heights in rooms appropriate (same as for chair)		
9. Toilet height in rooms appropriate (ratio of toilet height to lower leg length of average older adults [15.45 inches] between 80% and 120%)		
10. Evidence of cues in the environment to encourage functional activity		
11. Access to age-appropriate exercise equipment		
12. Evidence of poor lighting[a]		
13. Evidence of slippery floors[a]		
14. Evidence of uneven surfaces[a]		
15. Evidence of items that could cause a trip[a]		
16. Availability of safe footwear		

[a]Negative components of the environment.

In addition to the physical environment, it is helpful to consider other resources within settings that can motivate individuals to engage in function and physical activity. This might include signs that serve as reminders (e.g., "Use the Stairs!") or murals along hallways that measure out walking distances. Alternatively, access to pedometers or other type of activity monitoring can be a useful source of encouragement and motivation to remain engaged in physical activity (De Greef, Deforche, Tudor-Locke, & De Bourdeaudhuij, 2010). Other types of interventions within the environment include establishing pleasant and fun destinations sites that can be used as motivational incentives to walk. For example, a coffee shop or a little store with groceries or gifts (Mitchell, Goodman, Alter, Oh, & Faulkner, 2014; Resnick, Galik, Gruber-Baldini, & Zimmerman, 2011) are all useful ways to alter the environment and provide incentives for physical activity.

The last component to be considered within the Social Ecological Model is the evaluation of policies and/or culture within the setting of care. Policies can facilitate access to opportunities for physical activity by establishing a culture in which physical activity is expected. For example, a policy that requires that stairs be well lit, open, carpeted, and pleasant to walk in would encourage its use and physical activity. Table 13.5 provides a guide for how to evaluate policies and cultures within settings of care.

THE FOUR-STEP APPROACH TO IMPLEMENTING FUNCTION FOCUSED CARE

To optimally integrate a Function Focused Care philosophy into all care settings, a four-step approach can be used. Ideally, the facility or setting of care should identify a champion to facilitate the implementation process and ensure that the steps are completed and that staff in the settings are engaged in providing this type of care. The steps, which include (a) environment and policy/procedure assessments; (b) education of staff, residents, and families; (c) developing function-focused goals for residents; and (d) mentoring and motivating staff, older adults, families, and other caregivers, are described in Table 13.6.

SPECIFIC CHALLENGES AND SOLUTIONS TO IMPLEMENTING FUNCTION FOCUSED CARE BY SETTING

Acute Care Settings

Given that the focus and goals of acute care are on the management of acute medical problems rather than long-term impact of disease, integrating a Function Focused Care philosophy is particularly challenging. Challenges include patient factors, the acute care environment, medical and nursing interventions, and regulatory and reimbursement systems that do not encourage physical activity (Boltz, Resnick, Capezuti, Shuluk, & Secic, 2012; Brown et al., 2009; Brown, Williams, Woodby, Davis, & Allman, 2007; Buttery & Martin, 2009;

TABLE 13.5
Function Focused Care Assessment of Policy/Protocols

Item	Present	Not Present	Not Applicable
1. Evidence of policy regarding physical restraints that optimizes function and physical activity			
2. Evidence of policy regarding Foley catheters that optimizes function and physical activity			
3. Evidence of policy related to use of free space (corridors, kitchens) that optimizes function and physical activity			
4. Evidence of policy around ambulation that optimizes function and physical activity			
5. Evidence of policy associated with transportation (in sites) that optimizes function and physical activity			
6. Evidence of policy associated with bed/chair/toilet height that optimizes function and physical activity			
7. Evidence of policy change associated with "hand-off" communication that optimizes function and physical activity			
8. Evidence of policy associated with discharge instructions that optimizes function and physical activity			

(*Continued*)

TABLE 13.5

Function Focused Care Assessment of Policy/Protocols (*Continued*)

Item	Present	Not Present	Not Applicable
9. Evidence of policy associated with pressure ulcer prevention that optimizes function and physical activity			
10. Evidence of policy associated with fall prevention that optimizes function and physical activity			
11. Evidence of policy associated with nursing assessment that addresses and optimizes function and physical activity			
12. Evidence of policy associated with change in patient condition that addresses and optimizes function and physical activity			
13. Evidence of policy associated with evaluation of nursing competencies to address function and physical activity of patients			
14. Evidence of policy associated with documentation of function and physical activity			
15. Evidence of policy associated with patient/family information that optimizes function and physical activity			

TABLE 13.6

Four Steps Associated With Implementing a Function Focused Care Philosophy Across Any Setting

Step	Description of Step Activity	Examples of Interventions Within Each Step
I. Environmental and policy assessments	• Champions evaluate the environment and policy using the assessment tools provided in Tables 13.3 and 13.4. • Interventions can be implemented as appropriate to decrease negative aspects of the environment and negative policies and increase positive components of the environment and alter policies so that they facilitate function and physical activity.	• Providing chairs to sit in that are the appropriate height in acute care hospital rooms. This can encourage patients to get out of bed and at least sit in the chair. • Providing resources for activities in assisted living that encourage physical activity such as age-appropriate weights, dance music, or a physical activity bingo game.
II. Education	• Basic education of all caregivers, families, and older individuals about the Function Focused Care philosophy and benefits associated with facilitating this type of approach to care.	• The webpage www.functionfocusedcare.org can be used to access materials for education of all types of staff, family, and older individuals. In addition, there are six short 3-minute video coaching sessions that can be used during staff training. These sessions provide ways in which to overcome challenging interactions with older individuals and facilitate their engagement in functional tasks and physical activity programs.

(Continued)

TABLE 13.6

Four Steps Associated With Implementing a Function Focused Care Philosophy Across Any Setting (*Continued*)

Step	Description of Step Activity	Examples of Interventions Within Each Step
III. Establishing Function Focused Care goals for residents	• Utilizing resources from the www.functionfocusedcare.org webpage (e.g., the Physical Capability Assessment) or talking with an older individual and/or the family, goals should be developed that identify what functional tasks and/or engagement in physical activity the individual can and should do.	• Setting clear and simple goals for what the individual can and should do. This might be walking to at least one meal a day; going to an exercise class three times a week; washing one's face; or dressing the upper body.
IV. Mentoring and motivating	• The champion provides ongoing motivational interventions for staff and residents and families to support engagement in functional and physical activity.	• Examples of motivational interventions include such things as contests between units, settings, or among individuals within a family in terms of who walks the most steps or who comes up with the most innovative way in which to incorporate physical activity into a holiday celebration.

Hopkins & Spuhler, 2009). Patient factors specific to the acute environment focus on the acute medical problem and associated fatigue, delirium, pain, depression, impaired nutritional status, sedation, and polypharmacy. Furthermore, patients generally believe that rest and lying in bed when experiencing an acute event will facilitate recovery.

Environmental challenges are also noted. The acute care environment generally provides limited opportunity for physical activity. The bed is often the only furniture in the hospital room and the height of the bed or chairs may limit the patient's ability to transfer. In addition, there are often no pleasant areas for walking or pleasant destination sites. Patients are often restricted from engaging in physical activity as part of ongoing care as they are not allowed to walk or self-propel to tests or procedures and are even escorted out of the hospital in a wheelchair. Basic environmental changes are commonly needed in acute care settings to provide the resources necessary for patients to perform functional and physical activity. Simple interventions such as making sure there are appropriate chairs in the rooms to sit on versus only a bed to lie in, access to appropriate size toilets, and clear pathways in rooms and hallways to ambulate can be implemented without excessive resources (Burkett, Hippensteel, Penrod, & Resnick, 2013).

Medical factors limiting physical activity and contributing to functional decline include the tethering effects of such things as indwelling urinary catheters, sequential compression devices, continuous monitoring (e.g., cardiac; pulse oximetry) and intravenous infusions; prescribed bed rest; sedating medications; insufficient management of pain; and tests and procedures that limit food/fluid intake (Leditschke, Green, Irvine, Bissett, & Mitchell, 2012; Thomsen, Snow, Rodriguez, & Hopkins, 2008; Zelada, Salinas, & Baztan, 2007). The culture and philosophy of care in acute care further impacts patient activity. Nurses in these settings tend to focus on and are rewarded for task completion (e.g., administering medications, monitoring vital signs, or arranging tests and procedures) and not on interventions that optimize patient function and physical activity. Perceptions continue to persist that it is quicker if the task is simply completed without any patient involvement (e.g., pull the patient up in bed, put him or her on a bedpan). Moreover, the nurses conceptualize their roles as "watching over" patients to protect them from falls and other adverse events (Leditschke, Green, Irvine, Bissett, & Mitchell, 2012; Schmidt, 2003) and encourage what are believed to be risk-free activities such as staying in bed (Dykes, Carroll, Hurley, Benoit, & Middelton, 2009; Laybourne, Biggs, & Martin, 2011; Lindquist & Sendelbach, 2007). This protective, custodial, task-oriented care facilitates functional decline, decreases physical activity, and contributes to deconditioning and disability.

In addition to using the four-step approach to implementing a Function Focused Care philosophy in acute care, it is critical to engage all members of the team including those who provide administrative oversight. Unlike other health care settings, interdisciplinary team members such as surgeons, physical and occupational therapists, case management as well as many layers of administration including charge nurses, clinical specialists, and directors of nursing can all influence the direct staff to change their approach to care. Furthermore, educating family caregivers about the importance of encouraging, motivating, and helping the patient be as physically active as possible will reinforce these efforts. Finally, ongoing reinforcement of care activities that increase patient time in function and physical activity is needed and should be overseen to make sure that function is encouraged during all care interactions.

Nursing Home Settings

Nursing homes provide personal care and skilled nursing care on a 24-hour per-day basis. Nursing homes are anticipated to be able to handle medical problems, disability, and behavioral problems in older adults that cannot be handled by caregivers in other care settings. In 1987, the Nursing Home Reform Act was passed. This law states that nursing homes "must provide services and activities to attain or maintain the highest practicable physical, mental, and psychosocial well-being of each resident in accordance with a written plan of care." To participate in Medicare and Medicaid, nursing homes must comply with this law. Furthermore, in the United States, a comprehensive assessment, referred to as the Minimum Data Set (Centers for Medicare and Medicare Services, 2013), is used to evaluate residents quarterly and when there is a change in condition. Other countries have similar assessment tools that are likewise regularly monitored (Habjanič, Saarnio, Elo, Turk, & Isola, 2012; Katz, 2011; Netten et al., 2010).

Despite federal guidelines to maintain function, it is unlikely that this is truly achieved, given the marked decline in function noted among those living in these settings (Carpenter, Hastie, Morris, Fries, & Ankri, 2006). There is repeated evidence, however, that Function Focused Care can be successfully implemented in these settings (Resnick, Galik, & Boltz, 2013). As with the acute care setting, there are specific challenges unique to the nursing home that must be considered. Environments may vary in nursing homes and thus individual consideration is necessary to determine how the environment can and should be optimized to best facilitate Function Focused Care activities. Traditionally, nursing home environments have been institutionally designed with wide-open hallways that can be used for safe ambulation. There is an increasing push toward settings that are more homelike in nature and these settings, unfortunately, have been shown to be less likely to facilitate physical activity (Pomeroy, Resnick, & Scherer, 2007). In homelike settings, there is often more clutter such as plants, fish tanks, bird cages, and other positive types of décor. This unfortunately impacts free movement. There is also a tendency to have very comfortable recliner-type chairs and easy and close access to one's television, the dining area, and other daily needs. The goal with regard to pleasant homelike environments is to balance what may be perceived as pleasant and homelike with assuring environments that can help optimize function and physical activity. Such things as access to age-appropriate exercise equipment, pleasant pathways for walking, and outdoor access can and should be incorporated into homelike settings.

Residents in nursing homes tend to be defined as frail and have multiple chronic illnesses and high levels of cognitive and functional impairment (Congressional Budget Office, 2013; Lapane, Quilliam, Chow, & Kim, 2012; The National Center for Health Statistics Data Brief No. 91, 2010). In addition to multiple physical comorbidities, approximately 50% of long-stay nursing home residents have dementia, 11% have a diagnosis of anxiety, and 40%, a diagnosis of depression (Lapane et al., 2012). This leads to challenges in terms of staff being able to know what the resident is actually able to do functionally, setting appropriate goals, and knowing how to overcome cognitive and behavioral issues to facilitate the resident's engagement in function and physical activity.

To overcome these challenges at the individual level (intrapersonal and interpersonal issues), we work with staff to do a quick evaluation of the residents' capability using the Physical Capability Measure (Resnick, Boltz, Galik, & Wells, 2013). This measure guides caregivers in determining if residents are able to follow a step command (one, two, or three steps) verbally or visually with cueing, whether or not they are able to come to a stand and maintain adequate sitting or standing balance, whether or not they have full range of motion across all major joints, and whether or not they are able to march in place. Goals can then be developed based on these findings. For example, if the individual is able to range his or her upper extremity independently after receiving a verbal command, then he or she should be expected to functionally (aside from swallowing issues) eat independently with verbal cueing or role modeling. If he or she can only range his or her extremities with passive assistance, then hand-over-hand feeding would be needed.

Another major challenge associated with optimizing function and physical activity among nursing home residents is associated with the fear of falling among residents, family, and staff (Resnick, Galik, Gruber-Baldini, & Zimmerman, 2012). Although the majority of falls do not result in trauma, the potential risk of fracture and head trauma outweighs the overall risks of trauma actually occurring. For staff, the implications are rooted in concerns about liability and survey penalties. The Code of Federal Regulations (CFR; Nursing Home Alert, 2014) requires that facilities "ensure that the resident receives adequate supervision and assistive devices to prevent accidents (42 CFR §483.25)." Thus, falls are closely scrutinized during annual or sporadic surveys. While it is recognized that all falls cannot be prevented, the survey process and evaluation of the fall and events around the fall are extremely stressful for all involved. There is evidence that physical activity is critical to fall prevention; there seems to be a *U*-shaped relationship. Specifically, the risk for falls is reduced among physically active people, but there is an increased risk among the most active and inactive individuals (Bergland, 2012; Moayyeri, 2008; Stenhagen, Ekström, Nordell, & Elmståhl, 2014). Furthermore, despite repeatedly demonstrating that engaging residents in function and physical activity does not increase the risk of falls (Galik et al., 2014; Gruber-Baldini, Resnick, Hebel, Galik, & Zimmerman, 2011), staff, families, and residents continue to believe that any activity will result in a fall.

As mentioned earlier, another commonly noted challenge to implementing Function Focused Care in nursing home settings is with regard to the cognitive impairment noted among individuals living in these settings. Innovative approaches are needed to engage these individuals and help the staff evaluate and implement appropriate techniques. Moreover, there is a major focus on behavioral symptoms and a current mandate to decrease inappropriate use of medications such as antipsychotics (Centers for Medicare and Medicaid Services, 2014) as well as increase a person-centered approach to care. Unfortunately, facilities may exclusively focus on approaches that are comfort inducing but provide limited opportunity for physical activity. This results in a persistent decrease in physical activity and functional decline. For example, if a resident with cognitive impairment and behavioral symptoms resists personal care such as bathing or dressing, the caregiver's approach might be to avoid the care interaction or try to bathe and dress the individual later in the day. This is in contrast to a Function Focused Care approach that alters the environment and provides the necessary cueing for the individual to bath and dress himself or herself and have staff help as needed. Depending on the level of the individual, this might simply include giving the individual a washcloth and role model washing one's face. Often these individuals will mimic the behavior. The webpage www.functionfocusedcare.org provides examples in short video coaching sessions to demonstrate how to approach cognitively impaired residents in a way that facilitates their performance of the activity and avoids behavioral symptoms such as resistance to care, hitting, or screaming.

Assisted Living Settings

Residents in assisted living settings can be quite similar to those living in the nursing home, with the exception that in assisted living, they tend to have fewer medical problems and functional impairment (Resnick & Galik, 2015). Individuals in assisted living settings need help with activities of daily living for physical or for cognitive reasons and this help is provided by DCWs who may or may not be certified nursing assistants. It is very much task-focused care as the

DCWs have a set amount of time in which to provide the care in order to meet the needs of all residents. Furthermore, depending on the assisted living setting, daily rates may be based on the amount of care needed and provided. Thus, it is critical to address and overcome the task-focused philosophy while implementing Function Focused Care. From the facility perspective, decreasing care needs of residents is financially advantageous, even in a payment model in which care is not bundled. Less care needs of residents means that fewer staff may be needed within the facility, thus providing a cost savings. To the individual, greater independence and less care needs can mean a decrease in their monthly payments.

Given that the individuals living in assisted living settings tend to be less functionally impaired, implementing Function Focused Care in these settings tends to include a greater emphasis on integrating physical activity into the programing and activities provided in the setting. For example, instead of playing trivia or bingo, an afternoon activity might be attending an exercise or dance class. Depending on setting size and resources, there may or may not be an activity director. If there is no designated activity director, a DCW or the assisted living manager will likely serve in this capacity and can be used as the contact person to help facilitate change. Generally, based on residents' preferences, most of the activities offered are for entertainment and involve sedentary activities such as playing trivia, bingo, or word games, cooking, or listening to music or watching movies. Revising activities to offer such things as activity bingo, walking programs, music and dance classes, as well as walk-to-dine programs and holiday dance parties in which residents dance rather than observe dancing can all help to integrate physical activity into the daily lives of the residents. Our webpage www.functionfocusedcare.org provides over a hundred examples of activities to increase physical activity among residents in assisted living settings.

The environments in assisted living settings are also very variable, depending on size and type of facility. There are many small assisted living settings that are incorporated into residential home settings and have short, narrow hallways, small rooms, and limited space to ambulate either indoors or outdoors. Innovative ways to utilize these spaces to facilitate function and physical should still be considered. For example, making outdoor areas safe for ambulation by clearing pathways and placing chairs along the path to allow for rest periods or making stairways safe and pleasant to walk up and down (e.g., assure there is appropriate lighting, handrails, and markings on the stairs) are some of the ways in which to encourage physical activity.

Home Settings

Implementing Function Focused Care in home settings with caregivers has some challenges and advantages not found in the other institutional settings. Although it is important to evaluate the home culture and the relationship between the care recipient and caregiver, the home setting does not have to adhere to the same policies and regulations found in the other settings of care. One of the first things to explore is whether the caregiver takes a task completion approach (i.e., "doing for" the care recipient) versus an enabling approach, that is, helping the care recipient optimize his or her performance across all activities of daily living and time spent in physical activity. Helping caregivers plan out time to ensure care tasks are completed when needed (e.g., getting ready to go to the day care or to an appointment) or helping the caregiver set up the environment to facilitate self-care aspects of bathing or dressing for the care recipient are useful interventions. Most important is to help the caregiver see that a function-focused philosophy of care will help the care recipient maintain optimal health and quality of life and will be of benefit to him or her as well. Caregivers in home settings may have to manage behavioral symptoms as well and should be encouraged to view the videos for care techniques on the www.functionfocusedcare.org webpage.

As with assisted living facilities, the home environment may require some innovative interventions to provide the care recipient with opportunities to engage in functional tasks such as walking and other types of physical activity. In the home setting, there is no access to activity programs to facilitate function. Thus, the caregiver will need to work with the care recipient to establish realistic activities that they can do together. For example, a daily walk either within the home setting or around the block or as far as the care recipient can tolerate can be set as a routine daily activity. Alternatively, setting short 10-minute blocks to dance and engage in aerobic activity throughout the day is another cost-neutral activity. Community-based resources can also be explored such as going to a local exercise class at a senior center.

SIGNIFICANCE OF FUNCTION FOCUSED CARE ACROSS ALL SETTINGS

Multiple studies have been done testing Function Focused Care approaches in nursing homes and assisted living, with less work testing this approach in home and acute care environments. Consistently, across all settings, we have demonstrated that we can teach caregivers (nurses, nursing assistants, and family caregivers) how to provide Function Focused Care to older adults (Burkett et al., 2013; Galik et al., 2014; Pretzer-Aboff, Galik, & Resnick, 2011; Resnick, Galik, Enders, et al., 2011; Resnick, Galik, Gruber-Baldini, et al., 2011; Resnick, Gruber-Baldini, Galik, et al., 2009).

The outcomes following exposure to Function Focused Care approaches for older adults vary, based on the setting and participants involved. Table 13.7

TABLE 13.7

Function Focused Care Outcomes for Older Adults Across Settings

Outcome	Nursing Home	Assisted Living	Acute Care	Home
Function	Increased ability to walk 50 feet in treatment versus decline in control at 12 months (Resnick, Gruber-Baldini, Zimmerman et al., 2009); increased overall function (activities of daily living) in treatment versus control at 3 months (Galik et al., 2014).	Less decline in function among residents in treatment sites versus control (Resnick, Galik, Gruber-Baldini, et al., 2011).	When patients in acute care were provided with Function Focused Care, there was less decline in function during the hospital stay than when no Function Focused Care was provided (Boltz et al., 2012). When family caregivers in the acute care setting provided Function Focused Care, patients improved with regard to function during the hospital stay and up to 2 months after hospitalization (Boltz, Resnick, Capezuti, & Shuluk, 2014).	Older adults with Parkinson's disease who were exposed to Function Focused Care by their home caregivers improved functionally over a 6-month period.

(*Continued*)

TABLE 13.7
Function Focused Care Outcomes for Older Adults Across Settings (*Continued*)

Outcome	Nursing Home	Assisted Living	Acute Care	Home
Physical activity	Increased counts of physical activity at 6 months in treatment versus control (Galik et al., 2014).	Increase in counts of activity and times spent in physical activity at 6 or 12 months in treatment sites versus control (Resnick, Galik, Gruber-Baldini, et al., 2011; Resnick, Galik, Gruber-Baldini, & Zimmerman, 2009).		Older adults with Parkinson's disease who were exposed to Function Focused Care by their home caregivers increased the time they spent in physical activity over a 6-month period.
Mood	No change in mood over time in treatment versus control.	No change in life satisfaction over time (Resnick, Galik, Gruber-Baldini, & Zimmerman, 2010).		No change in mood over a 6-month period.

provides an overview of the findings. In nursing home settings, residents exposed to Function Focused Care showed less of a functional decline over time and were noted to maintain walking ability better than those exposed to routine care (Galik et al., 2014; Galik et al., 2008; Resnick, Gruber-Baldini, Zimmerman et al., 2009). The nursing home residents exposed to Function Focused Care also increased the amount of physical activity they engaged in based on actigraphy data (Galik et al., 2014). There was no change in mood or behavior among those exposed to Function Focused Care. It was noted, however, that there was less resistance to care (Galik et al., 2014).

In assisted living settings, we similarly found that there was an increase in the amount of physical activity older individuals performed when exposed to Function Focused Care (Resnick, Galik, et al., 2009; Resnick, Galik, Gruber-Baldini, et al., 2011) and less decline in function among these individuals (Resnick, Galik, Gruber-Baldini, et al., 2011). There was no change in quality of life or life satisfaction following exposure to Function Focused Care (Resnick, Galik, et al., 2009; Resnick, Galik, Gruber-Baldini, et al., 2011). The work that has been done in acute care suggests that those who are exposed to Function Focused Care either by nurses or family caregivers have better functional outcomes (Boltz et al., 2012), suggesting that there is benefit to this approach when hospitalized. Finally, in home settings, functional benefits and increased time in physical activity have also been noted when home caregivers expose older adults with Parkinson's disease to Function Focused Care.

Overall, there is sufficient evidence to indicate that across all of these settings, there are benefits to providing Function Focused Care. Moreover, there is no evidence that Function Focused Care approaches increase the risk of falls or adverse events (Gruber-Baldini et al., 2011; Resnick et al., 2012). Rather in some studies, we have shown that there are fewer falls and hospital transfers in settings that implement Function Focused Care approaches (Galik et al., 2014; Resnick, Galik, Gruber-Baldini, Zimmerman, 2013; Resnick, Galik, & Vigne, 2014).

CONCLUSION

Maintaining function and physical activity across all settings of care is critical if we are to help older adults remain at their highest level of functioning. The tendency among nursing and other caregivers is to provide care rather than facilitate self-care, as this is much of how nurses and other caregivers are trained. Disuse and deconditioning occur when individuals stop ranging their extremities during activities of daily living or in exercise and limit time standing or walking. The focus of care and education of caregivers needs to be geared to prevention and focused on helping all older adults achieve their highest level of function and physical activity.

REFERENCES

American College of Sports Medicine and the American Heart Association. (2013). *Guidelines for physical activity*. Retrieved from http://www.heart.org/HEARTORG/GettingHealthy/PhysicalActivity/StartWalking/American-Heart-Association-Recommendations-for-Physical-Activity-in-Adults_UCM_307976_Article.jsp

Bandura, A. (1997). *Self-efficacy: The exercise of control*. New York, NY: W.H. Freeman and Company.

Bergland, A. (2012). Fall risk factors in community-dwelling people. *Norweigan Journal of Epidemiology, 22*, 151–164.

Blair, S. (2009). Physical inactivity: The biggest public health problem of the 21st century. *British Journal of Sports Medicine, 43*(1), 1–2.

Boltz, M., Resnick, B., Capezuti, E., & Shabbat, N. (2011). Function-focused activity and changes in physical function in Chinese and non-Chinese hospitalized older adults. *Rehabilitation Nursing, 36*(6), 233–240.

Boltz, M., Resnick, B., Capezuti, E., & Shuluk, J. (2014). Activity restriction versus self-direction: Hospitalized older adults' response to fear of falling. *International Journal of Older People Nursing, 9*(1), 44–53.

Boltz, M., Resnick, B., Capezuti, E., Shuluk, J., & Secic, M. (2012). Functional decline in hospitalized older adults: Can nursing make a difference? *Geriatric Nursing, 33*(4), 272–279.

Brown, C. J., Redden, D. T., Flood, K. L., & Allman, R. M. (2009). The underrecognized epidemic of low mobility during hospitalization of older adults. *Journal of the American Geriatrics Society, 57*(9), 1660–1667.

Brown, C. J., Williams, B. R., Woodby, L. L., Davis, L. L., & Allman, R. M. (2007). Barriers to mobility during hospitalization from the persepctive of the patient, their nurses and physicians. *Journal of Hospital Medicine, 2*, 305–331.

Burkett, T., Hippensteel, N., Penrod, J., & Resnick, B. (2013). Pilot testing of the Function Focused Care intervention on an acute care trauma unit. *Geriatric Nursing, 34*(3), 241–246.

Buttery, A. K., & Martin, F. C. (2009). Knowledge, attitudes and intentions about participation in physical activity of older post acute hospital inpatients. *Physioltherapy, 95*(3), 192–198.

Carpenter, G. I., Hastie, C. L., Morris, J. N., Fries, B. E., & Ankri, J. (2006). Measuring change in activities of daily living in nursing home residents with moderate to severe cognitive impairment. *Biomedical Central Geriatrics, 6*, 7. Retrieved June 27, 2015 from http://www.ncbi.nlm.nih.gov/pmc/articles/PMC1522014/

Centers for Disease Control. (2014). *Physical activity and health*. Retrieved June 27, 2015 from http://www.cdc.gov/nccdphp/sgr/pdf/olderad.pdf

Centers for Medicare and Medicare Services. (2013). *MDS database*. Retrieved June 27, 2015 from http://www.cms.gov/apps/mds/

Centers for Medicare and Medicaid Services. (2014). *National Partnership to Improve Dementia Careexceeds goals to reduce unnecessary antipsychotic medications in nursing homes*. Retrieved June 27, 2015 from http://www.cms.gov/Newsroom/MediaReleaseDatabase/Fact-sheets/2014-Fact-sheets-items/2014-09-19.html

Chung, G. (2012). Understanding nursing home worker conceptualizations about good care. *The Gerontologist, 53*(2), 246–254.

Clegg, A., Barber, S., Young, J. B., Forster, A., & Iliffe, S. J. (2012). Do home-based exercise interventions improve outcomes for frail older people? Findings from a systematic review. *Reviews in Clinical Gerontology, 22*(1), 68–78.

Congressional Budget Office. (2013). *Rising demand for long-term services and supports for elderly people*. Retrieved June 27, 2015 from http://www.cbo.gov

Cornelissen, V. A., & Fagard, R. H. (2005). Effect of resistance training on resting blood pressure: A meta-analysis of randomized controlled trials. *Journal of Hypertension, 23*(2), 251–259.

Cress, M., Buchner, D., Prohaska, T., Rimmer, J., Brown, M., & Macera, C. (2005). Best practices for physical activity programs and behavior counseling in older adult populations. *Journal of Aging and Physical Activity, 13*(1), 61–74.

De Greef, K., Deforche, B., Tudor-Locke, C., & De Bourdeaudhuij, I. (2010). A cognitive-behavioural pedometer-based group intervention on physical activity and sedentary behaviour in individuals with type 2 diabetes. *Health Education Research, 25*(5), 724–736.

Desveaux, L., Beauchamp, M., Goldstein, R., & Brooks, D. (2014). Community-based exercise programs as a strategy to optimize function in chronic disease: A systematic review. *Medical Care, 52*(3), 216–226.

Dolansky, M., Stepanczuk, B., Charvat, J., & Moore, S. (2010). Women's and men's exercise adherence after a cardiac event: Does age make a difference? *Research in Gerontological Nursing, 3*(1), 30–38.

Dykes, P., Carroll, D., Hurley, A., Benoit, A., & Middelton, B. (2009). Why do patients in acute care hospitals fall? Can falls be prevented? *The Journal of Nursing Administration, 39*(6), 299–304.

Ferrer, R., Cruz, I., Burge, S., Bayles, B., & Castilla, M. (2014). Measuring capability for healthy diet and physical activity. *Annals of Family Medicine, 12*(1), 46–56.

Galik, E. M., Resnick, B., Gruber-Baldini, A., Nahm, E. S., Pearson, K., & Pretzer-Aboff, I. (2008). Pilot testing of the restorative care intervention for the cognitively impaired. *Journal of the American Medical Directors Association, 9*(7), 516–522.

Galik, E., Resnick, B., Hammersla, M., & Brightwater, J. (2014). Optimizing function and physical activity among nursing home residents with dementia: Testing the impact of Function Focused Care. *The Gerontologist, 54*(6), 930–943.

Gregson, J., Foerster, S., Orr, R., Jones, L., Benedict, J., & Clark, B. (2003). System, environment and policy changes: Using the Social Ecological Model as a framework for evaluating nutrition eductaion and social marketing programs with low income audiences. *Journal of Nutrition Education, 33*, S4–S15.

Gruber-Baldini, A., Resnick, B., Hebel, J., Galik, E., & Zimmerman, S. (2011). Adverse events associated with the Res-Care Intervention. *Journal of the American Medical Directors Association, 12*(8), 584–589.

Habjanič, A., Saarnio, R., Elo, S., Turk, D., & Isola, A. (2012). Challenges for institutional elder care in Slovenian nursing homes. *Journal of Clinical Nursing, 21*, 2579–2589.

Hawley-Hague, H., Horne, M., Campbell, M., Demack, S., Skelton, D., & Todd, C. (2014). Multiple levels of influence on older adults' attendance and adherence to community exercise classes. *The Gerontologist, 54*(4), 599–610.

Hopkins, R., & Spuhler, V. J. (2009). Strategies for promoting early activity in critically ill mechanically ventilated patients. *AACN Advanced Critical Care, 20*, 277–289.

Horne, M., & Tierney, S. (2012). What are the barriers and facilitators to exercise and physical activity uptake and adherence among South Asian older adults: A systematic review of qualitative studies. *Preventive Medicine, 55*(4), 276–284.

Hyman, B., Oden, G., & Wagner, M. (2010). The aging process: Physiological changes and implications for educators and practitioners. *Activities, Adaptation & Aging, 34*(2), 148–153.

Janssen, I., Dugan, S., Karavolos, K., Lynch, E., & Powell, L. (2014). Correlates of 15-year maintenance of physical activity in middle-aged women. *International Journal of Behavioral Medicine, 21*(3), 511–518.

Katz, P. (2011). An international perspective on long term care: Focus on nursing homes. *Journal of the American Medical Directors Association, 12*(7), 487–492.

Król-Zielińska, M., Kusy, K., Zieliński, J., & Osiński, W. (2011). Physical activity and functional fitness in institutionalized vs. independently living elderly: A comparison of 70–80-year-old city-dwellers. *Archives of Gerontology & Geriatrics, 53*(1), e10–e16.

Kumar, A., & Carpenter, H., Cook, J., Skelton, D. A., Stevens, Z., Haworth, D., et al. (2014). Exercise for reducing fear of falling in older people living in the community: A cochrane systematic review. *Age and Ageing, 42*(Suppl. 2), ii17.

Kuo, Y. (2013). The influence of chair seat height on the performance of community-dwelling older adults' 30-second chair stand test. *Aging and Clinical Experimental Research, 25*(3), 305–309.

Lapane, K., Quilliam, B. J., Chow, W., & Kim, M. (2012). The association between pain and measures of well being among nursing home residents. *Journal of the American Medical Directors Association, 13*(4), 344–349.

Laybourne, A., Biggs, S., & Martin, F. C. (2011). Predicting habitual physical activity using coping strategies in older fallers engaged in falls prevention exercise. *Journal of Aging and Physical Activity, 19*, 189–200.

Leditschke, A., Green, M., Irvine, J., Bissett, B., & Mitchell, I. A. (2012). What are the barriers to mobilizing intensive care patients? *Cardiopulmonary Physical Therapy Journal, 23*(1), 26–29.

Lindquist, R., & Sendelbach, S. E. (2007). Maximizing safety of hospitalized elders. *Critical Care Nursing Clinics of North America, 19*(3), 277–284.

Mitchell, M., Goodman, J., Alter, D., Oh, P., & Faulkner, G. (2014). 'Will walk for groceries': Acceptability of financial health incentives among Canadian cardiac rehabilitation patients. *Psychology & Health, 29*(9), 1032–1043.

Moayyeri, A. (2008). The association between physical activity and osteoporotic fractures: A review of the evidence and implications for future research. *Annals of Epidemiology, 18*(11), 827–835.

Moody, J., Hale, L., & Waters, D. (2012). Perceptions of a water-based exercise programme to improve physical function and falls risk in older adults with lower extremity osteoarthritis: Barriers, motivators and sustainability. *New Zealand Journal of Physiotherapy, 40*(2), 64–70.

Netten, A., Beadle-Brown, J., Trukeschitz, B., Towers, A., Welch, E., & Forder, J. (2010). Measuring the outcomes of care homes: Final report. *Personal Social Services Research Unit.* Retrieved June 27, 2015 from www.pssru.ac.uk

Netz, Y., Wu, M. J., Becker, B. J., & Tennenbaum, G. (2005). Physical activity and psychological well being in advanced age: A meta-analysis of intervention studies. *Psychology and Aging, 20*(2), 272–284.

Nursing Home Alert. (2014). *Federal nursing home regulations and state laws.* Retrieved June 27, 2015 from http://www.nursinghomealert.com/federal-nursing-home-regulations-and-state-laws

Pomeroy, S., Resnick, B., & Scherer, Y. (2007). Person-Environment Fit (PE-FIT) and functioning among older adults in a long-term care setting. *The Gerontologist, 47*(1), 671.

Pretzer-Aboff, I., Galik, E., & Resnick, B. (2011). Testing the impact of res-care parkinson's disease. *Nursing Research, 60*(4), 276–283.

Rana, B. K., Darst, B. F., Bloss, C., Shih, P. B., Depp, C., Nievergelt, C. M., et al. (2014). Candidate SNP associations of optimism and resilience in older adults: Exploratory study of 935 communty dwelling adults. *American Journal of Geriatric Psychiatry, 22*(10), 997–1006.

Resnick, B., Boltz, M., Galik, E., & Wells, C. (2013). Reliability and validity of the physical capability assessment. *Clinical Nursing Research, 22*(1), 7–29.

Resnick, B., & Galik, E. (2015). Impact of care settings on residents' functional and psychosocial status, physical activity and adverse events. *International Journal of Older Persons.* Retrieved September 25, 2015, from http://onlinelibrary.wiley.com/doi/10.1111/opn.12086/abstract

Resnick, B., Galik, E., & Boltz, M. (2013). Function Focused Care approaches: Literature review of progress and future possibilities. *Journal of the American Medical Directors Association, 14*(5), 313–318.

Resnick, B., Galik, E., Enders, H., Sobol, K., Hammersla, M., Boltz, M., et al. (2011). Functional and physical activity of older adults in acute care settings: Where we are and where we need to go. *Journal of Nursing Care Quality, 26*(2), 169–177.

Resnick, B., Galik, E., Gruber-Baldini, A. L., & Zimmerman, S. (2009). Implementing a restorative care philosophy of care in assisted living: Pilot testing of Res-Care-AL. *Journal of the American Academy of Nurse Practitioners, 21*(2), 123–133.

Resnick, B., Galik, E., Gruber-Baldini, A., & Zimmerman, S. (2010). Satisfaction with assisted living: The unexplored role of physical activity. *Geriatric Nursing, 31*(3), 197–205.

Resnick, B., Galik, E., Gruber-Baldini, A., & Zimmerman, S. (2011). Testing the impact of function focused care in assisted living. *Journal of the American Geriatrics Society, 59*(12), 2233–2240.

Resnick, B., Galik, E., Gruber-Baldini, A., & Zimmerman, S. (2012). Falls and fall related injuries associated with Function Focused Care. *Clinical Nursing Research, 21*(1), 43–63.

Resnick, B., Galik, E., Gruber-Baldini, A., & Zimmerman, S. (2013). Understanding dissemination and implementation of a new intervention in assisted living settings: The case of Function Focused Care. *Journal of Applied Gerontology, 32*(3), 280–301.

Resnick, B., Galik, E., & Vigne, E. (2014). Translation of Function Focused Care to assisted living facilities. *Family and Community Health, 37*(2), 155–165.

Resnick, B., Gruber-Baldini, A., Galik, E., Pretzer-Aboff, I., Russ, K., Hebel, J., & Magaziner, J. (2009). Changing the philosophy of care in long-term care: Testing of the restorative care intervention. *The Gerontologist, 49*(2), 175–184.

Resnick, B., Gruber-Baldini, A., Zimmerman, S. I., Galik, E., Pretzer-Aboff, I., Russ, K., et al. (2009). Nursing home resident outcomes from the Res-Care intervention. *Journal of the American Geriatrics Society, 57*(7), 1156–1165.

Sangster, J., Furber, S., Phongsavan, P., Allman-Farinelli, M., Redfern. J., & Bauman, A. (2013). Where you live matters: Challenges and opportunities to address the urban-rural divide through innovative secondary cardiac rehabilitation programs. *Australian Journal of Rural Health, 21*(3), 170–177.

Schepens, S., Sen, A., & Painter, J., & Murphy, S. L. (2012). Relationship between fall-related efficacy and activity engagement in community-dwelling older adults: A meta-analytic review. *American Journal of Occupational Therapy, 66*(2), 137–148.

Schmidt, L. (2003). Patients' perceptions of nursing care in the hospital setting. *Journal of Advanced Nursing, 44*(4), 393–399.

Shinichi, D., & Takayoshi, Y. (2007). Height of chair seat and movement characteristics in sit to stand by yound and elderly adults. *Perceptual and Motor Skills, 104*, 21–31.

Siceloff, E., Coulon, S., & Wilson, D. (2014). Physical activity as a mediator linking neighborhood environmental supports and obesity in African Americans in the path trial. *Health Psychology, 33*(5), 481–489.

Silva, R., Eslick, G., & Duque, G. J. (2013). Exercise for falls and fracture prevention in long term care facilities: A systematic review and meta-analysis. *Journal of the American Medical Directors Association, 14*(9), 685–689.

Singh, M. (2002). Exercise comes of age: Rationale and recommendations for a geriatric exercise prescription. *Journal of Gerontology a Biolological Sciences Medicine and Science, 57*(5), M262–M282.

Stenhagen, M., Ekström, H., Nordell, E., & Elmstahl, S. (2014). Both deterioration and improvement in activities of daily living are related to falls: A 6-year follow-up of the general elderly population study Good Aging in Skane. *Clinical Interventions in Aging, 9*, 1839–1846.

Stubbs, B., Binnekade, T., Soundy, A., Schofield, P., Huijnen, I., & Eggermont, L. (2013). Are older adults with chronic musculoskeletal pain less active than older adults without pain? A systematic review and meta-analysis. *Pain Medicine, 14*, 1316–1331.

The National Center for Health Statistics Data Brief No. 91. (2010). *Data from the 2010 National Survey of Residential Care Facilities*. Retrieved June 27, 2015 from www.ahcancal.org/ncal/resources/Pages/ResidentProfile.aspx

Thomsen, G. E., Snow, G. L., Rodriguez, L., & Hopkins, R. G. (2008). Patients with respiratory failure inrease ambulation after transfer to an intesive care unit where early activity is a priority. *Crical Care Medicine, 36*(4), 1119–1124.

Trinh, L., Wilson, R., Williams, H., & Sum, A. (2012). Physicians promoting physical activity using pedometers and community partnerships: A real world trial. *British Journal of Sports Medicine, 46*, 284–290.

Tudor-Locke, C., Craig, C. L., Aoyagi, Y., Bell, R. C., Croteau, K. A., De Bourdeaudhuij, I., et al. (2011). How many steps/day are enough? For older adults and special populations. *International Journal of Behavior Nutrition and Physical Activity, 8*(1), 80.

Tung, Y., Cooke, M., & Moyle, W. (2013). Sources older people draw on to nurture, strengthen and improve self-efficacy in managing home rehabilitation following orthopaedic surgery. *Journal of Clinical Nursing, 22*(9/10), 1217–1225.

Whear, R., Coon, J., Bethel, A., Abbott, R., Stein, K., & Garside, R. (2014). What is the impact of using outdoor spaces such as gardens on the physical and mental well-being of those with dementia? A systematic review of quantitative and qualitative evidence. *Journal of the American Medical Directors Association, 15*(10), 697–705.

Windle, G., Hughes, D., Linck, P., Russell, I., & Woods, B. (2010). Is exercise effective in promoting mental well-being in older age? A systematic review. *Aging & Mental Health, 14*(6), 652–669.

World Health Organization. (2014). *Physical activity*. Retrieved June 27, 2015 from http://www.who.int/dietphysicalactivity/pa/en/

Zelada, M., Salinas, R., & Baztan, J. (2007). Reduction of functional deteroiration during hospitalization in an acute geriatric unit. *Archives of Gerontology & Geriatrics, 48*, 35–39.

Index

Note: Page references followed by "*f*" and "*t*" denote figures and tables

www.ingramcontent.com/pod-product-compliance
Ingram Content Group UK Ltd.
Pitfield, Milton Keynes, MK11 3LW, UK
UKHW021845100926
8556IPUK00019B/1068

9 780826 198150